AF531674

BIOLOGY OF CANCER

ENCYCLOPAEDIA OF CANCER

Vol. I

BIOLOGY OF CANCER

By

Dr. Amita Sarkar

Dept. of Zoology
Agra College
Agra (U.P.)
(India)

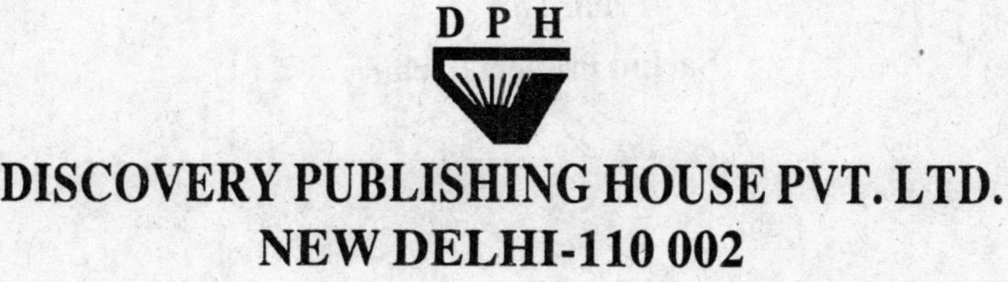

DISCOVERY PUBLISHING HOUSE PVT. LTD.
NEW DELHI-110 002

First Published-2008

ISBN 978-81-8356-356-7 (Set)

Published by:

DISCOVERY PUBLISHING HOUSE PVT. LTD.

4831/24, Ansari Road, Prahlad Street,
Darya Ganj, New Delhi-110002 (India)
Phone: 23279245 • Fax: 91-11-23253475
E-mail: dphbooks@rediffmail.com
dphtemp@indiatimes.com
Website: www.discoverypublishinghouse.com

Printed at:

Sachin Printers, Delhi

Preface

Over the past 20 years, technological advances in molecular biology have proven invaluable to the understanding of the pathogenesis of cancer. The application of molecular technology to the study of cancer has not only led to advances in tumor diagnosis, but has also provided markers for the assessment of prognosis and disease progression. The aim of *Encyclopaedia of Cancer* is to provide a comprehensive collection of the most up-to-date techniques for the detection of molecular changes in cancer.

This book is intended to provide a relatively short overview of important concepts and notions on the molecular biology of human cancers, including many facts essential to find one's way in this field. It is, however, not meant to be compreshensive and probably cannot be, as our knowledge is rapidly growing.

The salient feature of this book is that it covers a wide range of molecular techniques and provides a source of information to readers at all levels. Although several books on cancer have been published in the last decade, most of either very shallow or cover few areas in depth. Rarely do they cover the broad spectrum of topics which would provide enough information for understanding the subject or provide simple protocols for execution of molecular change. In my opinion, this book can help the reader to easily understand the subject and also excecute the experiments very efficiently.

There can be no claim to originality except in the manner of treatment and much of the information has been obtained from the books and scientific journals available in the different libraries.

The author expresses his thanks to his friends and colleagues whose continue inspirations have initiated him to bring out this book.

The author is painfully aware of the shortcomings, errors and misprints that have crept in, and shall be greateful to receive suggestion for improvement of the next edition from all the readers.

The author expresses his gratitude to Mr. Wasan and staff of M/s Discovery Publishing House for their whole hearted co-operation in the publication of this book.

Author

Contents

1

Introduction

Roughly one person in five, in the prosperous countries of the world, will die of cancer. Heart disease causes more deaths, and in the world as a whole, other health problems, such as malnutrition and parasitic infections, are more serious. In the context of cell biology, however, cancer has a unique importance, for the family of diseases grouped under this heading reflect disturbances of the most fundamental rules of behavior of the cells in a multicellular organism. To understand cancer and to devise rational ways to treat it, we have to understand both the inner workings of cells and their social interactions in the tissues of the body. Thus the cancer research effort has profoundly benefited a much wider area of medical knowledge than that of cancer alone.

Cancer as a Microevolutionary Process

The body of an animal can be viewed as a society or ecosystem whose individual members are cells, reproducing by cell division and organized into collaborative assemblies or tissues. In our earlier discussion of the maintenance of tissues, our concerns were similar to those of the ecologist: cell births, deaths, habitats, territorial limitations, the maintenance of population sizes, and the like. The one ecological topic conspicuously absent was that of natural selection: we said nothing of competition or mutation among somatic cells. The reason is that a healthy body is in this respect a very peculiar society, where self-sacrifice, rather than competition, is the rule: all somatic cell lineages are committed to die, leaving no progeny but dedicating their existence to support of the germ cells, which alone have a chance of survival. There is no mystery in this, for the body is a clone, and the genome of the somatic cells is the same as the genome of the germ cells; by their self-sacrifice for the sake of the germ cells, the somatic cells help to propagate copies of their own genes.

Thus, unlike free-living cells such as bacteria, which compete to survive, the cells of a multicellular organism are committed to collaboration. Any mutation that gives rise to selfish behavior by individual members of the cooperative will jeopardize the future of the whole enterprise. Mutation, competition, and natural selection operating within the population of somatic cells are the basic ingredients of cancer: it is a disease in which individual mutant cells begin by prospering at the expense of their neighbors but in the end destroy the whole cellular society and die.

In this section we discuss the development of cancer as a microevolutionary process. This process occurs on a time scale of months or years in a population of cells in the body, and it is dependent on the same principles of mutation and natural selection that govern the long-term evolution of all living organisms.

Cancers Differ According to the Cell Type from Which they Derive

Cancer cells are defined by two heritable properties: they and their progeny (1) reproduce in defiance of the normal restraints and (2) invade and colonize territories normally reserved for other cells. It is the combination of these features that makes cancers peculiarly dangerous. An isolated abnormal cell that does not proliferate more than its normal neighbors does no significant damage, no matter what other disagreeable properties it may have; but if its proliferation is out of control, it will give rise to a tumor, or ***neoplasm***- a relentlessly growing mass of abnormal cells. As long as the neoplastic cells remain clustered together in a single mass, however, the tumor is said to be benign, and a complete cure can usually be achieved by removing the mass surgically. A tumor is counted as a cancer only if it is malignant, that is, only if its cells have the ability to invade surrounding tissue. Invasiveness usually implies an ability to break loose, enter the bloodstream or lymphatic vessels, and form secondary tumors, or metastases, at other sites in the body. The more widely a cancer metastasizes, the harder it becomes to eradicate.

Cancers are classified according to the tissue and cell type from which they arise. Cancers arising from epithelial cells are termed carcinomas; those arising from connective tissue or muscle cells are termed sarcomas. Cancers that do not fit in either of these two broad categories include the various leukemias, derived from hemopoietic cells, and cancers derived from cells of the nervous system. Each of the broad categories has many subdivisions according to the specific cell type, the location in the body, and the structure of the tumor; many of the names used are fixed by tradition and have no modern rational basis. In parallel with the set of names for malignant tumors, there is a related set of names for benign tumors: an *adenoma*, for example, is a benign epithelial tumor with a glandular organization, the corresponding type of malignant tumor being an *adenocarcinoma*; a *chondroma* and a *chondrosarcoma* are, respectively, benign and malignant tumors of cartilage. About 90% of human cancers are carcinomas, perhaps because most of the cell proliferation in the body occurs in epithelia or perhaps because epithelial tissues are most frequently exposed to the various forms of physical and chemical damage that favor the development of cancer.

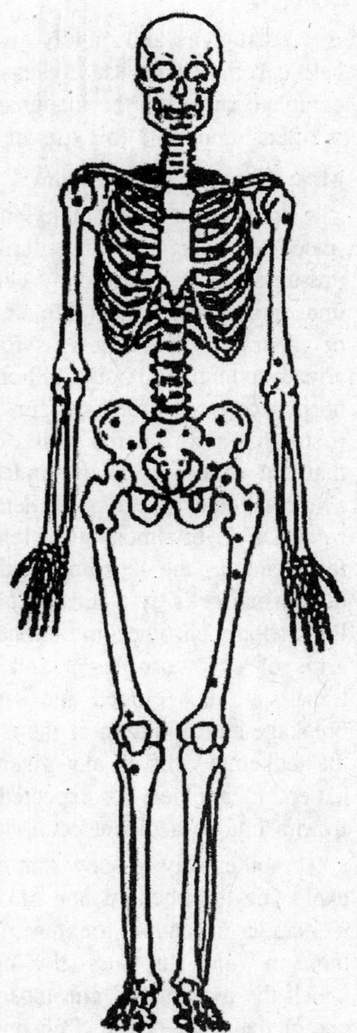

Fig. 1.1. Metastasis. Malignant tumors typically dive rise to metastases, making the cancer hard to eradicate.

Each cancer has characteristics that reflect its origin. Thus, for example, the cells of an epidermal *basal-cell carcinoma*, derived from a keratinocyte stem cell in the skin, will generally continue to synthesize cytokeratin intermediate filaments, whereas the cells of a *melanoma*, derived from a pigment cell in the skin, will often (but not always) continue to make pigment granules. Cancers originating from different cell types are, in general, very different diseases. The basal-cell carcinoma, for example, is only locally invasive and rarely forms metastases, whereas the melanoma is much more malignant and rapidly gives rise to many metastases. The basal-cell carcinoma is usually easy to remove by surgery, leading to complete cure; but the malignant melanoma, once it has metastasized, is often impossible to extirpate and consequently fatal.

Most Cancers Derive from a Single Abnormal Cell

Even when a cancer has metastasized, its origins can usually be traced to a single primary tumor, arising in an identified organ and presumed to be derived by cell division from a single cell that has undergone some heritable change that enables it to outgrow its neighbors. By the time it is first detected, however, a typical tumor already contains about a billion cells or more, often including many normal cells - fibroblasts, for example, in the supporting connective tissue that is associated with a carcinoma. What evidence do we have that the cancer cells are indeed a clone descended from a single abnormal cell? One type of demonstration comes from analysis of the cells' DNA. In almost all patients with *chronic myelogenous leukemia*, for example, the leukemic white blood cells are distinguished from the normal cells by a specific chromosomal abnormality (the so-called Philadelphia chromosome, created by a translocation between the long arms of chromosomes 9 and 22). When the DNA at the site of translocation is cloned and sequenced, it is found that the site of breakage and rejoining of the translocated fragments is identical in all the leukemic cells in any given patient but differs slightly from one patient to another, as expected if each case of the leukemia arises from a unique accident occurring in a single cell.

Another way to show that a cancer has a monoclonal origin is by exploiting the phenomenon of X-chromosome inactivation. A normal woman is a random mixture, or mosaic, of two classes of cells - those in which the paternal X chromosome is inactivated and those in which the maternal X chromosome is inactivated. The inactivation of one or the other of the X chromosomes occurs at random in each cell early in embryonic development, but once the choice has been made it is irreversible, so that when a cell divides it passes on its own state of X-inactivation to its daughters. Consequently, the state of X-chromosome inactivation - maternal or paternal - can be used as a heritable marker to trace the lineage of cells in the body. In the great majority of tumors that have been analyzed - both benign and malignant - all the tumor cells have been found to have the same X chromosome inactivated, strongly suggesting that they are derived from a single deranged cell.

Most Cancers are Probably Initiated by a Change in the Cell's DNA Sequence

If a single abnormal cell is to give rise to a tumor, it must pass on its abnormality to its progeny: the aberration has to be heritable. A first problem in understanding a cancer is to discover whether the heritable aberration is due to a genetic change - that is, an alteration in the cell's DNA sequence - or to an *epigenetic* change - that is, a change in the pattern of gene expression without a change in the DNA sequence. Heritable epigenetic changes, reflecting cell memory, are a familiar feature of normal development, as manifest in the stability of the differentiated state and in such phenomena as Xchromosome inactivation; and there is no obvious a priori reason why they should not be involved in cancer. For one rare and extraordinary type of cancer - the teratocarcinoma - the evidence does favor an epigenetic origin.

There are, however, good reasons to think that most cancers are initiated by genetic change. Thus cells of a given cancer car often be shown to have a shared abnormality in their DNA sequence, as we have just seen for chronic myelogenous leukemia; many other examples are discussed in the second half of this chapter. Further evidence that genetic change can be a *cause* of cancer comes from a study of agents known to give rise to the disease. A correlation between carcinogenesis (the generation of cancer) and *mutagenesis* (the production of a change in the DNA sequence) is clear for three classes of agents: chemical carcinogens (which typically cause simple local changes in the nucleotide sequence), ionizing radiation such as x-rays (which typically cause chromosome breaks and translocations), and viruses (which introduce

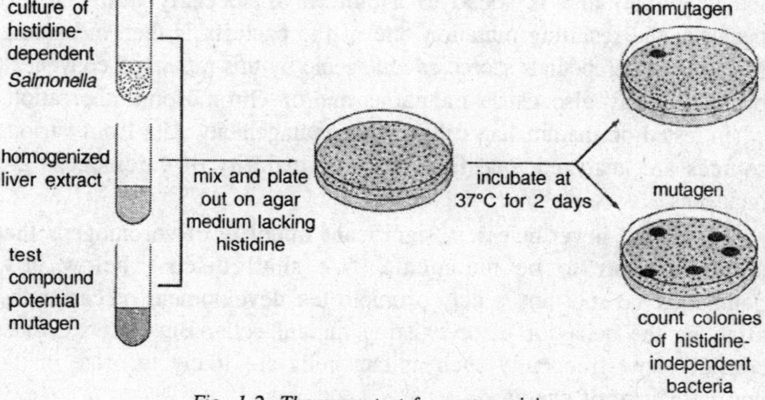

Fig. 1.2. The ames test for mutagenicity.

foreign DNA into the cell). The role of viruses in cancer is discussed later; we pause here to discuss chemical carcinogens.

In general, a given cancer cannot be blamed entirely on a single event or a single cause: as we shall see, cancers as a rule result from the chance occurrence in one cell of several independent accidents, with cumulative effects. There are, however, some unusually carcinogenic agents that increase the likelihood of the critical events to the point where it becomes virtually certain, given a high enough dosage, that at least one cell in the body will turn cancerous. The compound 2-naphthylamine, used in the chemical industry in the early part of this century, is one notorious example: in one British factory, all of the men who had been employed in distilling it (and were thereby subjected to prolonged exposure) eventually developed bladder cancer.

Many quite disparate chemicals have been shown to be likewise carcinogenic when they are fed to experimental animals or painted repeatedly on their skin. Some of these carcinogens act directly on the target cells; many others take effect only after they have been changed to a more reactive form by metabolic processes - notably by a set of intracellular enzymes known as the cytochrome P-450 oxidases. These enzymes normally help to convert ingested toxins and foreign lipid-soluble materials into harmless and easily excreted compounds, but they fail in this task with certain substances, converting them instead into direct carcinogens. Although the known chemical carcinogens are very diverse, most of them have at least one property in common - they cause mutations. In one popular test for mutagenicity, the carcinogen is mixed with an activating extract prepared from rat liver cells (to mimic the biochemical processing that occurs in an intact animal) and is added to a culture of specially designed test bacteria; the resulting mutation rate of the bacteria is then measured. Most of the compounds scored as mutagenic by this rapid and convenient bacterial assay also cause mutations and/or chromosome aberrations when tested on mammalian cells. When mutagenicity data from various sources are analyzed, one finds that the majority of carcinogens are mutagens.

There is, nevertheless, a significant minority of carcinogens that do not appear to be mutagenic. We shall discuss below how nonmutagenic substances may promote the development of cancer by affecting the behavior of preexisting mutant cells. But first we must consider how frequently such mutant cells are likely to arise in the normal course of events.

Single Mutation is not Enough to Cause Cancer

Something on the order of 10^{16} cell divisions take place in a human body in the course of a lifetime; in a mouse, with its smaller number of cells and its shorter life-span, the number is about 10^{12}. Even in an environment that is free of mutagens, mutations will occur spontaneously at an estimated rate of about 10^{-6} mutations per gene per cell division - a value set by fundamental limitations on the accuracy of DNA replication and repair. Thus, in a lifetime, every single gene is likely to have undergone mutation on about 10^{10} separate occasions in any individual human being, or about 10^{6} occasions in a mouse. Among the resulting mutant cells one might expect that there would be many that have disturbances in genes involved in the regulation of cell division and that consequently disobey the normal restrictions on cell proliferation. From this point of view, the problem of cancer seems to be not why it occurs but why it occurs so infrequently.

Evidently, a single mutation is not enough to convert a typical healthy cell into a cancer cell that proliferates without restraint, or we would not be viable organisms. Many lines of evidence indicate that the genesis of a cancer as a rule requires that several independent rare accidents occur together in one cell. One such indication comes from epidemiological studies of the incidence of cancer as a function of age. If a single mutation were responsible, occurring with a fixed probability per year, the chance of developing cancer in any given year should be independent of age. In fact, for most types of cancer the chance goes up very steeply with age - typically as the third, fourth, or fifth power. From such statistics it has been estimated that somewhere between three and seven independent random events, each of low probability, are typically required to turn a normal cell into a cancer cell; the smaller numbers apply to leukemias, the larger to carcinomas.

Now that specific mutations responsible for the development of cancer have been identified, it has become possible to test the effects of the mutant genes in transgenic mice; as we see later, the results give additional and more direct evidence for the hypothesis that a single mutation is insufficient to cause cancer. The hypothesis is also supported by many older studies of the phenomenon of tumor progression, whereby an initial mild disorder of cell behavior evolves gradually into a full-blown cancer. These observations of how tumors develop, moreover, provide insight into the nature of the multiple changes that must occur for a normal cell to become a cancer cell and into the factors that control their occurrence.

Cancers Develop in Slow Stages from Mildly Aberrant Cells

For those cancers that have a discernible external cause, there is almost always a long delay between the causal event(s) and the onset of the disease: the incidence of lung cancer does not begin to rise steeply until after 10 or 20 years of heavy smoking; the incidence of leukemias in Hiroshima and Nagasaki did not show a marked rise until about 5 years after the explosion of the atomic bombs, and it did not reach its peak until 8 years had elapsed; industrial workers exposed for a limited period to chemical carcinogens do not usually develop the cancers characteristic of their occupation until 10, 20, or even more years after the exposure; and so on. During this long incubation period, the prospective cancer cells undergo a succession of changes. Chronic myelogenous leukemia, mentioned earlier, provides a clear and simple example. This disease begins as a disorder characterized by a nonlethal overproduction of white blood cells and continues as such for several years before changing into a much more rapidly progressing illness that usually ends in death within a few months. In the chronic early phase the leukemic cells in the body are distinguished simply by their possession of the chromosomal translocation mentioned previously. In the subsequent acute phase of the illness, the hemopoietic system is overrun by cells that show not only this chromosomal abnormality but also several others. It appears as though members of the initial mutant clone have undergone further mutations that make them proliferate more rapidly (or divide more times before they die or terminally differentiate), so that they come to outnumber both the normal hemopoietic cells and their cousins that have only the primary disorder.

Carcinomas and other solid tumors are thought to evolve in a similar way. Although most such cancers in humans are not diagnosed until a relatively late stage, in a few cases it is possible to observe the early steps in the development of the disease. Another example is provided by cancers of the *uterine cervix* (the neck of the womb). These cancers derive from the multilayered cervical epithelium, which has an organization similar to that of the epidermis of the skin. Normally, proliferation occurs only in the basal layer, generating cells that then move outward toward the surface, differentiating into flattened, keratin-rich, nondividing cells as they go, and finally being sloughed off from the surface. When many specimens of this epithelium from different women are examined, however, it is not unusual to find patches of dysplasia, where dividing cells are no longer confined to the basal layer and there is some disorder in the process of differentiation. Cells are sloughed from the surface in abnormally early stages of differentiation, and the presence of the dysplasia can be detected by scraping a sample of cells from the surface and viewing it under the microscope (the "*Pap smear*" technique). Left alone, the dysplastic patches will often remain harmless or even regress spontaneously; more rarely, however, they may progress, over a period of several years, to give rise to patches of so-called *carcinoma in situ*. In these more serious lesions (somewhat misleadingly named, since they are not yet fully malignant), the usual pattern of cell division and differentiation is much more severely disrupted, and all the layers of the epithelium consist of undifferentiated proliferating cells, which are often highly variable in size and karyotype; the abnormal cells are still confined, however, to the epithelial side of the basal lamina. At this stage it is still easy to achieve a complete cure by destroying or removing the abnormal tissue surgically. Without such treatment the abnormal patch may still remain harmless or regress; but in an estimated 20-30% of cases it will develop, again over a period of several years, to give rise to a truly malignant cervical carcinoma, whose cells break out of the epithelium by crossing the basal lamina and begin to invade the underlying connective tissue. Surgical cure becomes progressively more difficult as the invasive growth spreads.

Tumor Progression Involves Successive Rounds of Mutation and Natural Selection

As illustrated by the examples just discussed, cancers in general seem to arise by a process in which an initial population of slightly abnormal cells, descendants of a single mutant ancestor, evolves from bad to worse through successive cycles of mutation and natural selection. This evolution involves a large element of chance and usually takes many years; most of us die of other ailments before cancer has had time to develop. To understand the causation of cancer, it is essential to understand the factors that may speed up the process.

In general, the rate of evolution, whether in a population of cells exploiting the opportunities for cancerous behavior in the body or in a population of organisms adapting to a new environment on the surface of the earth, would be expected to depend on four main parameters: (1) the *mutation rate*, that is, the probability per gene per unit time that any given member of the population will undergo genetic change; (2) the number of individuals in the population; (3) the rate of reproduction, that is, the average number of generations of progeny produced per unit time; and (4) the selective advantage enjoyed by successful mutant individuals, that is, the ratio of the number of surviving fertile progeny they produce per unit time to the number of surviving fertile progeny produced by nonmutant individuals. Experimental studies on the induction of cancer in animals illustrate these evolutionary principles.

The Development of a Cancer can be Promoted by Factors that do not Alter the Cell's DNA Sequence

The stages by which an initial mild lesion progresses to become a cancer can be most easily observed in the skin. Skin cancers can be elicited in mice, for example, by repeatedly painting the skin with a mutagenic chemical carcinogen such as benzo[a]pyrene (a constituent of coal tar and tobacco smoke) or the related compound dimethylbenz[a]anthracene (DMBA). A single application of the carcinogen, however, usually does not by itself give rise to a tumor or any other obvious lasting abnormality. Yet it does cause latent genetic damage, and this can be detected through a greatly increased incidence of cancer when the cells are exposed either to further treatments with the same substance or to certain other, quite different, insults. A carcinogen that sows the seeds of cancer in this way is said to act as a tumor initiator. Simply wounding skin that has been exposed once to such an initiator can cause cancers to develop from some of the cells at the edge of the wound. Alternatively, repeated exposure over a period of months to certain substances known as tumor promoters, which are not themselves mutagenic, can cause cancer selectively in skin previously exposed to a tumor initiator. The most widely studied tumor promoters are *phorbol esters*, such as *tetradecanoylphorbol acetate* (TPA), which we have already encountered in another context as artificial activators of protein kinase C. These substances cause cancers at high frequency only if they are applied *after* a treatment with a mutagenic initiator.

As one might expect for genetic damage, the hidden changes caused by a tumor initiator are irreversible: thus they can be uncovered by treatment with a tumor promoter even after a long delay. The immediate effect of the promoter is apparently to stimulate cell division (or to cause cells that would normally undergo terminal differentiation to continue dividing instead), and in the region that had previously been exposed to the initiator, this results in the growth of many small, benign, wartlike tumors called *papillomas*. The greater the prior dose of initiator, the larger the number of papillomas induced; it is thought that each papilloma (at least for low doses of the initiator) consists of a single clone of cells descended from a mutant cell that the initiator has engendered. Both wounding and the application of the promoter probably act by inducing the expression of some of the genes that directly or indirectly affect cell proliferation. Such genes may remain quiescent in the resting epithelium, so that any mutations they have undergone in response to the initiator go undetected; by inducing expression of the mutated genes, the promoter or the stimulus of wounding may enable them to begin influencing cell proliferation.

A typical papilloma might contain about 10^5 cells. If exposure to the tumor promoter is stopped, almost all the papillomas regress, and the skin regains a largely normal appearance - as expected from the hypothesis. In a few of the papillomas, however, further changes occur that enable growth to continue in an uncontrolled way, even after the promoter has been withdrawn. These changes seem to originate in occasional single papilloma cells, at about the frequency expected for spontaneous mutations. In this way a small proportion of the papillomas progress to become cancers. Thus the tumor promoter apparently favors the development of cancer, in this system at least, by expanding the population of cells that carry an initial mutation: the more such cells there are and the more times they divide, the greater the chance that at least one of them will undergo another mutation carrying it one more step along the road to malignancy. Although naturally occurring cancers do not necessarily arise through the specific sequence of distinct initiation and promotion steps just described, their evolution must be governed by similar principles. They too will evolve at a rate that depends both on the frequency of mutations and on influences affecting the survival, proliferation, and spread of certain types of mutant cells once they have been created.

Most Cancers Result from Avoidable Combinations of Environmental Causes

The development of a cancer generally involves many steps, each governed by multiple factors, some dependent on the genetic constitution of the individual, others dependent on his or her environment and way of life. By changing our surroundings or our habits, therefore, we should, in principle, be able to reduce drastically our chance of developing almost any given type of cancer. This is demonstrated most clearly by a comparison of cancer incidence in different countries: for almost every cancer that is common in one country, there is another country where the incidence is several times lower; and migrant populations tend to take on the pattern of cancer incidence typical of the host country, implying that the differences are due to environmental, not genetic, factors. From such data it is estimated that 80- 90% of cancers should be avoidable. Unfortunately, different cancers have different environmental risk factors, and a country that happens to escape one such danger is no more likely than other countries to escape the rest; thus the incidence of all cancers combined (among individuals of a given age) is similar from country to country. There are, however, some subgroups whose abstinent way of life does seem to reduce the total cancer death rate.

While such epidemiological observations indicate that cancer can be avoided, it remains difficult to identify the specific environmental risk factors or to establish how they act. Some certainly operate as mutagenic tumor initiators, directly provoking genetic change; others presumably serve as tumor promoters that help to enlarge the population of cells liable to progress, through further mutation, to full-blown cancer. The carcinogens in tobacco smoke, like the aflatoxin on tropical peanuts, probably belong mostly in the first category, while the reproductive hormones that circulate in a woman's body at different stages of her life may belong in the second category. The importance of these hormones is indicated by the striking correlations that exist between a woman's reproductive history and her risk of developing breast cancer; the hormones presumably affect cancer incidence through their influence on cell proliferation in the breast. It is possible that some factors act in still other ways - for example, by causing heritable epigenetic changes. Of course, it is not necessary to understand how cancer-causing agents act in order to identify them and show how to avoid them. In this task cancer epidemiology has had some notable successes and promises more to come. Simply by revealing the role of smoking, it has shown a way to reduce the total cancer death rate in North America and Europe by as much as 30%. The prevention of cancer is not only better than cure but seems also, given our present state of knowledge, to be much more readily attainable.

Search for Cancer Cures is Hard but Not Hopeless

The difficulty of curing a cancer is like the difficulty of getting rid of weeds. Cancer cells can be removed surgically or destroyed with toxic chemicals or radiation; but it is hard to eradicate every single one of them. Surgery can rarely ferret out every metastasis, and treatments that kill cancer cells are generally toxic to normal cells as well. If even a few cancerous cells remain, they can proliferate to produce a resurgence of the disease; and unlike the normal cells they may evolve resistance to the poisons used against them. Yet the outlook is not hopeless. In spite of the difficulties, effective cures using anticancer drugs have been devised for some formerly highly lethal cancers (notably Hodgkin's lymphoma, testicular cancer, choriocarcinoma, and some leukemias and other cancers of childhood). For several of the more common cancers, moreover, appropriate surgery or local radiotherapy enables a large proportion of patients to recover if the illness is diagnosed at a reasonably early stage. Effective treatments can sometimes be based on an understanding of the causes of a specific type of cancer. Estrogens, for example, appear to act as natural tumor promoters in cancer of the breast, and treatment with an estrogen antagonist, such as the drug *tamoxifen*, is effective in many breast cancer patients in preventing or delaying recurrence of the disease. Even for types of cancer where a cure at present seems beyond our reach, there are treatments that will prolong life or at least relieve distress.

A great deal of clinical cancer research centers on the problem of how to kill cancer cells selectively. For the most part, current methods exploit relatively subtle differences between normal and neoplastic cells with respect to proliferation rate, metabolism, and radiosensitivity, and they have unpleasant toxic side effects. A few types of cancer cells are especially vulnerable to selective attack because they depend on specific hormones or because their surfaces have unusual chemical features that can be recognized by antibodies. In general, however, progress with the vexing problem of anticancer selectivity has been slow - a matter of trial and error and guesswork as much as rational calculation.

In the search for better ways of curbing the survival, proliferation, and spread of cancer cells, it is important to examine more closely the strategies by which they thrive and multiply.

Cancerous Growth Often Depends on Deranged Control of Cell Differentiation or Cell Death

We have so far emphasized that cancer cells defy the normal controls on cell division: this is their central property. But there are other requirements too, if a tumor is to grow without limit. The tumor cells must, for example, stimulate the development of blood vessels to bring the nutrients and oxygen they require for growth. Moreover, many tissues are organized in such a way that even an uncontrolled increase in the frequency of cell division will not by itself produce a

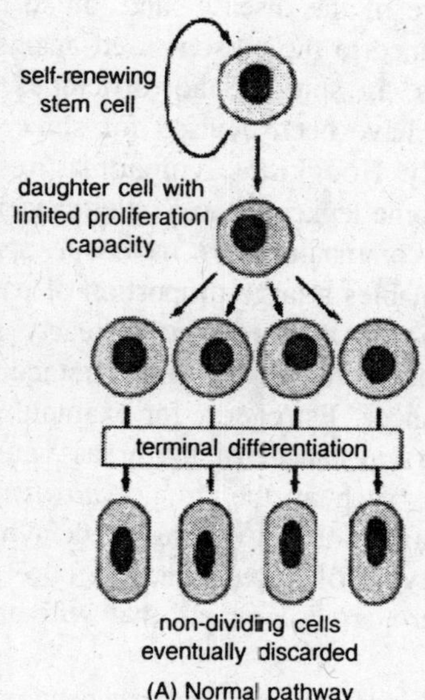

(A) Normal pathway

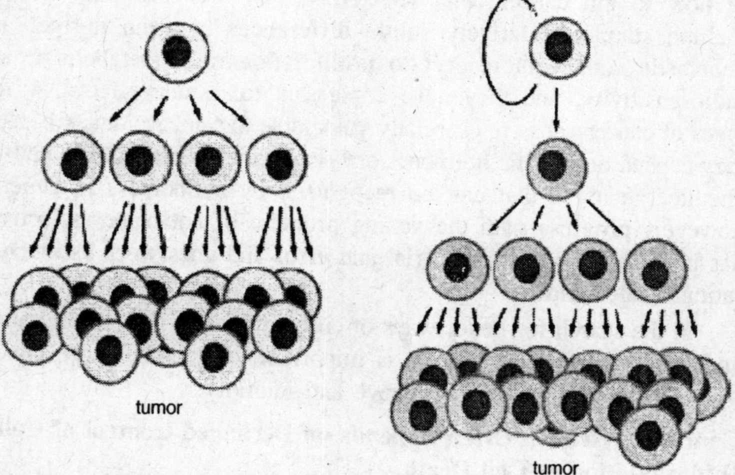

(B) Stem cell fails to produce one non-stem-cell daughter in each division and thereby proliferates to form a tumor

(C) Daughter cells fail to differentiate normally and therapy proliferate to form a tumor

Fig. 1.3. Normal and deranged control of cell production from stem cells.

steadily growing tumor. Like the epidermis of the skin and many other epithelia, the epithelium of the uterine cervix normally renews itself continually by shedding terminally differentiated cells from its outer surface and generating replacements from stem cells in the basal layer.

On average, each normal stem cell division generates one daughter stem cell and one cell that is condemned to terminal differentiation and a cessation of cell division. If the stem cell simply divides more rapidly, terminally differentiated cells will be produced and shed more rapidly, and a balance of genesis and destruction will still be maintained. Thus if a transformed stem cell is to generate a steadily growing clone of progeny, the basic rules must be upset: either more than 50% of the daughter cells must remain as stem cells or the process of differentiation must be deranged so that daughter cells embarked on this route retain an ability to carry on dividing indefinitely and avoid dying or being discarded at the end of the production line.

Presumably, the development of such properties underlies the progression from a mild dysplasia of the uterine cervix to carcinoma *in situ* and malignant cancer. Similar considerations apply to the development of cancer in other tissues that rely on stem cells, such as the skin, the lining of the gut, and the hemopoietic system. Several forms of leukemia, for example, seem to arise from a disruption of the normal program of differentiation, such that a committed progenitor of a particular type of blood cell continues to divide indefinitely, instead of differentiating terminally in the normal way and dying after a strictly limited number of division cycles. In general, changes that block the normal maturation of cells toward a nondividing, terminally differentiated state or prevent normal programmed cell death must play an essential part in many cancers. In the treatment of cancer, therefore, there is some prospect that drugs that promote cell differentiation may turn out to be a useful alternative to drugs that simply kill dividing cells.

Metastasize, Cancer Cells must be able to Cross Basal Laminae

It is the ability to metastasize that makes cancers hard to eradicate surgically or by localized irradiation. To disseminate widely in the body, the cells of a typical solid tumor must be able to loosen their adhesion to their original neighbors, escape from the tissue of origin, burrow through other tissues until they reach a blood vessel or a lymphatic vessel, cross the basal lamina and endothelial lining of the vessel so as to enter the circulation, make an exit from the circulation elsewhere in the body, and survive and proliferate in the new environment in which they find themselves. Each of these steps requires different properties. For example, in a variety of carcinomas that have been studied, loss of adhesion to neighboring cells in an epithelium depends on loss of expression of the epithelial cell-cell adhesion molecule *E-cadherin*, but the ability to burrow through tissues seems to depend on the production of proteolytic enzymes that can break down extracellular matrix. The final steps in metastasis are probably the most difficult: many tumors release large numbers of cells into the circulation, but only a tiny proportion of these cells succeed in founding metastatic colonies.

A few types of normal cells - notably white blood cells - already have some or all of the properties needed to disseminate through the body, but for most cancers the ability to metastasize probably requires additional mutations or epigenetic changes. Such transformations, like the others involved in the development of cancer, are thought to occur at random in the initial tumor population: only those few cells that acquire the properties needed for metastasis and that happen to land in a suitable environment will be able to produce secondary tumors. In accordance with this concept of evolution through random variation and natural selection, one finds that the cells of a single tumor are heterogeneous in metastatic capacity.

An understanding of the molecular mechanisms of metastasis should eventually allow the design of treatments to block it. Some progress is being made along these lines. It has been shown, for example, that for tumor cells to cross a basal lamina they must have appropriate integrins to act as laminin receptors, which enable the cells to adhere to the lamina, and they must carry on their surface type-IV collagenase, which helps them digest the lamina. Antibodies or other reagents that block either laminin attachment or the activity of type-IV collagenase have been found to block metastasis in experimental animals. It remains to be seen whether human cancer patients can be helped by similar treatments.

Mutations that Increase the Mutation Rate Accelerate the Development of Cancer

As we have emphasized, the incidence of tumors and their rate of progression toward malignancy depends on the frequency of mutations. The mutation rate may be high because of mutagens in the environment or because of intracellular defects in the machinery governing replication, recombination, and repair of DNA. People with the rare genetic disorder *xeroderma pigmentosum*, for example, have a defect in the system of enzymes required to repair the type of damage done to DNA by ultraviolet irradiation; as a result, the slightest exposure of the skin to sunlight is liable to provoke skin cancers. A more general predisposition to cancer due to faults in DNA repair and replication occurs in the relatively common *HNPCC syndrome*, and in *Bloom's syndrome*, *Fanconi's anemia*, and *ataxia-telangiectasia*. In all these rare genetic disorders the abnormality is inherited through the germ line and is therefore present in all the cells of the body. Similar genetic defects in DNA metabolism can also arise, however, through mutations originating in somatic cells. In fact, mutations that increase the mutation rate appear to be an important factor in the development of many cancers. Some of these mutations facilitate small local changes of DNA sequence. Others, especially common, facilitate gross disturbances of the genome.

Cancer cells often display an abnormal variability in the size and shape of their nuclei and in the number and structure of their chromosomes; indeed, abnormal nuclear morphology is one of the key features used by pathologists to diagnose cancer. When cancer cells are grown in culture, they are often found to have an extraordinarily unstable karyotype: genes become amplified or deleted and chromosomes become lost, duplicated, or translocated with a far higher frequency than in normal cells in culture. Such chromosomal variability suggests that the cells have some heritable fault in the machinery or control of chromosome replication, repair, recombination, or segregation. Such a fault, arising by somatic mutation, would be liable to increase the likelihood of subsequent mutations in other classes of genes and so to provide a short cut to the accumulation of the multiple mutations required for cancerous behavior. Molecular genetic studies have revealed one mechanism for this destabilization of the karyotype in cancer cells.

Enhanced Mutability of Cancer Cells Helps them Evade Destruction by Anticancer Drugs

Because of the abnormally high mutability of many cancer cells, most malignant tumor cell populations are heterogeneous in many respects and capable of evolving at an alarming rate when subjected to new selection pressures. This aggravates the difficulties of cancer therapy. Repeated treatments with drugs that are selectively toxic to dividing cells can be used to kill the majority of neoplastic cells in a cancer patient, but it is rarely possible to kill them all. Usually some small proportion are drug-resistant, and the effect of the treatment is to favor the spread and evolution of cells with this trait.

To make matters worse, cells that are exposed to one drug often develop a resistance not only to that drug, but also to other drugs to which they have never been exposed. This phenomenon of multidrug resistance is frequently correlated with a curious change in the karyotype: the cell is seen to contain additional pairs of miniature chromosomes - so-called *double minute chromosomes* - or to have a *homogeneously staining region* interpolated in the normal banding pattern of one of its regular chromosomes. Both these aberrations consist of massively amplified numbers of copies of a small segment of the genome. The amplified DNA often contains a specific gene, known as the *multidrug resistance* (*mdr1*) gene, which codes for a plasma-membrane-bound transport ATPase that is thought to prevent the intracellular accumulation of certain classes of lipophilic drugs by pumping them out of the cell. The amplification of other types of genes can also give the cancer cell a selective advantage: thus the gene for the enzyme dihydrofolate reductase (DHFR) often becomes amplified in response to cancer chemotherapy with the folic-acid antagonist methotrexate, and *myc* proto-oncogenes, whose products stimulate cell proliferation, are similarly amplified in some cancers.

While defects in DNA replication, recombination, or repair may help cancer cells to evolve by increasing their mutability, they may also make the cells more vulnerable to certain types of attack. This may explain the observation - exploited in therapy - that the cells of many tumors are killed more easily than normal cells by irradiation or by exposure to specific drugs that interfere with DNA metabolism. As we learn more about the molecular mechanisms regulating DNA replication, recombination, and repair, it is beginning to be possible to pinpoint defects in these functions in individual cases of cancer. By using such information, we may be better able to kill the delinquent cells by designing drugs that exploit their particular weaknesses.

2

GENETIC DISEASE

Cancer cells typically contain multiple alterations in the number and structure of genes and chromosomes. The majority of genetic alterations found in cancer cells are acquired by mutations in somatic cells. A few cancers in children and young adults are caused by genetic or epigenetic defects acquired during fetal development. Germ-line mutations underlie familial cancer syndromes. These can be inherited in an recessive or in a dominant fashion.

The mutations causing inherited cancer syndromes increase the risk of cancers by orders of magnitude. Overall, they are relatively rare. In contrast, less dramatic inherited variations (*'polymorphisms'*) in a large number of genes influence cancer risk only slightly to moderately, but are highly prevalent. Such genes encode, e.g., proteins involved in the metabolism of carcinogens and in protection against cell damage, in the regulation of immunity and inflammation, and in the metabolism of hormones and growth factors.

Many different genetic alterations are observed in cancer cells. Individual genes display point mutations such as base changes, insertions and deletions, or can be affected by chromosomal translocations or inversions. These changes lead to the expression of altered gene products, to decreased or increased gene expression, or to novel gene products like fusion proteins. Moreover, cancer cells are often aneuploid exhibiting numerical and/or structural alterations of chromosomes. These comprise loss or gain of chromosomes or chromosomal parts as well as rearrangements and recombinations. The consequences for individual genes range from complete loss by homozygous deletion through decreased copy numbers and increased gene dosage to gene amplification. At polymorphic loci, loss of heterozygosity may occur as a consequence of deletions or recombination.

In certain cancers, infection by DNA viruses and retroviruses alter the composition of the genome, adding new sequences and mutating existing ones as a consequence of insertion or induced deletions and rearrangements. These diverse types of genetic alterations occur to different extents in different types of cancers and even in cancers of the same type. So, in some cancers point mutations may prevail, while in others predominantly chromosomal aberrations are found.

The diverse types of genetic changes result in altered patterns of gene expression and altered gene products in cancer cells. Changes in gene expression are compounded by epigenetic mechanisms. Epigenetics in general designates the stable inheritance of alterations in gene expression without changes in the DNA sequence. Two particular important classes of genes affected by genetic and epigenetic alterations in cancer cells are oncogenes and tumor suppressor genes. Oncogenes contribute to tumor development by increased or misdirected activity. In the case of tumor suppressors, conversely, insufficient or lost function supports tumor development. Typically, in human cancers activation of oncogenes and inactivation of tumor suppressor genes are both observed. Multiple genetic as well as epigenetic changes accumulate during the development of malignant tumors, of which many are necessary. To accumulate so many changes, cancer cells may need to acquire a '*mutator phenotype*' during tumor initiation or progression. Indeed, cancer cells typically show defects in genome stability which lead to increased rates of fixed point mutations or chromosomal alterations or both.

Cancer as a Genetic Disease

The characteristic properties of cancer cells are to a large extent the consequences of genetic changes in the tumor cells. Indeed, genomic instability is one of the properties defining cancer and the aberrant structure of the nucleus seen in many cancer cells is an obvious morphological consequence of their altered genome. It is plausible that every cancer cell contains structural or numerical alterations of its genome. The number of alterations is not precisely known, and certainly varies with cancer type and stage of progression. Systematic DNA sequencing has yielded estimates of hundreds to thousands of point mutations in some tumors. Screening by arbitrary PCR has suggested an even higher number of alterations for some cancers. Certainly, 20 or more chromosomal aberrations detectable by cytogenetic techniques are not unusual in an advanced carcinoma.

It is therefore very appropriate to regard cancer as a genetic disease. Still, a few points must be kept in mind:

1. Only a minority of cancers are caused by mutations inherited in the germline. Rather, the vast majority of genetic alterations found in cancers develop during the life of a patient in somatic cells. Thus, cancer is almost always a disease caused by '*somatic mutations*'. Even in cancers which are passed on over several generations in a family, the initial inherited mutations are complemented by additional somatic mutations. Likewise, cancers arising in young children or adolescents are often caused by mutations originating de novo in their parents' germ cells or during intra-uterine development. A typical cancer of this kind is Wilms tumor, but similar circumstances apply to testicular cancer and certain childhood leukemias.
2. The relationship between mutant genotype and disease phenotype is not straightforward in cancer, which per se is not so unusual for genetic diseases. However, in cancer the relationship is extremely complex. Cancer cells as a rule contain many different mutations which each may contribute to various extents to the properties of the tumor.
3. Not all properties of cancer cells may result from genetic defects. Many stable changes in cancer cells may be set up by regulatory loops without alterations in the sequence or the amount of DNA. Such changes are designated as '*epigenetic*'. They can occur within a cancer cell or concern its interaction with other cell types.

Genetic Alterations in Cancer Cells

Many different types of genetic alterations can be observed in human tumor cells by molecular or cytogenetic methods. Some alterations affect single or only a few genes. The DNA sequence of an individual gene can be altered by point mutations, smaller or larger deletions or insertions, or by rearrangements, with a wide array of potential consequences. Larger deletions can affect several genes at once. Rearrangements can lead to the creation of novel genes from others.

Point Mutations

Point mutations are due to base exchanges in the DNA. These are categorized as transitions (pyrimidine→pyrimidine or purine→purine) or transversions (pyrimidine→purine or purine→pyrimidine). They can have very different effects, even if one considers only those occurring within the coding region of a gene. Silent mutations lead to a different codon encoding the same amino acid. They therefore do not change the coding potential of the mRNA, but they may affect its stability. The same effect can be elicited by mutations in the 3'- or 5'-UTR (untranslated region). Missense mutations lead to a change in the amino acid sequence. The resulting altered protein may possess increased, decreased or even unchanged activity. Therefore, the evaluation of the functional impact of a missense mutation detected in a tumor cell requires a biochemical or cellular assay for the function of the encoded protein. Nonsense mutations are more easy to evaluate since they lead to a truncated, often unstable protein product. Moreover, nonsense mutations occurring between the ATG start codon and the next splice site, i.e. in the first or second exon of a gene, destabilize its mRNA by making it prone to '*nonsense-mediated decay* (NMD)', a cellular quality control mechanism. Importantly, point mutations in principle can be activating or inactivating. However, the spectrum of mutations that lead to increased activity of a gene product is normally much narrower than that decreasing its activity. For instance, mutations activating RAS oncogenes are restricted to three codons, while mutations inactivating the tumor suppressor gene TP53 are distributed across the gene.

Splice Mutations

Splicing requires specific consensus sequences at the exon - intron junctions and also in the intron. The efficiency of splicing is also influenced by sequences within the exon. Mutations of sequences required for splicing may alter the protein product or the expression level of a gene more or less subtly. Mutations disrupting a 5'-splice site may lead to skipping of an exon, whereas mutations affecting a 3'-splice site may lead to an elongation of an exon until the next recognizable splice site. In both cases, an altered protein may result that lacks amino acids or contains additional amino acids. If the reading frame in the following exons is changed, the ensuing protein product is often truncated and/or unstable. With similar consequences, point mutations in introns or exons may create novel splice sites from '*cryptic splice sites*', i.e. sequences resembling proper splice consensus signals.

Alternative Splicing

The issue of altered splicing in human tumors is rendered difficult by the vagaries of splicing in normal mammalian cells. According to current estimates the average human gene generates about five different mRNA variants by differential splicing, alternative promotor usage and use of alternate termination signals. This can make it very difficult to decide, whether altered splicing found in tumors is relevant or not, and to determine whether it is caused by mutations in the affected gene or perhaps by mutations in a splice regulator. Several important genes display variations in splicing in human cancers that are probably functional relevant, but whose causes are unknown. Among them are relatives of the tumor suppressor *TP53*, called *TP73L* and *TP73*. They encode several different proteins with different functions, the prototypic forms being designated p63α and p73α respectively.

Mutations in Regulatory Sequences

Even more complicated is the issue of mutations in non-coding sequences that regulate transcription. The regulatory sequences for a gene are often spread out over several 10 kb. In addition to the basal promoter, they comprise enhancers and silencers that may be located upstream and downstream of the gene as well as in introns and boundary elements. They are not well characterized for many human genes, and the effect of point mutations or even larger changes can only be judged by tedious experiments. As a consequence, many investigations of human cancers have focussed on mutations in coding sequences only, considering at most exon/intron junctions. It is therefore generally assumed that in many cancers mutations occur outside the coding regions of genes, but their frequency and their functional impact is impossible to assess at present. Moreover, many mutations are documented outside of actual genes, e.g., in microsatellite repeats, whose functional importance is also uncertain.

Deletions

In addition to base changes, smaller or larger deletions or insertions in tumor cells disrupt the coding regions of genes or destroy their regulatory elements. Small deletions become evident in PCR-based analyses, while very large deletions can be detected by cytogenetic methods. Intermediate-sized deletions in the kb range are more easily detected and charted in tumor cell lines than in tumor tissues, because PCR methods amplify residual alleles from tumor cells or non-tumor cells in the tissue. Therefore, it is not quite clear to what extent deletions contribute to loss of gene function in human tumors. In some cases, deletions affect both copies of a gene, e.g. through an internal deletion in one chromosome and loss of the second corresponding chromosome. This case is called '*homozygous deletion*'. Charted homozygous deletions in tumor cells sometimes extend across several Mbp.

Insertions

Insertions in the genomes of tumor cells can comprise one to several bps. In the coding sequence of a gene, they typically lead to frame-shift mutations and/or change the stability of its mRNA. Insertions can arise by several mechanisms. Some are in fact duplications, e.g., in short repetitive sequences such as genomic polyA-tracts, caused by unrepaired slipping of DNA polymerases. Others may arise during repair of DNA strand breaks. Insertions as well as deletions can also be caused by viruses or endogenous retroelements. Somewhat surprisingly, in human cancers, transposition of endogenous retroelements appears to be relatively rare, even though a few active retrotransposons, all from the LINE-1 class, exist in the human genome.

Viral Genomes

Viruses add extra genetic material to cells and often change the genome of the host cell. In human cancers, DNA viruses are more prevalent than retroviruses and contribute to the development of several human cancers by expression of specific viral proteins. They normally replicate as episomes, but in cancer cells integrates are not unusual. These insertions typically disrupt genes and are often associated with partial losses of the viral genomes and altered expression patterns of the viral genes. Importantly, the integrates are often unstable and therefore induce chromosomal breaks with losses and rearrangements. Retroviral insertions in particular also often affect gene expression near the insertion site substantially, and cause over-expression. In human cancer, retroviral insertions seem to be rare, but the DNA virus HBV may sometimes act in a similar manner.

Chromosomal Translocations

Alterations in the structure or expression of specific genes can also be caused by chromosomal translocations, which are most evident in hematological and soft tissue cancers. Obviously, a translocation may simply destroy and inactivate genes at the translocation sites. However, the opposite outcome is not infrequent and is important in human cancers. A translocation may separate inhibitory regulatory elements from the coding region of a gene and/or place it under the influence of activating regulatory elements from another gene. In either case, over-expression or deregulation ensue. This mechanism accounts, e.g., for the activation of the MYC gene in Burkitt lymphoma. A third possible outcome is the generation of novel genes by translocations appositioning two genes to each other. Typically, the product of the novel gene is a fusion protein which contains N-terminal sequences

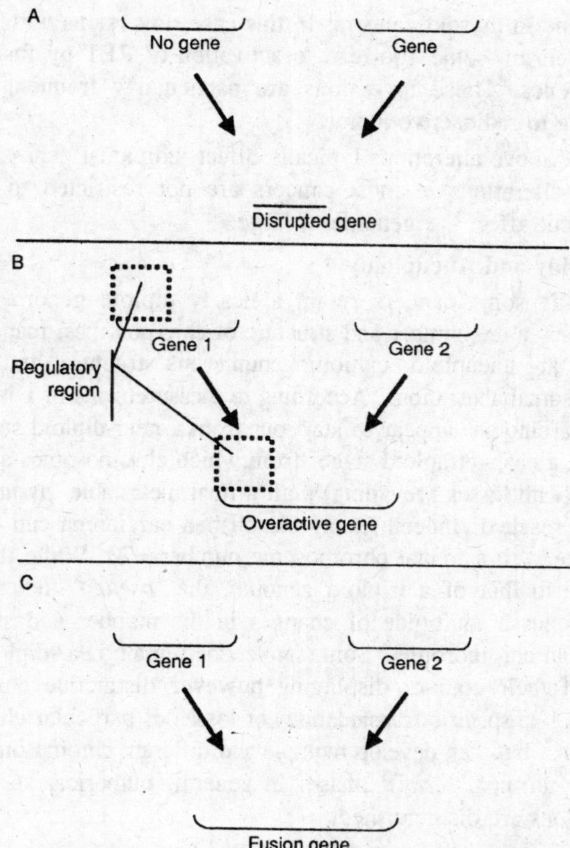

Fig. 2.1. Effects of chromosomal translocations in human cancers.

from one fusion partner and C-terminal sequences from the other. If a balanced translocation occurs, two fusion genes and proteins may be formed. The fusion proteins can possess properties that differ significantly from those of the original proteins. Two infamous proteins of this type are BCR-ABL and PML-RARα.

Chromosomal Inversions

Chromosomal inversions can basically have the same consequences as translocations, since they are essentially translocations within one chromosome. If they are not evident from the karyotype or from the analysis of a particular gene, they are difficult to detect because many molecular or cytogenetic methods in use do not distinguish the orientation of a sequence on a chromosome. Their prevalence is therefore difficult to ascertain. A prominent example concerns the

RET gene in thyroid cancers. In this case, inversions within the long arm of chromosome 10q lead to activation of RET by fusing it with other genes. These inversions are particularly frequent following exposure to radioactive iodine.

The above alterations typically affect individual genes. However, genetic alterations in most cancers are not restricted to individual genes, but affect the genome at large.

Polyploidy and Aneuploidy

While some cancers retain a nearly diploid genome with few alterations in the number and structure of chromosomes, many advanced cancers are aneuploid, exhibiting numerous structural and numerical chromosomal aberrations. According to measurements of DNA content, many carcinomas appear to start out from a near-diploid stage and go through a near-tetraploid stage, from which chromosomes are lost and gained (with losses prevailing) until a final metastable '*pseudo-triploid*' state is reached. Indeed, many established carcinoma cell lines show this state with a modal chromosome number ≈70. While this number is close to that of a triploid genome, the '*pseudo*' indicates that it often belies a multitude of changes in the number and structure of individual chromosomes. Some leukemias remain near-diploid through most of their course, displaying however distinctive chromosomal changes like specific translocations or losses of particular chromosomal fragments, but then develop multiple and different chromosomal changes in their terminal '*crisis*' phase. In general, numerical and structural aberrations are distinguished.

Numerical Chromosomal Aberrations

In aneuploid cells, the numbers of chromosomes or chromosome arms deviate from the total number of complements present, e.g., three chromosomes of one kind may be found in a diploid cell. These numerical aberrrations imply an altered gene dosage for the affected genes. The copy of one gene in a tumor cell therefore may range from zero (i.e. homozygous deletion) to very high. However, even in a tumor cell it is unusual to have more than 5 or 6 chromosomes of one kind.

Gene Amplification

Higher copy numbers of genes are reached by amplification of smaller chromosomal regions called amplicons, which may range from several hundred kbs to several Mbp in size. This size implicates that amplifications may contain several genes, of which one or several can be over-expressed and be relevant for the tumor phenotype. If sufficiently large, amplified regions contained in a chromosome can become cytogenetically detectable as *homogeneously staining regions* (HSR). Amplicons in tumor cells can also be episomal, typically as small DNA circles presenting as small speckles in cytogenetic analyses. These are designated '*double minutes*'. Double minutes replicate autonomously, but do not possess kinetochores and are randomly distributed to daughter cells. Accordingly, their numbers vary. Moreover, they may be in a dynamic exchange with corresponding HSR from which they may originate and into which they may reintegrate by recombination. Copy numbers of genes on double minutes can run up to thousands per cell. Gains or losses of whole chromosomes may result from missegregation at mitosis. However, amplifications presuppose structural changes.

Structural Chromosomal Aberration

Structural chromosomal aberrations in tumor cells include the translocations and inversions discussed above, but also internal deletions of various sizes. Classical cytogenetic methods have identified '*marker*' chromosomes in many cancer cells that are composed of fragments from several different chromosomes. Modern cytogenetic analyses reveal that in addition many chromosomes appearing grossly normal in cancer cells also harbor deletions, inversions or are also composed from parts of several chromosomes.

Numerical chromosomal changes can be brought about by mitotic non-disjunction. If a chromosome does not attach properly to the mitotic spindle, one daughter cell may end up with an additional chromosome and the other with one less. The origin of structural chromosomal changes is probably more complicated. Some may result from double-strand breaks in the involved chromosomes which may lead to deletions or recombinations. Another mechanism are breakage-fusion-bridge cycles initiated by strand breaks or telomeric fusions.

The multitude of structural changes in chromosomes reveals a high degree of illegitimate recombination in tumor cells. While some of them are evident, others may not be detectable at the cytogenetic level, especially, if they result in the exchange of genetic material rather than net loss or gain or translocations. Indeed, molecular analyses of polymorphic DNA sequences reveal that tumor cells often contain identical copies of a DNA sequence that is heterozygous in normal cells of the patient. This is called loss of heterozygosity. It can be caused by deletions of one allele, but also by recombination.

The various types of genetic alterations discussed in this section do not each occur to the same extent in every human cancer. Rather, in different tumors particular types of mutations tend to predominate. In some cancers point mutations are most prevalent, whereas chromosomal aberrations seem to be responsible for the majority of the genetic changes in others. In some cancers, distinct subtypes can be distinguished by this difference, e.g. in colon carcinomas. Further differences may be more subtle. For instance, some cancers tend to lose or gain whole chromosomes, whereas others tend to delete, gain or rearrange chromosomal fragments. The reasons underlying such differences are the subject of a very active area of current research.

Inherited Predisposition to Cancer

Although most genetic alterations in tumor cells develop during the life-time of a patient, the predisposition to cancers can be inherited. Three different types of inheritance can be distinguished.

In some families cancers are very frequent and occur (essentially) in each generation. This is a general hallmark of autosomal-dominant inherited diseases with high penetrance. The families may be plagued by specific cancers, rarer ones such as retinoblastoma, or common cancers such as breast cancer, or by various types of cancer, such as in Li-Fraumeni-syndrome. Typically, cancers manifest at a lower than average age of onset and also unusually often at multiple sites or bilaterally in paired organs, such as the eyes, kidney and breast. These are two further criteria pointing to inherited cancers. In some cases, cancer predisposition is associated with developmental defects, e.g. in the Gorlin and Cowden syndromes. This is a fourth, although not as strict criterion. The increased risk in cancer families with an autosomal-dominant mode of inheritance is caused by an inherited mutation in a single gene. The affected genes are usually tumor suppressor genes and more rarely oncogenes. The inherited mutations are likely not sufficient to cause cancer, but they provide the first mutation of several that are required.

In some families predisposition to cancer is inherited in a recessive mode. More often than in the dominantly inherited cases, cancer predisposition is found in the context of rare inherited syndromes. So, the affected patients are initially afflicted by other symptoms and cancers appear later, but still at a relatively early age. Syndromes in this category include Xeroderma pigmentosum, Ataxia telengiectasia, Fanconi anemia, Nijmegen breakage-syndrome as well as the Bloom and Werner syndromes. These syndromes differ in the extent of the cancer risk and the predominant cancer types, but at least one type of cancer is substantially more prevalent than in the general population. In these syndromes, predisposition to cancer is evidently caused by mutations inactivating both copies of the same gene. The genes affected are usually involved in cell protection and DNA repair. In general, the inherited defects in DNA repair favor genetic alterations in somatic cells that lead to cancer.

Inheritance of mutated genes in autosomal-dominant or recessive cancer syndromes carries a greatly enhanced risk of developing cancer during a human's lifetime which may approach 100%, whereas the life-time risk of '*sporadic*' cases in the general population may be minimal. Even in those cancers, like that of the skin, where the life-time risk is high in the general population, the risk to develop a cancer up to a certain age is strongly increased in persons with an inherited predisposition. Fortunately, cancer predisposition of this kind is infrequent. All high-risk mutations in dominantly and recessively inherited cancer syndromes together may account for less than 10% of all human cancers. Nevertheless, an individual's cancer risk may be strongly influenced by the genotype. About one in a thousand base pairs differs between individual humans. Differences that occur in more than 0.5% of the population are called '*polymorphisms*' and are thereby distinguished from rare changes considered as true mutations. Polymorphisms are found in coding regions of genes as well as in regulatory sequences and in non-coding sequences throughout the genome. These differences comprise *single nucleotide polymorphisms* (SNPs) and differences in the size of micro- and minisatellite repeats, but also insertions or deletions of various sizes.

For instance, up to 50% individuals in some European populations lack the gene for GSTM1, a glutathione transferase enzyme metabolizing xenobiotics. This is called a '*null-allele*' because no enzyme activity is present. Other polymorphisms have more subtle effects. Polymorphisms in genes involved in the metabolism of drugs and other exogenous compounds modulate the risk of cancer in people exposed to them. For instance, detoxification of carcinogenic benzopyrene metabolites is in general more efficient in individuals with GSTM1 compared to those lacking the enzyme. Since benzopyrene is one of the carcinogens in tobacco smoke, the risk of GSTM1$^{-/-}$ smokers to develop cancer of the lung (and other organs) is increased. Even if the risk of lung cancer were only two-fold enhanced by the lack of the enzyme, this increase would apply to up to 50% of the smoking population in some European populations. Clearly, such polymorphisms may have profound effects at the population level, even if they modulate the risk for each individual only slightly. It is also important to note that the effect of a polymorphism in a drug metabolism gene depends not only on the extent to which it alters the function of the gene, but also on the dose and the type of exposure. For instance, the product of another gene from the GST superfamily, GSTT1, also protects against carcinogens in general, but activates small chlorinated alkenes, such as trichloro-ethylene, to highly mutagenic compounds.

Other polymorphisms modulating cancer risks have been identified in genes involved in immunity, inflammation, hormone metabolism, and nucleotide metabolism. As with drug metabolism genes, the risk conferred by the polymorphic forms of these genes is contingent on non-genetic factors such as exposure or nutrition. Also, the differences in risk are always moderate, i.e. within one order of magnitude.

A complicated situation is posed by polymorphisms in high-risk cancer genes. For instance, several polymorphisms are known in the gene mutated in Li-Fraumeni-syndrome, *TP53*. At least one of these may be associated with only a small and more specific increase in cancer risk. An even more difficult problem concerns mutations in the *ATM* gene, which lead to a high risk of cancer when present in a homozygous state (in fact, often different high-risk mutations combine, so precisely this is a '*compound*' homozygosity). Homozygosity is fortunately rare, but heterozygosity for mutations like 7271T→G could be as frequent as 1:200 in some populations (so, one would have to consider this as a polymorphism). Whether persons with polymorphisms are at increased risk, is a hotly debated issue.

Since one characteristic of inherited tumors is their precocious appearance compared to sporadic cases, the question arises to which extent childhood tumors are inherited. This is evidently so when tumors arise in the context of inherited syndromes, e.g. childhood brain tumors in Li-Fraumeni-syndrome families. Indeed, some childhood tumors occur as familial as well as sporadic cases, e.g. retinoblastoma and Wilms tumor. Even though these are tumors of young children, the average onset is slightly earlier in familial cases.

Other cases of Wilms tumor, however, are caused by developmental defects in a parent's germ cell or during early development as a consequence of genetic or epigenetic changes. A similar situation holds for testicular germ cell cancers, which are derived from germ cells that due to mutations acquired in the fetus have not completed their maturation properly. A few of these cancers become evident in young children, but most start to expand under the influence of rising androgen levels during puberty, leading to a peak in incidence in the third decade of life. In the same vein, studies on twin children coming down with leukemia indicate that the responsible chromosomal translocations have likely taken place very early during fetal development, although the disease manifests roughly a decade later. So, while these cancer may be suspected to be inherited, they are more precisely considered as '*congenital*'.

Cancer Genes

In the cell of a cancer at a late stage of progression, several hundred genes may be mutated or rearranged and for many the dosage and accordingly as a rule their expression levels may be changed. Indeed, expression profiling of tumor cells by array techniques has revealed thousands of genes whose expression is increased or decreased. Moreover, expression changes cannot only be due to primary changes such as altered gene dosage or mutation, but also be secondary to mutations in regulatory genes or to epigenetic mechanisms. So, it is not immediately obvious which changes are essential for tumor development, which contribute to the phenotype of the cancer without being essential, and which are coincidental and irrelevant. Several different kinds of genes can be distinguished that are relevant in human cancers.

Tumor Suppressor Genes

The genes mutated in dominantly inherited cancers are obviously central to cancer development. Most of these belong to a class named '*tumor suppressor genes*'. Typically, their function is strongly diminished or obliterated in cancers by mutations or by epigenetic silencing. Not unexpectedly, these same genes are often found mutated in sporadic cases of the same cancer types and even in other types. Some genes of this kind are only found inactivated in sporadic cancers, but their inactivation can be shown to be essential for tumor development.

Oncogenes

A few responsible genes in dominantly inherited cancers, such as RET in hereditary endocrine cancers and MET in hereditary renal papillary carcinoma are activated by mutations instead of being inactivated like tumor suppressor genes. For a larger number of genes, activation by specific mutations or by overexpression as a consequence of gene amplification, or by other mechanisms, is found consistently in sporadic cancers. Some of these genes are related to those genes in oncogenic retroviruses known to cause cancers in animals. These genes are therefore called *oncogenes*.

DNA Repair and Checkpoint Genes

Most oncogenes and many tumor suppressor genes directly control cell proliferation, differentiation, and/or survival. Many genes inactivated by mutations in recessive cancer syndromes are not directly involved in this type of regulation. Instead, defects in these genes increase the rate of mutations, of which some alter the function of genes directly involved in the development of tumors. In fact, mutations in genes of this type underlie certain cancer predispositions inherited in a dominant fashion. This type of tumor suppressor gene is sometimes called a '*caretaker*' and those directly involved in growth regulation are called '*gatekeepers*'. Mutations in some caretaker genes are also found in some sporadic human cancers.

Risk Modulating Genes

A related group of relevant genes is even less directly involved in cancer development. The products of genes in this group, exemplified by the GSTs, modulate the development of cancer, e.g., by influencing the level of active carcinogens, the reaction of the immune system to cancer cells, or the level of hormones and growth factors that stimulate tumor cell proliferation. Very often, their importance depends on environmental factors such as exposure to carcinogens. Once a cancer is established, they are not absolutely necessary.

Execution Genes

In contrast, another group of genes only becomes important after the cancer is established. These genes may be activated by mutations, but are more often induced as a consequence of activation of oncogenes or inactivation of tumor suppressor genes. They may not be necessary for survival of the cancer cells, but for their sustained growth and specifically for invasion and metastasis. These complex processes appear to require a relatively well coordinated program of gene expression which can be initiated by mutations in a limited number of genes, but requires the activity of a much larger number for its execution.

So, it is, in fact, anything but trivial to define a '*cancer gene*'. There are some clear-cut cases, e.g. almost every retinoblastoma displays inactivation of the gene *RB1*, and every Burkitt lymphoma shows activation of the gene *MYC*, showing these are clearly tumor suppressor and oncogenes, respectively. However, such bonafide oncogenes and tumor suppressor genes apparently represent the extreme end of a continuum of more or less relevant cancer genes.

Accumulation of Genetic and Epigenetic Changes in Human Cancers

Advanced human cancers usually contain a multitude of genetic changes, and often epigenetic alterations. In human cancers, it is rarely possible to determine, at which stage of tumor progression they were acquired. Most data, however, suggest that they gradually accumulate during tumor progression. A gradual accumulation of multiple genetic changes would explain why most cancers appear at older age and would fit with epidemiological data suggesting 4 to 5 essential '*hits*' to be necessary for cancer development. The genes affected by such crucial mutations are likely oncogenes and tumor suppressor genes. Indeed, advanced human carcinomas typically contain mutations in several genes of both types. Genetic and epigenetic changes in further genes may modulate the tumor phenotype. Most genetic changes are the result of somatic mutations, but an inherited predisposition to cancer can be caused by one crucial mutation passed on in the germ-line, with further mutations occuring somatically.

Alternatively, inherited predisposition to cancer can be due to germ-line mutations in DNA repair genes or '*caretaker*' genes. These defects appear to favor cancer development by increasing the probability of crucial mutations in oncogenes and tumor suppressor genes, but are associated with additional mutations that are more or less important for tumor progression. For instance, cancers with defects in DNA mismatch repair contain a large number of mutations, some in oncogenes and tumor suppressor genes, but others in irrelevant microsatellite repeats.

So, tumors arising on that background exhibit a '*mutator phenotype*'. Depending on the type of defect, a mutator phenotype can manifest as an increase in point mutations or as various kinds of chromosomal instability. The multitude of genetic alterations observed in many advanced human cancers suggests that they have developed a sort of '*mutator phenotype*', leading to an increased rate of point mutations, to chromosomal instability, or even to frequent epigenetic alterations. While the existence of genomic instability in advanced cancers seems evident, an interesting question is whether it is required for their development. In other words, can the accumulation of genetic alterations required for an advanced cancer be achieved by random mutations at a normal rate, or does it require the establishment of a '*mutator phenotype*' at some stage of progression? This is a hotly debated question with ramifications for tumor therapy as well as tumor prevention.

3

CANCER CELLS

What happens to a cell when it becomes cancerous, when it loses its identity and stops caring about the community that it lives in? When Robert Louis Stevenson wrote *The Strange Case of Dr. Jekyll and Mr. Hyde,* in 1886, he was trying to illustrate the complex nature of the human psyche, which seems to be a mixture of good and bad intentions. Dr. Jekyll was a good and honest man, but his experiments turned him into the very bad Mr. Hyde, a crazy man who cared for nothing. Today, we know that human insanity can be traced to a disturbance in brain biochemistry. Likewise, the insanity of a cancer cell can now be traced to a disturbance in the biochemistry of the cell cycle and cellular communication. A deranged cell cycle can sometimes have a dramatic effect on a cell's lifespan.

CANCER CELLS ARE IMMORTAL

The difference between cancer cells and normal cells is profound, not only because of the way they look and the way they behave, but because of the radical difference in their lifespans. Placed in tissue culture, cancer cells can live forever. Normal cells, on the other hand, die after about 50 generations. The best proof of cancer cell immortality comes from HeLa cells, a cultured cancer cell line that was established in 1951 from a cervical tumor that was isolated from a woman named Henrietta Lacks. The HeLa cell line has been growing well ever since, and cultures of these cells are maintained for research purposes by laboratories around to world. Henrietta Lacks, a native of Baltimore, Maryland, was 31 years old when the tumor was discovered. She died of cervical cancer eight months later. It may seem odd to think that the achievement of immortality is a bad thing. There is a tendency to believe that if a cell becomes immortal, it might immortalize the entire organism. But an animal's body is designed around the principle of regulated cell division for the good of the community. Most cells in an adult's body are post-mitotic, a condition that guarantees a stable organ size and shape. Some cells, such as skin and bone marrow, are allowed to divide, but only a limited number of times. The only immortal cells in the body are the germ cells (sperm and eggs), although even they will die out if the individual never has children. This is not to say that such an arrangement can never be tampered with. Stem cells can also proliferate for years in

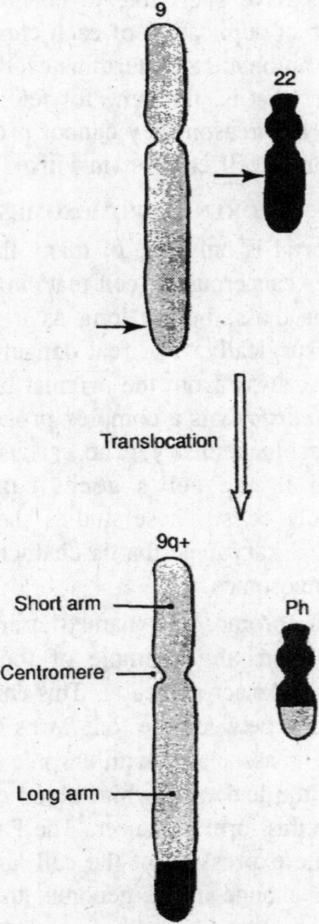

Fig. 3.1. The Philadelphia chromosome (Ph) is produced by a translocation between the long arms of chromosomes 9 and 22. The short arrows mark the fragmentation point. The chromosomes are aligned at the centromeres.

culture (although we do not yet know if they are truly immortal) and their use in medical therapies may make it possible to extend the human lifespan, but for now, the acquisition of immortality by a *somatic cell* always leads to trouble. For 40 years scientists struggled to understand the mechanism by which cancer cells are immortalized. Throughout the 1990s attention was drawn to a special DNA sequence called a telomere, located at the tips of the chromosomes. Each time the DNA is replicated during the S phase of the *cell cycle*, the telomeres shrink, but they are later restored by a special enzyme called *telomerase*. By carefully studying the mechanics of DNA replication, scientists have been able to conclude that telomeres are essential for the correct duplication of each chromosome. A failure to duplicate the DNA automatically terminates the cell cycle. Normal cells lack telomerase (that is, the gene for telomerase is turned off in adult cells), and for this reason they cannot proliferate indefinitely in the body (in vivo) or in cell culture (in vitro).

Broken Chromosomes

Becoming immortal is only one of many things that must happen before a cell becomes cancerous. A cell that simply divides indefinitely can produce a tumor mass, but as long as it remains benign it can usually be removed surgically. The real danger occurs when some of the cancer cells break away from the original tumor to colonize other parts of the body. *Metastasis* is a complex process that involves many changes in the cell's biochemistry. The earliest indication that these changes are rooted in the cell's genes came from histological examinations of cancer cells. These studies showed that most cancer cells have an abnormal karyotype that is characterized by the presence of many broken chromosomes.

The Philadelphia chromosome (named after the city where it was first discovered) is a striking example of the relationship between genetic abnormality and cancer induction. This chromosomal abnormality involves a translocation between the long arms of chromosomes 9 and 22. This abnormality is associated with chronic myelogenous leukemia and can be found in the leukemic white blood cells of virtually every patient suffering from this form of cancer. The Philadelphia chromosome alters the normal gene expression of the cell and is one example of a somatic mutation, or change in the genome, that can lead to cancer.

Failure to Communicate

When normal cells are placed in culture they can proliferate long enough to cover the bottom of the dish in a single layer, or *monolayer*, of cells. When the monolayer is established, the cells stop growing due to a phenomenon known as *contact inhibition*. The cells in the monolayer know they are in contact with other cells and this information is enough to signal an end to proliferation, to ensure that the cells do not pile up on each other. Cancer cells, in culture, do not respond to contact inhibition. Instead, they continue growing, often forming large clumps of cells on the plate.

The failure of contact inhibition in cancer cells is a failure to communicate, and is due to an abnormal glycocalyx. In normal cells, the glycocalyx contains many cell surface glycoproteins that act like sensory *antennae*. When those antennae make contact with the glycocalyx of another cell, the information is relayed to the interior of the cell by a signaling pathway that tells the cell to stop growing. It may also activate other pathways that stimulate the formation of physical connections between the cells. None of this works in cancer cells. The antennae are either gone or are no longer linked to the proper signaling pathway. As a consequence, cancer cells grow over the top of one another, and the only thing that limits their growth, in vivo and in vitro, is the availability of oxygen and nutrients. As they pile up, forming a large clump, the cells in the middle stop dividing and may even die for want of food and air.

THEY GO WHERE THEY PLEASE

The corrupted communication channels that are characteristic of cancer cells account for their apparent lack of manners and their tendency to crowd each other when grown in culture; it also accounts for the ability of cancer cells to colonize tissues that are normally reserved for other cells. A normal heart cell would never try to colonize the brain or the liver. Conversely, brain cells would never try to invade the skin, bone, or any other type of tissue.

If a normal cell should accidentally break loose from its parent tissue or organ and find itself in foreign territory, it would quickly receive and process signals from the surrounding cells that would cause it to commit suicide. Cell suicide is called *apoptosis*, and it is regulated by specific communication pathways. Cancer cells will not commit suicide. They either ignore the signals from cells around them, or the pathways regulating apoptosis are dysfunctional. In either case, the loss of the death signal makes it possible for cancer cells to grow in any environment.

However, the ability to ignore an order to commit suicide is only one element in the complex process known as metastasis. For cancer cells to invade other territory, they must break loose from the tumor mass, travel through the tissue or organ until they reach a blood vessel, penetrate the vessel wall, and then, after being carried along in the circulating blood, exit the vessel in some other part of the body. Once they have colonized fresh territory and begin forming a tumor they must activate angiogenesis, the growth of blood vessels into the tumor, in order to receive oxygen and nutrients. This may appear to be an unlikely scenario, depending as it does on so many processes, but cancer cells are capable of coordinating all of these events, and when they do, they are free to go where they please.

One Mutation Is Not Enough

Cancer cells are genetic mutants; this is clear from their abnormal karyotype and the apparent distortions in their communication pathways. These changes produce a standard behavior pattern for cancer cells that consists of the following:

1. They ignore signals that regulate proliferation.
2. They sidestep built-in limitations to their own reproduction.
3. They are genetically unstable.
4. They escape their parent tissue.
5. They colonize foreign tissue.
6. They avoid suicide.

This list is a good indication that more than one defective gene is required to produce a cancer cell. The actual number of genetic mutations that must occur to produce a cancer cell is unknown, but may involve 10 to 20 genes. The mutations occur slowly over time in a sequential fashion and may account for the age-related onset of brain tumors, breast cancer, and prostate cancer. This fits with many observations over the past 10 years concerning tumor progression, whereby a mildly abnormal cell gives rise to a colony of cells that gradually evolves into metastatic cancer.

The driving force behind the evolution of a cancer appears to be the genetic instability that is characteristic of these cells. Normal cells are vigilant and constantly check the accuracy of their products by monitoring the behavior of their own machinery. When the DNA is duplicated in preparation for cell division, regulators, monitors, and repair enzymes are on guard to make sure no mistakes occurred when the daughter strand was made. If an error is detected, the cell does not divide until the damage is repaired. If the damage cannot be repaired, the cell will either commit suicide voluntarily or be forced to do so by the immune system. Repair enzymes and monitors also check to ensure the chromosomes segregate properly (that is, are portioned out equally to the daughter cells). If segregation is abnormal, one daughter cell will end up with too many chromosomes, while the other cell will have too few. When this happens, apoptosis is activated by the monitoring system, so that both cells commit suicide.

Cancer cells behave as though they have an absolute disdain for quality control. If an error is made during DNA synthesis, they do not bother making repairs before continuing through the cell cycle. If chromosomes fail to segregate normally or develop an abnormal karyotype, the two daughter cells do not commit suicide. In this way, the abnormal cell line accumulates many genetic abnormalities until it becomes malignant, or until it is destroyed by the immune system. In a bizarre sense, cancer cells are trying to establish a situation in which genetic variability is maximized, with a subsequent increase in the rate at which they evolve.

The accumulation of mutations through genetic instability is acted upon by natural selection. Most of the cells in the original tumor will be so abnormal they will be incapable of providing for themselves and will eventually die out. In many cases this will lead to the disappearance of the entire tumor mass. But it can also happen that an abnormal cell will appear within the original tumor that has just the right combination of mutated genes, mutations that turn a benign tumor into a malignant cancer.

4

ONCOGENESIS

What could cells have been thinking, all those long years as they climbed out the primordial ooze to produce the stunning array of creatures that now inhabit the Earth? They dealt with obstacles that would have killed the faint of heart, noxious atmospheres that would make us choke, heat that would curl or straighten our hair, and storms that would make us quake in our boots. All these hurdles were brushed aside, like a bit of dust in the air, as cells refined their structure and expanded their communities to such an extent that they tamed the Earth and made its atmosphere fit for modern creatures to breathe.

But all along, as they went from one triumph to the next, their free-living carefree life-style set the stage for trouble to come. *Oncogenesis* (cancer development) is an unfortunate legacy of our protozoan ancestry. Paradoxically, cancer as we know it does not exist for modern-day protozoans. If any of those cells becomes abnormal, it is of no great consequence; that crazy cell, with a mangled genetic composition, simply dies because of its weirdness, without taking a virtual universe of cells with it. Perhaps this is why our single-cell ancestors never found a way to fully protect themselves from cancer: it simply did not matter to them. Abnormal cells occurred, but they never threatened the survival of other cells.

Our protozoan ancestors were not only free-living, but like economists, they were firm believers in the principle of continual growth. Those cells never became *postmitotic* but divided every half-hour or so and kept it up for as long as they could. To this extent, protozoans and their bacterial ancestors are immortal creatures that have existed for millions of years. But in order to produce multicellular organisms, protozoans had to come to some kind of mutual understanding, which limited the reproductive ability of some of the cells, forcing them to become postmitotic, while allowing others to divide for the life of the organism.

For the postmitotic crowd, the arrangement may have seemed impossible, as they were being asked to do something that went against their very nature. Genes that regulated their reproduction, which had undergone millions of years of adaptive evolution to ensure the cells could divide rapidly, were now being asked to shut down and remain silent. For the mitotic crowd, the agreement meant that each cell division had to be tightly controlled; no variation in the daughter cells would be allowed as it might have been with their free-living ancestors. When a human cell becomes cancerous it is simply reawakening its ancestral urge for unlimited growth and the carefree attitude that comes with it. The immortal life-style of protozoans depends on special genes that regulate the cell cycle and communication with the outside world. In that context, those genes are the cell's most prized possession, but when a cell in an animal's body becomes cancerous, those same cherished genes begin to fail and ultimately become a liability.

Cancer and the Cell Cycle

Evolution of cells has always been marked by two competing forces: the need for change, so the cell can evolve, and the need to stay the same, so daughter cells can inherit whatever genetic advantage the parent cell had. In the short term, cells work a very long day to make sure their daughter cells are as much like the original as possible. Cell cycle monitors, consisting of many different enzymes, check to make sure that everything is going well each time a cell divides, and if it is not, those monitors stop the cell from dividing until the problem is corrected. If the damage cannot be repaired, a protozoan remains stuck in midstream for the remainder of its life. If this happens to a cell in an animal's body, the cell is forced to commit suicide, in a process called apoptosis, by other cells in the immediate neighborhood or by the immune system.

The cell cycle consists of four stages or phases: *cell division* (M phase, for mitosis); a gap immediately after M phase, called G_1; DNA synthesis (S phase); followed by another gap, called G_2. The cycle includes three checkpoints: the first is a DNA damage checkpoint that occurs in G_1. The monitors check for damage that may have occurred as a result of the last cell cycle or were caused by something in the environment, such as UV radiation or toxic chemicals. If damage is

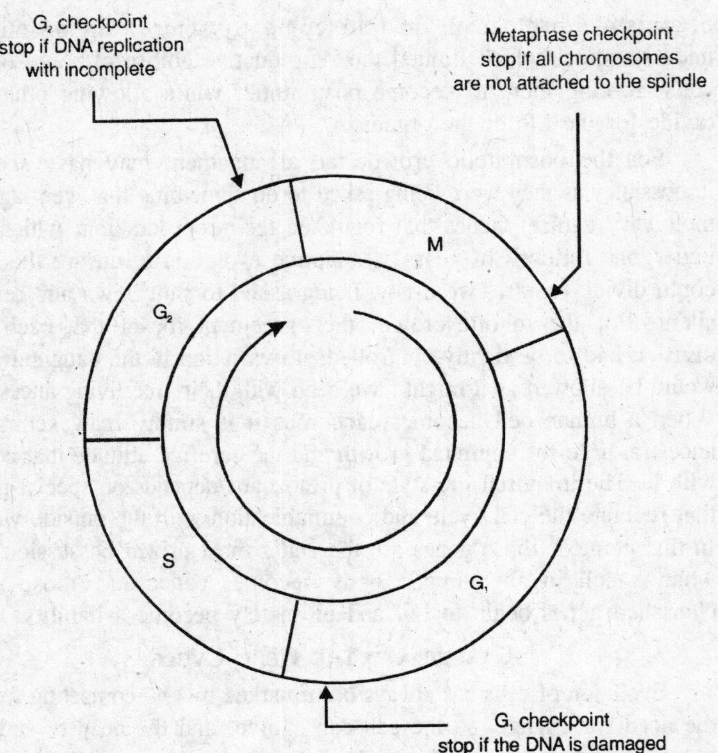

Fig. 4.1. Cell cycle check points. The cell is equipped with three checkpoints to ensure that the daughter cells are identical and that there is no genetic damage. The circular arrow indicates the direction of the cycle.

detected, DNA synthesis is blocked until it can be repaired. The second checkpoint occurs in G_2, where the monitors make sure errors were not introduced when the chromosomes were duplicated during the S phase. The G_1 and G_2 checkpoints are sometimes referred to collectively as DNA damage checkpoints. The third and final checkpoint occurs in M phase, to ensure that all of the chromosomes are properly attached to the spindle. This checkpoint is intended to prevent gross abnormalities in the daughter cells with regard to chromosome number. If a chromosome fails to attach to the spindle, one daughter cell will end up with too many chromosomes, while the other will have too few.

Typically, cancer cells lose one or more of their checkpoint monitors, so they divide whether things are right or not. This is the reason they develop an abnormal genome and physical appearance. Corrupting the genome in this way may seem to spell certain death for a cell, but it is really the means by which cancer cells reinvent themselves. The checkpoints are intended to maintain the status quo; without them the genetic profile of a cell, including which genes are on or off and which are mutated, can change very quickly and radically.

The T cells of our immune system can detect abnormal, potentially dangerous cells, and when they do they order those cells to commit suicide. The gross changes in a cancer cell's genetic structure, however, often knock out its ability to respond to those signals. When this happens, the cancer cell has gained immunity to apoptosis and is well on its way to fulfilling its quest for immortality and assuming the life-style enjoyed by its protozoan ancestors.

Disease of the Genes

It may seem odd that our genes can make us sick, and even kill us, for they are, in a sense, our most trusted ally. Their evolution, stretching back 3.5 billion years, made life what it is today: vigorous, diverse, and perfectly adapted to Earth's many environments. At the cellular level, dozens of enzymes devote themselves to tending the chromosomes and the genes they contain, like worker bees tending their queen. When genes are damaged, the enzymes repair them; when the genes need to divide, the enzymes carefully copy each chromosome into an exact duplicate; and when it is time for the cell to divide, the enzyme attendants move the chromosomes into position, attach them to the spindle, and gently send them on their way.

A gene giving us cancer is like a queen bee stinging a caretaker drone to death. When a tumor forms, some of our genes cross the line from a good gene that codes for an important cellular protein to a bad gene that produces a protein capable of sending us to an early grave. Fortunately for us, the number of cancer-causing genes is small compared with the 30,000 we possess. Genes that cause cancer do so by gaining a new function or by losing their normal function. The gain-of-function cancer genes are called *oncogenes*, and their normal counterparts are called *proto-oncogenes*. The loss-of-function cancer genes are called *tumor suppressor genes* (TSGs), because their normal job is to keep the cell from dividing inappropriately.

Tumor Suppressor Genes

Three genes, called *rb, p53,* and *p21,* code for proteins (RB, P53, and P21) that act as *tumor suppressor genes* (TSGs), and all of them are required for the G_1 checkpoint to work properly. The *rb* gene, the first tumor suppressor gene to be identified, was discovered in a study of retinoblastoma, a rare childhood cancer of the eye. Subsequent studies have shown that *rb* codes for a protein that is involved in blocking DNA synthesis when the G_1 checkpoint detects a problem and is expressed in all cells of the body. The function of this gene is now known to be abnormal, or simply lost, in many kinds of cancers, including carcinomas of the lung, breast, and bladder.

Table 4.1. Examples of cancer genes

Gene	*Type*	*Function*	*Tumor*
p53	Tumor suppressor	G_1 checkpoint/apoptosis	Carcinoma
rb	Tumor suppressor	G_1 checkpoint	Carcinoma
p21	Tumor suppressor	G_1 checkpoint	Carcinoma
ras	Oncogene	G-protein	Sarcoma
src	Oncogene	Tyrosine kinase	Sarcoma
myc	Oncogene	Transcription factor	Carcinoma

The *p53* gene (named after the weight of the gene's protein product) may be the most important cancer-causing gene known, as its loss of function is associated with more than half of all known cancers. This gene, like *rb,* blocks progression through S phase when DNA damage is detected. It does this indirectly by activating the synthesis of P21, which binds to the DNA to block replication. In addition, *p53* mediates external requests (primarily from T cells) for the cell to commit suicide. Consequently, cancer cells lacking a functional *p53* gene can divide without restraint, and they are no longer under the control of the immune system or inhibiting signals from neighboring cells, meaning they are immune to apoptosis.

Tumor suppressor genes (TSGs) lose their normal function as a consequence of a point mutation (a change affecting single nucleotide), leading to a defective protein. The mutation may occur spontaneously, or it may be induced by radiation, such as UV light, X-rays, or radioactivity, or by noxious chemicals, such as pesticides, industrial pollutants, or those found in tobacco smoke.

Oncogenes and Proto-oncogenes

An oncogene is produced when its normal counterpart, the proto-oncogene, is altered in some way. Research in many laboratories over the past 20 years has shown that the conversion of proto-oncogenes to oncogenes (a PO conversion) occurs by essentially two methods: a point mutation, occurring as described above for TSGs, and insertional mutagenesis. If the mutation occurs within the gene's promoter (the

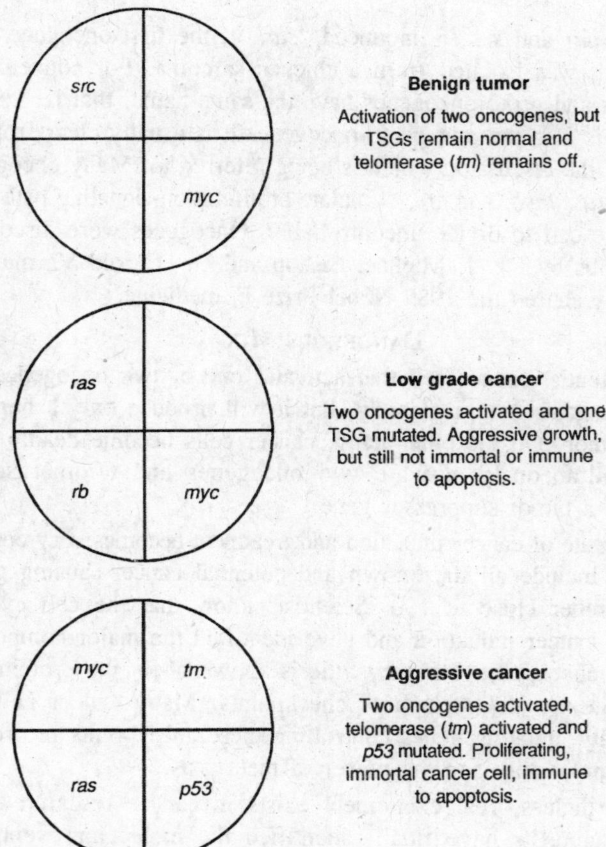

Fig. 4.2. A dangerous mix of gases. The deadliness of cancer cell depends on the mix of genes it can turn on or off.

genetic element that turns a gene on or off), the protein product will be the same before and after the conversion, but the amount of the protein will be different. More commonly, the mutation occurs within the coding region, in which case the protein still functions, but it does its job in a much different way. It is for this reason that oncogenes are referred to as gain-of-function cancer genes. In the second method of PO conversion, insertional mutagenesis, a retrovirus inserts itself into a chromosome as part of its own life cycle.

Oncogenes have names that are derived from the type of cancer they induce or are associated with. For example, the *ras* (rhymes with "*gas*") oncogene was originally isolated from a rat sarcoma; *myc* (pronounced "*mick*") is often expressed in a leukemia called *myelocytoma*; and *src* (pronounced "*sark*"), the first oncogene to be discovered, was isolated from a chicken sarcoma. For convenience, oncogenes and proto-oncogenes have the same name; that is, the *myc* oncogene is also the *myc* proto-oncogene. It is usually clear from the context of the discussion which is being referred to. Many oncogenes, including *ras, myc,* and *src,* stimulate proliferation-signaling pathways, forcing the cell to divide uncontrollably. Oncogenes were discovered in the 1980s by Dr. J. Michael Bishop and Dr. Harold Varmus, for which they shared the 1989 Nobel Prize in medicine.

Dangerous Mix

A potential cancer cell that activates one or two oncogenes may be able to grow inappropriately, but it will produce only a harmless benign tumor. On the other hand, cancer cells become deadly when they simultaneously activate two oncogenes and telomerase and deactivate a tumor suppressor gene.

The issue of cancer induction and treatment becomes very complex when we include all the known and potential cancer-causing genes, which number close to 100. Scientists know that the cell cycle is central to cancer induction and have identified the major components of the G_1 checkpoint, but very little is known about the proteins that manage the G_2 and metaphase checkpoints. Many cancer cells are undoubtedly mutating genes controlling these checkpoints in order to acquire immortality and the power of metastasis.

Nevertheless, real excitement exists in cancer research today, because scientists have finally identified the molecular events that lead to some of the deadliest forms of cancer, such as those affecting the pancreas, liver, and colon. Perhaps for the first time in 20 years, since the war on cancer began, we may feel confident that cures for these terrible diseases are close at hand.

Genes Involved in Hepatocellular Carcinoma

Hepatocellular carcinoma (HCC) accounts for 80–90% of all liver cancers and is one of the most frequently occurring carcinomas worldwide. Clinical and molecular medical analyses yielded a considerable amount of information about liver carcinogenesis. Many genes undergo somatic aberrations with a tendency to cluster at genes involved in cell cycle regulation, in the p53 and Wnt/catenin pathways of signal transduction and cellular adhesion and also in the *transforming growth factor*-beta (TGF-β)/*insulinlike growth factor* (IGF) axis. Because HCC may arise in cirrhotic and noncirrhotic livers, one may speculate that different pathways in hepatocarcinogenesis may exist. Recent results of high-output gene analysis using *complementary deoxyribonucleic acid* (cDNA) microarrays support the idea of different genetic alterations in HCC with or without cirrhosis. However, molecular diagnosis of HCC has—until now—been of limited clinical value in routine surgical pathology. There are no specific markers with diagnostic sensitivity to exclude other types of liver tumors.

As is true in other types of cancers, the etiology and carcinogenesis of HCC is *multifactorial* and *multistage*. The multistep process of HCC may be divided into several steps: chronic liver injury, which produces inflammation, cell death, cirrhosis, and regeneration; epigenetic/genetic DNA damage; dysplasia; and HCC. In general, specific genetic or epigenetic changes have been identified for some of these stages. These genetic changes include gene amplification (leading to activation of proto-oncogenes), gene deletion or mutation (leading to inactivation of tumor-suppressor genes), and reactivation of telomerase activity. The high number of genes involved in HCC may indicate that different etiologic factors affect different sets of genes in hepatocytes. This etiologically defined genetic heterogeneity of HCC results in the phenotypic heterogeneity of these tumors. In other words, distinct but related genetic pathways are altered during hepatocarcinogenesis as a result of different etiologic factors. Given the facts that 60–80% of all HCCs arise in liver cirrhosis and that the risk of development of HCC increases up to 1–5% per year in patients with cirrhosis, cirrhotic nodules are apparently premalignant lesions of HCC, and they may already contain genetic aberrations. Because a number of somatic gene and protein changes have been investigated in HCC, we discuss the main regulatory pathways that are altered in HCC. It is emphasized that these pathways are related one to another, and the genetic events should not be considered as independent and separate pathways. Furthermore, because of the etiologic heterogeneity, differences in the genetic alterations of HCC arising in cirrhosis compared to those without cirrhosis will be described.

Allelic Imbalance and Microsatellite Instability

Chromosomal instability is characterized by allelic losses and *aneuploidy*. Most of the genes mutated in HCC are tumor-suppressor genes, and frequent allelic losses (*loss of heterozygosity* [LOH]) leading to the biallelic inactivation have been described. By comparative genomic hybridization, chromosomes 1q, 8q, and 17q showed gene dosage increase, whereas chromosomes 1p, 4q, 8p, 9p, 13q, 16p, 16q, and 17p showed gene dosage loss. Consistently, frequent LOH, or more comprehensive *allelic imbalance* (AI), was observed on chromosomes 1p, 4q, 6p, 8p, 13q, 16q, and 17p by whole-genome allelotyping. The chromosome regions with gene dosage increase may contain critical oncogenes, whereas those with gene dosage loss may contain tumor-suppressor genes. For chromosomes 17p, 13q, 9p, 6q, and 16p, LOH could be related to p53, *retinoblastoma* 1 (RB1), p16, and IGF2R inactivation, respectively.

Although the genes causing chromosomal instability or AI remain unknown, *microsatellite instability* (MSI) is caused by inactivation of a DNA mismatch repair gene (predominantly hMLH1 or hMSH2). It has been shown that most tumors in patients with *hereditary nonpolyposis colorectal cancer* (HNPCC) harbor MSI. This phenotype was linked to defects in the DNA mismatch repair genes MSH2 and MLH1 located on chromosomes 2 and 3. In HCC these chromosomal regions are not frequently affected by allelic losses. Furthermore, no mutation in the repeated sequences in *Bax, IGF-IIR,* or *MLH* genes has been detected so far in HCC. These findings indicate that, in contrast to AI, defective mismatch repair does not contribute significantly to hepatocellular carcinogenesis.

Cell Cycle Regulation

The RB gene is one of the best-studied tumor-suppressor genes in HCC. Mutations of RB are observed in ~15% of HCC. At chromosome 13q, where RB is located, LOH is frequently observed in HCC with a prevalence of 25–48%. An overexpression of cyclins has been observed in ~10–13% of all HCC. Cyclin D1, for example, is a known oncogene and a key regulator of cell cycle progression. Amplification of the cyclin D1 gene and its overexpression has been associated with aggressive forms of HCC. It has been shown in a transgene mouse model that overexpression of cyclin D1 is sufficient to initiate hepatocellular carcinogenesis. The transduction of anti-sense cyclin D1 inhibits tumor growth in a xenograft hepatoma model. Correcting alterations that have occurred in the G1-phase regulatory machinery may therefore provide a novel weapon to prevent and treat HCC.

Signaling through the *mitogen-activated protein kinase* (MAPK) cascade is transduced by *guanosine triphosphate* (GTP) loading of RAS leading to the activation of RAF kinase. In mammalian cells, there are three isoforms of RAF: A-*RAF,* B-*RAF,* and C-*RAF.* Although all three of the RAF isoforms share a common function with respect to

MEK phosphorylation, studies have shown that these proteins might be differentially activated by oncogenic *ras*. In 2003 we described that activating B-*RAF* mutations may play a role in the carcinogenesis of cholangiocarcinoma of the liver, but not in HCC.

Inactivation of p16, either as a result of LOH at chromosome 9p or *de novo* methylation of the promoter, is detected in up to 60% of all HCC examined; p14 alterations were found in ~15% of HCC. Our observations demonstrate that the INK4a-ARF/p53-pathway was disrupted in 86% of HCC, either by p53 mutations or by INK4a-ARF inactivation. It is interesting that an inverse relationship between p53 and p14 existed in our patients: Inactivation of p14 was nearly restricted to tumors with wild-type p53. Thus, the loss of p14 and mutations of p53 could be mutually exclusive events, suggesting that they may be functionally equivalent in hepatocarcinogenesis. The overall frequency of 9p21 alterations, including deletion and methylation, was 78%. Silencing of INK4a-ARF gene products (coding for critical regulators of cell cycle progression) is therefore one of the most frequent genetic defects in HCC.

p53 and homologues

The *p53* tumor-suppressor gene is frequently mutated in human cancers. Additionally, in many cancers, p53 function is altered through binding to viral oncoproteins or abrogation of p53 degradation by mdm-2/hdm-2 in concert with p14, as described earlier. The identification of two homologues, p63 and p73, revealed that p53 is a member of a family of related transcription factors. In contrast to *p53, p63* and *p73* genes are rarely mutated in human cancer. In HCC, p53 mutations were found in ~30% of HCC worldwide. The frequency of all p53 mutations varies between 20% in North America and 67% in Africa. Up to now, all reported mutations (mostly missense leading to stabilization of protein) are somatic, indicating that germline p53 mutations appear not to predispose for HCC. Both the frequency and the type of mutations are different depending on the geographic location and etiology of the tumors.

Specific-specific p53 mutations have been identified in several studies, linking the mutation pattern to suspected etiologic factors. A selective guanine-to-thymine transversion mutation in codon 249 (AGG to AGT leading to an arginine-to-serine substitution) of the p53 gene has been identified as a "*hotspot*" mutation for HCC. Epidemiologic and experimental evidence have suggested that in HCC this mutation is strongly associated with exposure to aflatoxin B1 in combination with a high level of chronic hepatitis B virus infection in the population. The presence of this "*hotspot*" mutation in HCC is extremely low in patients in Europe, United States, Japan, and Australia; only three mutations were identified among 664 patients with HCC. Patients who have not been exposed to aflatoxin B1 or hepatitis virus have a lower prevalence of p53 gene mutations, indicating other genes involved in the process of hepatocarcinogenesis.

For p73 and p63, no specific mutations have been described so far. However, an overexpression of p73 (wild type) has been described in a subset of HCC, indicating a poor prognosis of these patients. According to our data, p53 mutations in a given tumor are neither related to absence nor presence of p73 or p63.

Wnt pathway: APC, β-catenin, axin 1, and E-cadherin

Adenomatous polyposis coli (APC) protein has been thought to function as a tumor suppressor through its involvement in the Wnt/β-catenin signaling pathway. The APC/β-catenin pathway is highly regulated and includes molecules such as GSK3, CBP, Groucho, Axin, Conductin, and TCF. Furthermore, c-MYC and cyclin D1 have been identified as key transcriptional targets of this pathway, indicating a broad overlap between several tumor-permissive pathways. Wnt proteins are involved in a large number of events during tumor development, not only in HCC but also in other types of cancers. Activation of the Wnt pathway can be caused by β-catenin mutation or by an inactivating mutation of the *axin* gene.

In HCCs, somatic mutations of β-catenin were observed in 19–26%, mostly missense mutations and interstitial deletions of exon 3. These mutations that occur at the N-terminal region of β-catenin lead to a nuclear accumulation of aberrant β-catenin proteins that stimulate the activity of other transcription factors. Axin, an important regulator of β-catenin, is mutated in ~10% of HCC, leading to an activation of the Wnt pathway. However, mutations in the *axin* gene were identified only in HCC that lacked mutations in the β-*catenin* gene. It has been shown that transduction of the wild-type *Axin* gene (AXIN1) induces apoptosis in HCC cells, indicating that Axin 1 may be an effective growth suppressor of hepatocytes.

Somatic APC mutations are rare events in HCC, but it has been reported that biallelic inactivation of the APC gene contributed to the development of HCC in a patient with *familial adenomatous polyposis* (FAP) and a known germline mutation of the *APC* gene at codon 208. E-cadherin, the cytoplasmic anchor protein of β-catenin, is rarely mutated in HCC. However, loss of function because of LOH or *de novo* methylation occurred in ~30% of all HCCs.

Alterations of the transforming growth factor-β/insulin-like growth factor-axis

Both growth inhibition and apoptosis are induced by TGF-β in hepatocytes; TGF-β initiates signaling through heteromeric complexes of transmembrane type I and type II serine/threonine kinase receptors. Activated TGF-β type I receptor phosphorylates receptor-regulated Smads (2 and 3). However, genetic alterations of the TGF-β pathway are mediated by mutations of the *Smad2* and *Smad4* genes, which occur in ~10% of all HCCs. Mutations of the TGF-β receptor (TGF-β1RII) gene itself are detected in patients with HCC and may also abrogate TGF-β signaling. A potent activator of TGF-β is the mannose-6-phosphate/insulin-like growth factor 2 receptor (M6P/IGF2R). This receptor suppresses cell growth through binding to the IGF2 and latent complex of TGF-β. The deregulation of the IGF axis, including the autocrine production of IGFs, *IGF-binding proteins* (IGFBPs), IGFBP proteases, and the expression of the *IGF receptors* (IGFR), has also been identified in the development of HCC. Mutations of the M6P/IGF2R and LOH have been reported in ~30% of patients in North America with HCC. However, a recently published study from Japan failed to identify relevant alterations of the M6P/IGF2R gene. Increased expression of IGF-II, IGF-I receptor, alterations of IGFBP production, and the proteolytic degradation of IGFBPs result in an excess of bioactive IGFs. The previously mentioned defective function of the IGF degrading M6P/IGF2R may further potentiate the mitogenic effects of IGFs in the development of HCC.

PTEN/MMAC1/TEP1 (*PTEN*) is a tumor-suppressor gene that is located on chromosome band 10q23.3. Alterations, mainly mutations but also LOH, of PTEN have been reported in ~10% of HCCs. It has been demonstrated that PTEN significantly reduced IGF secretion and also expression of secretory and cellular *vascular endothelial growth factor* (VEGF) proteins in HCC cell lines and could therefore inhibit tumorigenicity. Taken together, these findings demonstrate that several genes of the complex growth regulatory TGF-β/IGF pathway could be altered during hepatocellular carcinogenesis. The situation is further complicated as a result of the observation that activation of TGF-β and IGF signaling is observed even in liver cirrhosis and that complex interactions may exist between hepatitis virus particles in a preneoplastic stage.

Distinct hepatocarcinogenic pathways in hepatocellular carcinoma with or without cirrhosis?

A number of genetic alterations have been described in HCC, and more than 20 genes within at least four carcinogenesis pathways have been shown to be altered in HCC. One of the most frequently affected genes in HCC is *p53,* and the INK4a-ARF pathway is most frequently altered in HCCs. This may be explained by different etiologic factors (hepatitis B or C virus, aflatoxin intake) leading to liver cirrhosis, which is present in up to 90% of all HCCs in high-incidence areas. In contrast, in low-incidence areas the incidence of HCC in a cirrhotic liver is much lower (~60%). In the current literature, these differences have not been discussed in detail, which may be because of a lack of patients having HCC without cirrhosis. Recent advances in DNA sequencing technology and the development of gene expression arrays have provided more powerful tools to study the expression of thousands of genes in HCC in a single experiment. Gene expression arrays are created by depositing unique cDNA fragments on a nylon filter or on glass slides. The filter is then hybridized with labeled cDNA from HCC tissue of interest. The readout is performed by high-throughput (phospho) imagers. Using this new technique in combination with bioinformatics, the first results indicate two different "*genetic makeups*" for HCC, depending on whether they arise in cirrhosis or in noncirrhotic liver. Despite our small number of patients (a total of 210), a trend toward a lower rate of p53 mutations (and p73 expression), higher prevalence of β-catenin mutations, p14 inactivation, and global gene methylation were observed in HCC without cirrhosis. Evidently, further studies on a larger number of patients are necessary to define distinct pathways of hepatocarcinogenesis more precisely.

Molecular markers in the differential diagnosis of hepatocellular carcinomas

The main differential diagnosis in liver nodules is benign liver tumors (focal nodular hyperplasia, liver cell adenoma, dysplastic nodules) and primary and secondary liver cancer. The histologic appearance of tumorlike nodules is, at least in most cases, typical, and the differential diagnosis is relatively easy in everyday practice. However, the differential diagnosis of *liver cell adenoma* (LCA) versus well-differentiated HCC may cause problems, at least in fine-needle biopsies. Molecular markers are of limited value in this setting because there are no clear "*cutoff*" data to differentiate between LCA and HCC. In LCA, genetic alterations are also present, e.g., hypermethylation of p16^{INK4a}. β-catenin and p53 mutations may occur in a subset of LCA, making these markers unsuitable for differential diagnosis. It may be difficult to exclude metastases from primary liver tumors in some cases. When there is doubt about the hepatocyte origin of the tumor, further evidence can be gained by immunohistochemical analysis of (polyclonal) carcino-embryonic antigen, liver cell cytokeratins 8 and 18, albumin, or fibrinogen. *In situ* hybridization may show albumin messenger ribonucleic acid in the tumor cells as evidence for hepatocellular origin. To exclude primary cholangiocarcinoma of the liver, immunohistochemical analysis of biliary cytokeratins 7 and 19, and epithelial membrane antigen may be useful because these markers are negative in HCC. The specificity of *alpha feto protein* (AFP) is high, but, unfortunately, the sensitivity of AFP staining in HCC tumor tissue is low. The expression pattern may be weak, and a specific staining may be detected only in ~30% of all HCCs. The proliferative activity of HCC is not of special value in the differential diagnosis of HCC. The expression of Ki-67 (MIB1) or proliferating cell nuclear antigen correlates with histologic grade of differentiation. In general, the proliferation rate in liver cirrhosis and LCA may be as high as in well-differentiated HCC.

Other proteins, such as p27, thrombospondin, MMPs, TGF-α and -β, cathepsin B, inhibin, or CD44 have also been shown to be expressed in HCC. However, they are of limited value in routine surgical pathology because they are not specifically expressed in HCC.

Role of p53 and ZBP-89 in Hepatocellular Carcinoma

Hepatocellular carcinoma (HCC) is one of the most common cancers in Africa and Asia, especially in sub-Saharan Africa, Southeast Asia, and China. Unlike in Western countries, ~90% of HCC in Asia is associated with *hepatitis B virus* (HBV) infection instead of *hepatitis C virus* (HCV) infection. According to the *Cancer Incidence and Mortality in Hong Kong* issued by the Hong Kong Cancer Registry of Hospital Authority, HCC is the second leading cause of cancer death in Hong Kong, with the crude mortality rate of 32.7 per 100,000 in men and 10.5 in women. Surgical resection of tumor is still the most effective treatment for HCC. However, ~70% of patients will die from recurrent tumor within 5 years after liver tumor resection. Furthermore, most patients with HCC are unresectable at the time of diagnosis because of widespread intrahepatic or extrahepatic involvement or limited hepatic reserves resulting from coexisting advanced cirrhosis. The median survival for patients with unresectable tumor is less than

3 months. Searching an early detection of cancer and a novel treatment for HCC has been challenging scientists and clinicians for years, and a reliable early detection tool and an effective remedy are yet to be established.

Over the past two decades, a great deal of effort has been made to reveal how HBV contributes to the development of HCC and how to prevent its formation. It is now known that HBV contains four overlapping open-reading frames that encode the structural and nonstructural viral proteins. Among them, the x protein (HBx) has been shown to play a central role in HBV infection and a causative role in liver oncogenesis. There is evidence for an important role of HBx in the expression and replication of viral *deoxyribonucleic acid* (DNA). Furthermore, transfection experiments have suggested that HBx can transform NIH3T3 immortalized fibroblasts and differentiate murine hepatocytes *in vitro*. The HBx gene is frequently integrated into the cellular genome and expressed in HCC and interferes with various tumor suppressor genes and other molecules related to cell proliferation and growth, such as p53, insulin-like growth factor 1, nuclear factor kappa B, and Bid.

The p53 tumor suppressor gene is the most frequent target for genetic alterations in human cancer. The wild-type p53 protein can exert a variety of anti-proliferative effects, including induction of cell cycle arrest and apoptosis. These effects are usually evident in cells exposed to DNA damage and other types of stress, which impinge on the otherwise latent p53 protein and cause its accumulation and biochemical activation. The therapeutic efficacy of anti-cancer agents depends strongly on their ability to trigger apoptosis in target tumor cells. Many physical and chemical DNA damaging agents used routinely in cancer therapy are potent apoptosis inducers via the p53-related pathway. Given the documented contribution of p53 to radiation-induced apoptosis, it is conceivable that cells maintaining functional p53 will be more prone to be killed by many anti-cancer agents. Numerous subsequent basic and clinical studies have provided further support for this notion. However, accumulation of certain mutant p53 may also enhance the sensitivity of tumor cells to chemotherapy. For example, paclitaxel or other DNA-damaging agents have been shown to be more effective against cancer cells with p53 mutations than those without. The mechanism responsible for the sensitivity of cancer cells with p53 mutations to therapeutic agents is unknown. However, wild-type p53 may enhance chemosensitivity by promoting apoptosis via transcription-independent mechanisms as well as transcriptional activation of proapoptotic genes such as Bax and transcriptional repression of anti-apoptotic genes such as Bcl-2. Drug-induced suicide mediated by the CD95/CD95 ligand system may also involve the p53-controlled pathway.

ZBP-89 is a four zinc-finger transcription factor that regulates the expression of several genes related to cell growth through binding to GC-rich DNA elements. It can function at the transcriptional level to regulate the expression of several genes and exert a negative effect on cell proliferation. Altered expression of ZBP-89 has been documented in malignant cells, and the inhibitory mechanism of ZBP-89 is now known to involve activation of $p21^{waf1}$ and stabilization of p53. It has been suggested that ZBP-89 stabilizes p53 through direct protein contact, which leads to retention of p53 in the nucleus.

Materials

1. ABC reagent (ABC-HRP or ABC-AP).
2. Antibodies: (1) normal serum (goat, rabbit or horse) for blocking; (2) primary antibody (monoclonal or polyclonal): rabbit polyclonal ZBP-89 antibody, which was raised against amino acids 1-521 of rat ZBP-89, mouse anti-p53 antibody; (3) secondary antibody (rabbit anti-mouse, goat anti-rabbit, etc.).
3. Antibody diluent: *phosphate buffer saline* (PBS) containing 0.1% *bovine serum albumin* (BSA) and 0.1% sodium azide. Store antibody at 4°C at working dilution.
4. Avidin/biotin blocking kit.
5. BCIP/NBT substrate.
6. Blocking serum: 1000 μl of blocking serum consists of 900 μl PBS, 100 μl of goat or rabbit or horse serum, and 4 drops of avidin D.
7. Citrate buffer, 0.01 M, (pH 6.0): (1) 1.05 g citric acid; (2) 2M NaOH. Dissolve citric acid in 450 ml distilled water and add enough NaOH until pH 6.0 is reached, then top up to 500 ml.
8. Diaminobenzidine tetrahydrochloride (DAB). To make a stock, take 5 g of DAB and add 100 ml distilled water. Using a magnetic stirrer, stir for 30 min in a fume hood until completely dissolved; then aliquot into small tubes and store at –20°C.
9. DPX mountant.
10. ECL kit: available from Amersham Biosciences.
11. Ethanol: 100%, 98%, 95%, and 70%.
12. Formalin: 10% neutral buffered.

13. Gill's hematoxylene.
14. Hematoxylene.
15. Hydrogen peroxide: stock solution: 30% aqueous (w/v), stored at 4°C.
16. Levamisole solution (100X).
17. Lysis buffer: 30 mM Tris-HCl, 150 mM NaCl, 1 mM PMSF, 1% Triton X-100, 10% glycerol, and a protease inhibitor cocktail.
18. Methanol 70% in PBS.
19. NovaRED.
20. OCT embedding medium.
21. PBS/BSA solution: add 1–2 mg thimerosal merthiolate and 0.1 g BSA in 1 L PBS, and use a stirrer to dissolve both.
22. PBS: (1) 8.7 g sodium chloride; (2) 0.272 g potassium dihydrogen phosphate; and (3) 1.136 g disodium hydrogen phosphate. Dissolve all salts separately in distilled water, then mix, make up to 1 L, and check pH is 7.2.
23. Protein A-Sepharose.
24. SDS-PAGE buffer (2X).
25. Thimerosal merthiolate.
26. Xylene.

METHODS

Handling of Liver Tissues

1. Wear gloves and use universal precautions when handling fresh tissue samples.
2. Liver tissue samples are normally collected at the time of surgical resection of tumors. After collection, samples should immediately stored in liquid nitrogen (–160°C) until use.
3. Liver tissues can be snap frozen by placing them in histocassettes or cryogenic tubes and dropping these cassettes or tubes in liquid nitrogen. Tissues can be stored indefinitely in liquid nitrogen. Alternatively, and preferably for reliable immunohistochemical staining, fresh tissue can be placed on a clean chuck layered with OCT embedding medium and cold embedded in a precooled cryostat. Freshly embedded tissue generally sections better than snap-frozen tissue, which is subsequently embedded. Tissues can be snap frozen in OCT for better histology, but keep in mind that OCT might interfere with molecular biology techniques requiring snap-frozen tissue. Therefore, snap freeze in OCT only if the tissue will be

used for histology. Otherwise, cut liver tissue in half and snap freeze it with and without OCT respectively.

4. Fix overnight fresh liver tissue or thawed tissue (from liquid nitrogen) in 10% neutral buffered formalin. Larger tissue sections require a longer period of time; the time of fixation will affect the characteristics of sectioning the tissue (crumbling or cracking of the tissue) and possibly antigen recognition.
5. After carrying out tissue processing through graded alcohol, xylene, and paraffin, the tissue is subjected to paraffin emedding. Tissue is sectioned at 4 μm thick and is adhered to the microscope slide previously treated with 3-aminopropyltriethoxysilane.

Immunohistochemical Staining of p53 or ZBP-89

1. Deparaffinization:
   (a) Incubate 2–3× in xylene for 3 min each.
   (b) Incubate 3× in 100% ethanol for 1 min each.
   (c) Hydrate by placing in 95% and 70% ethanol for 1 min each.
   (d) Place in tap water 2× for 2 min each.
2. Antigen retrieval:
   (a) Place the slides in the container containing citrate buffer and boil for 20 min using a microwave oven.
   (b) Leave at room temperature for 20 min to cool.
3. Rinsing
   (a) Rinse with distilled or Milliq water for 5 min, then wash with H_2O_2 + methanol solution (2 ml 30% H_2O_2 + 200 ml methanol) for 20–30 min.
   (b) Rinse with distilled water for 5 min.
   (c) Rinse with PBS for 5 min.
4. Equilibrate in PBS/BSA solution for ~5 min.
5. Blocking:
   (a) Wipe off excess liquid and surround the tissue with PAP PEN.
   (b) Add 100 μl of blocking serum to each slide.
   (c) Incubate at room temperature for 30 min.
6. Application of primary antibody:
   (a) Appropriately dilute primary antibody to a working concentration.
   (b) Add 4 drops of biotin for 1 ml of primary antibody.
   (c) Add 100 μl of primary antibody (with biotin) to each slide.

(d) Incubate for 1 hr at room temperature or overnight at 4°C.
(e) Tap off excess antibody and rinse slides in PBS/BSA solution for at least 5 min.

7. Application of secondary antibody (rabbit immunoglobulin G, or IgG)
   (a) Apply 100 μl of biotinylated secondary antibody (appropriate dilution in PBS) for 30 min at room temperature.
   (b) Rinse slides in PBS/BSA solution for at least 5 min.
8. Application of ABC-HRP reagent:
   (a) Add 20 μl of solution A (avidin DH) and 20 μl of solution B (biotinylated horseradish peroxidase H) to 1000 μl PBS/BSA solution and let it sit for at least 30 min at room temperature.
   (b) Apply 100 μl of the previously mentioned ABC reagent for each slide and leave for 30 min at room temperature.
   (c) Rinse in PBS/BSA solution for 5 min at room temperature. Do not dry the slides.
9. Application of DAB or NovaRED:
   (a) Apply 100 μl of DAB or NovaRED to each slide for equal time (each for 5 min).
   (b) Rinse in PBS or distilled water.
10. Counterstaining:
    (a) Counterstain with Gill's hematoxylin for 1 or 2 min.
    (b) Rinse in tap water until cleared from blue color (usually need 2 rinses).
11. Dehydration:
    (a) Place the slide in different concentrations of ethanol, starting with 70% ethanol for 1 min. Followed by 98% for 1 min and 100% 3× each for 1 min.
    (b) Incubate with xylene 2× for 3 min. Do not dry the slides.
12. Mounting:
    (a) Place the slides down with the section facing upward.
    (b) Add a drop of the DPX mount.
    (c) Cover the section with coverslip.

Dual-Immunohistochemical Staining to Detect ZBP-89 and p53 in the Same Cell

1. Stain the first antigen (ZBP-89) following Steps 1–9 listen in *Immunohistochemical staining of p53 or* ZBP-89.

2. Add 100 μl of blocking serum to each slide and incubate at room temperature for 30 min.
3. Application of the second primary antibody (anti-p53):
   (a) Appropriately dilute primary antibody to a working concentration.
   (b) Add 4 drops of biotin for 1 ml of primary antibody.
   (c) Add 100 μl of primary antibody to each slide.
   (d) Incubate for 1 hr at room temperature or overnight at 4°C.
   (e) Tap off excess antibody and rinse slides in PBS/BSA solution for at least 5 min.
4. Application of secondary antibody (horse anti-mouse IgG):
   (a) Apply 100 μl of secondary antibody (appropriate dilution in PBS) for 30 min at room temperature.
   (b) Rinse slides in PBS/BSA solution for at least 5 min.
5. Application of ABC-AP reagent
   (a) Add 20 μl of solution A (avidin DH) and 20 μl of solution B (biotinylated horseradish peroxidase H) to 1000 μl PBS/BSA solution and let it sit for at least 30 min at room temperature.
   (b) Apply 100 μl of the previously mentioned ABC reagent for each slide and leave for 30 min at room temperature.
   (c) Rinse in PBS/BSA solution for 5 min at room temperature. Do not dry the slides.
6. Application of BCIP/NBT substrate and levamisole solution (100X):
   (a) Add one drop of levamisole solution (100X) to 5 ml of BCIP/NBT substrate solution.
   (b) Apply 100 μl BCIP/NBT/levamisole to each slide for equal time (each for 20 min). Incubation time with BCIP/NBT/levamisole may need to be adjusted according to the degree of the molecule staining because too strong staining of the second antigen may affect the first antigen detection.
   (c) Rinse in PBS or water.
7. Follow Steps 10–12 listed in *Immunohistochemical* staining of p53 or ZBP-89.

Co-Immunoprecipitation of p53 and ZBP-89

1. Harvest cells, wash with PBS 1×, and transfer cells into microcentrifuge tubes.
2. Lyse cell samples in 1 ml lysis buffer for 10 min at 4°C with pipetting cells up and down extensively.

3. Spin down cell extracts at 14,000 rpm for 10 min at 4°C.
4. Add 10 μg of anti-p53 antibody to 1 ml of extract.
5. Incubate with end-over-end mixing for 2 hr at 4°C.
6. Add 50 μl protein A-Sepharose and incubate with end-over-end mixing for 1 hr at 4°C.
7. Wash immunoprecipates 3× with 1 ml of lysis buffer.
8. Add 50 μl of 2 X SDS-PAGE buffer and boil for 5 min.
9. Load onto a SDS-PAGE gel.
10. Western Blot to transfer proteins to membranes.
11. Probe the membrane with ZBP-89 antibody and detect signals using the ECL kit.

Notes:

1. Protocols for immunohistochemistry vary widely as a result of the differences between antigens and their recognition by antibody. Some epitopes are destroyed by the high temperatures and organic solvents used for paraffin embedding, whereas others cannot survive freezing and thawing. Each fixative is effective with a different mechanism, which may either help to uncover the epitope or may destroy it or make it less accessible. Some antibodies may even adhere to the blocking agent used, so that it causes rather than eliminates background.
2. *Negative control*: The simplest negative control is the absence of expression in tissues, in which the molecule of interest is known not to be expressed. A better negative control is the elimination of the signal by pre-incubating the antibody with an excess of the peptide or protein with which it is raised. A Western Blot can suggest specificity of the interaction if only one band is seen; nonetheless, the difficulty of optimizing conditions for a Western Blot should demonstrate the possibility that conditions in the immunohistochemistry reaction are less than optimal. However, there can also be doubts as to whether the antigen is visualized everywhere; in particular, one must determine whether the fixation protocol used actually permeabilizes the nuclear membrane to a sufficient degree for nuclear antigens to be fully visible.
3. *Positive control*: Cells or tissues known to express the protein molecule of interest can be used as positive control.
4. If there is a high level of background staining, try one of the following solutions:

(a) Dilute the primary antibody further, or reduce the antibody incubation time. The following problems are often caused by the use of excess antibody: (1) staining is excessively dark; (2) staining occurs throughout the section rather than in expected areas of antigen localization; (3) staining appears to fade, float, or leach off the section during or after substrate reaction; (4) color develops immediately after addition of substrate; and (5) particles of dye are scattered across the section after staining.

(b) Reduce substrate staining time. In some instances prolonged staining also inhibits nuclear counterstaining.

(c) Raise the pH, or increase the ionic strength of diluent buffers. Sodium chloride (0.1–0.5 M) added to the buffer diluent reduces nonspecific binding on endothelia and collagen fibers.

(d) Apply blocking protein before applying primary antibody. The blocking protein should be of the same species used in the link or enzyme labeled antibody diluent and should not be used in the primary antibody diluent.

(e) The addition of ethylene glycol, Tween 20, or other detergent to the antibody diluent and washes will help remove unbound antibodies and artifacts that contribute to nonspecific binding as well as remove excess dye from the section.

(f) Try an alternative enzyme system, such as alkaline phosphatase, horseradish peroxidase, or β-galactosidase.

(g) Factors related to tissue preparation and fixation are as follows: (1) Inadequate penetration of fixative can produce nonspecific staining. (2) Overfixation can destroy antigens contained within the tissue. (3) Tissue that has dried out can exhibit artifact and nonspecific staining. (4) Incomplete removal of paraffin from tissue sections will result in artifacts. (5) Poor dehydration causes smudging of the stain. (6) Thick sections may prevent adequate penetration of primary antibody, producing false reactions or uneven staining over the tissue surface.

Results and Discussion

In human tumors, the majority of p53 gene alterations are missense mutations, often within the conserved DNA binding core domain of the protein. The primary selective advantage of such mutations may well be the elimination of cellular wild-type p53 activity. However, at variance with the observations for several other tumor-suppressor

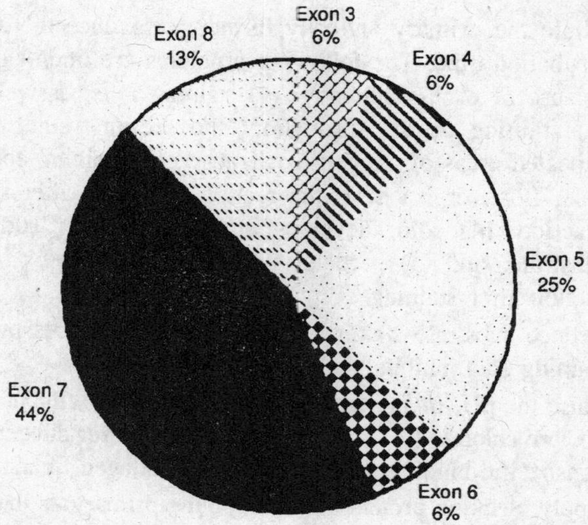

Fig. 4.3. The distribution of p53 mutations in the different exons.

genes, cells with p53 mutations typically maintain expression of full-length mutant protein, often at markedly elevated levels. This suggests that at least certain mutant forms of p53 may possess a gain of function. Multiple types of p53 mutations are known to possess distinct biological features, e.g., mutants deficient for transcriptional activation, but competent for induction of apoptosis, and vice versa. Many studies have shown that p53 is frequently mutated in human HCC and is correlated with advanced tumor grade, progression, therapy, and survival. It is believed that p53 may also play a role in recurrent HCC, which is the major factor contributing to the high mortality of HCC. Therefore, understanding the role of p53 in recurrent tumor

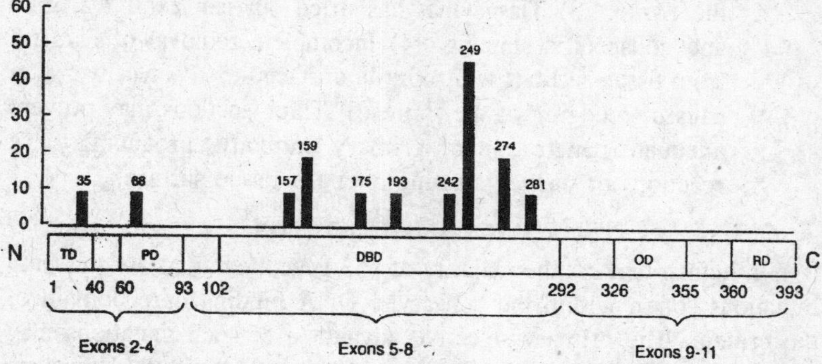

Fig. 4.4: Schematic outline of human p53 protein and p53 mutations in hepatocellular carcinoma (HCC).

may provide useful molecular information that can be of therapeutic significance. Very few reports have addressed the p53 status in recurrence of HCC. In our experiment, we found that mutations in the p53 gene were detected in 48.5% of recurrent HCC. Exon 7 of p53 gene may be considered a prevalent site of p53 mutation because it accounts for 44% of all alterations found.

The p53 nuclear import or retention is essential for its normal function in growth inhibition or induction of apoptosis. A defect in the regulation of p53 nuclear import or export may result in tumorigenesis. Dysfunctional transportation of p53 between the nucleus and cytoplasm is known to occur in a subset of human tumors, and in such a situation p53 is sequestered either in the cytoplasm or in the nucleus. In normal cells, wild-type p53 protein is kept at a low concentration by rapid degradation. Therefore, wild-type p53 protein is usually undetected or detected at very low levels. However, when there are mutations within the p53 gene, they result in a dysfunctional protein product with a prolonged half-life that enables them to accumulate in the cell. Accumulation of p53 protein either in the cytoplasm or in the nucleus is considered a pathologic index. In the case of recurrent HCC, nearly 58% (19/33) of patients showed nuclear localization of p53 protein and ~9% (3/33) are positive for p53 protein in the cytoplasm. Accumulation of p53 protein in the nucleus occurs in the cells either with or without a mutant p53 gene, whereas cytoplasmic p53 protein exists in all recurrent HCC with mutant p53 gene.

Mechanisms responsible for the sequestration of a particular mutant p53 protein in the nucleus or the cytoplasm are very complicated and not yet completely known. The nuclear localization signals are located within the carboxyl terminus of p53 (amino acids 293–393). Mutations in this nuclear signal region can affect the nuclear import or export of p53. However, none of the mutations detected in the HCC study are within this nuclear signal region. ZBP-89 protein can stabilize p53 through a direct protein contact leading to its retention in the nucleus. ZBP-89 can be co-localized with p53 in the nucleus in about 63% of HCC positive for the nuclear p53 protein, suggesting that ZBP-89 may play a role in the nuclear accumulation of p53 protein in a subset of HCC. Indeed, ZBP-89 is able to bind wild-type p53 and some forms of p53 mutants, as demonstrated by co-immunoprecipitation experiments. Mutation in N-terminal of p53 nonbinding domains retains the binding ability to ZBP-89, whereas mutation in DNA binding domain (after codon 175) abolishes the direct interaction between ZBP-89 and p53.

These p53 mutations may thus eliminate ZBP-89-mediated stabilization of p53.

In agreement with co-immunoprecipitation experiments, ZBP-89 is found to be co-localized not only with the wild-type p53 but also with mutant one. This further confirms that the ZBP-89-interaction domain in some mutant p53 remains intact. The co-localization of ZBP-89 and p53 in the nucleus may be clinically significant in certain types of patients who possess a functional p53. The function of p53 protein depends on the nuclear localization. With accumulation of p53 protein in the nucleus, tumor cells are liable to undergo apoptosis and thus more susceptible to radiotherapy and chemotherapy.

In conclusion, by co-localizing p53 protein, the expression of ZBP-89 may be clinically significant and may define a subgroup of recurrent HCC that is more suitable to receive radiotherapy and chemotherapy.

5

TUMOR

Cancers usually take a long time to develop. This is because, as pointed out in previous chapters, there must be a defect in more than one gene before a cell can make the switch. Potential cancer cells appear continuously throughout an individual's life, but most are destroyed by the immune system, and still others never manage to develop a lethal genetic profile. For a cancer to develop, all the "right" conditions must exist simultaneously in the same cell. This is the reason a tumor appears originally in only one part of the body and, over the years, spreads to other areas.

CANCERS DEVELOP FROM A SINGLE BAD CELL

Cancer cells within a tumor are like any other living community in that they are subject to the same laws of natural selection. Most cancer cells die spontaneously because their genome has been so badly corrupted that they are incapable of maintaining basic housekeeping functions. Of those that survive, one may have a genetic profile that favors rapid growth, so much so that it quickly becomes the only cell type within the tumor. This scenario has been confirmed experimentally by examining characteristics of cancer cells isolated from different regions of a single individual's body. For example, certain forms of leukemia are associated with the presence of the Philadelphia chromosome, created by a translocation between the long arms of chromosomes 9 and 22. Detailed sequence analysis of the DNA spanning the break site shows it is identical in all leukemic cells from a single patient, confirming a common ancestry. In other words, the leukemia cells in that particular patient are all derived from a single cancerous founder cell.

Switch from Benign to Malignant Tumors

Malignant cancer cells are those that have acquired the ability to leave the tumor of their origin and migrate throughout the body where they initiate the formation of new tumors. This process, called *metastasis*, requires the following conditions: First, the cancer cell must be able to break away from the tumor mass. Second, once it has broken free, it must be able to migrate throughout the intercellular space until it contacts a blood vessel; at this stage the cancer is locally invasive. Third, the cancer cell must be able to penetrate a blood vessel in order to enter general circulation, which carries the cell to a new location where it forms new tumors. Scientists believe each step in the development of invasiveness and metastasis is controlled by a separate group of genes, but so far no such genes have been identified.

However, it is possible to infer the identities of some of the genes, based on the requirements at each step. Separation of a cancer cell from the rest of the tumor requires the breaking of chemical bonds that normally hold cells together. The most important of these are mediated by cell surface proteins called *cadherins*, which project from every cell, allowing two or more cells to make physical connections. Disruption of these bonds may occur in cancer cells when the gene coding for a cadherin mutates, thus producing a defective protein. Metastasis, invasiveness, and penetration of blood vessels requires the activation of genes that make it possible for the cell to move, much like an amoeba or a macrophage of the immune system. Since more than 80 percent of all human cancers are carcinomas (cancers of stationary epithelial cells) the acquisition of motility is a crucial step. If it were possible to block this step, all cancers could be reduced to harmless benign tumors. One gene, called *Rho,* shows increased expression in aggressively metastatic cancers, and it is known that this gene is involved in regulating cell motility in protozoans and macrophages. It is hoped that with the completion of the human genome project it will soon be possible to identify other genes involved in metastasis.

Role of Sex Hormones

Hormones such as estrogen, progesterone, and testosterone prepare the human body for reproduction and stimulate the development of sexual characteristics as an individual passes through puberty. In women, estrogen stimulates development of the breasts, ovaries, uterus, and the general shape of the body. The cells of the uterine lining are stimulated to grow and divide every month as part of the woman's menstrual cycle. If a pregnancy occurs, progesterone, along with estrogen, helps maintain the uterine lining to support development of the fetus. In men, testosterone stimulates development of the testes, sperm production, and growth of facial hair and musculature.

The *sex hormones* exert their varied effects by promoting cell growth and cell division. As long as the cells in the target organs are healthy, with checkpoint monitors intact, there is no problem. But if a crucial gene or set of genes is defective, and the cell is being bombarded with signals to proliferate, the situation can become serious very quickly. This is the reason why cancers of the breast, uterus, ovaries, and prostate are so common and so dangerous. Cancers such as these are a natural consequence of reproductive physiology, and treatments often try to reduce the levels of sex hormones to withdraw the stimulus to the tumor cells. This approach is not a pleasant experience, involving as it often does the removal of the ovaries, to eliminate the synthesis of estrogen, or the testes, to block production of testosterone.

The relationship between steroid hormones and cancer production introduces serious concerns regarding hormone replacement therapy, particularly for women, to minimize bone loss in the elderly. Hormone replacement therapy can alleviate some of the symptoms of osteoporosis in men and women, but it may do so at the risk of developing cancer. Similar concerns exist in the sporting world, where steroids are used to enhance performance. While such treatments seem to be effective, the athlete who uses hormone supplements will likely pay a heavy price for it in later life by developing prostate, breast, or uterine cancer.

Aging and the Incidence of Cancer

Human cancer is primarily an age-related disease that strikes when an individual is 50 years of age or older. The age of the individual and the time element are important largely because the formation of a tumor is a multistep process that takes many years to complete. There are, however, many exceptions to the age-cancer relationship. Lung cancer brought on by cigarette smoke and childhood leukemias are the most notable examples. The chemicals in cigarette smoke are known to accelerate tumor formation, but the factors responsible for cancer acceleration in children are still unclear.

Cancers are age-related because our cells change with time, becoming more susceptible to genetic damage and less capable of dealing with the damage when it does occur. This problem is believed to be due, in large measure, to a reduction in the ability of our immune system to track down and destroy abnormal cells as they appear; the body's diminished immune response gives those cells time to evolve into a potentially lethal cancer.

The increased incidence of cancer in those age 50 and older is also coincidental with the onset of sexual senescence in both men and women. It is quite possible that the hormonal changes that occur during this period contribute to our increased susceptibility to cancer. Agerelated hormonal changes are primarily concerned with a shift in the ratio of estrogen to testosterone (ET ratio) in both men and women. Young women have a high estrogen/testosterone ratio (a lot of estrogen, very little testosterone), whereas young men have a low estrogen/testosterone ratio (a lot of testosterone, very little estrogen). Estrogen levels drop dramatically in women after menopause, and men show a similar decline in the level of testosterone at a corresponding age. As a consequence, men and women approach a similar ET ratio between the ages of 50 and 80, which is thought to influence the rate at which genetic instability occurs. In addition, many scientists believe the shift in the ET ratio is largely responsible for the weakening of our immune system, leading to the increased occurrence not only of cancer but of many other diseases as well.

Carcinogens

Many cancers are an unfortunate consequence of our physiology, biochemistry, and cellular ancestry, but an even greater number may be caused by chemicals or radiation in our environment. Cancer-causing agents such as these are called carcinogens. The *National Institutes of Health* (NIH) in the United States currently lists more than 200 known or suspected carcinogens. Radiation that can cause cancer is usually high doses of ultraviolet (UV) light, X-rays, and various forms of high-energy radiation produced by radioactive materials. The nature of chemical carcinogens is highly variable, ranging from industrial pollutants to the cooking grease used in fast-food restaurants, all of which are suspected of causing cancer. Surprisingly, there is very little evidence to support these suspicions. Of all the suspected cases of cancer induction from industrial sources, only two, asbestos and beta-napthylamine, have been confirmed as carcinogens in epidemiological studies (studies of a disease and the factors affecting its occurrence).

Asbestos is a generic name given to a group of six naturally occurring fibrous silicate minerals. Asbestos minerals possess a number of desirable properties that were useful in commercial applications, including heat stability and thermal and electrical insulation. Although asbestos use dates back at least 2,000 years, modern industrial use began in about 1880, reaching a peak in the late 1960s and early 1970s when more than 3,000 industrial applications or products were listed. This material has been used primarily in roofing, production of plastics, and thermal and electrical insulation.

Beta-naphthylamine, also known as 2-naphthylamine, occurs as colorless or white-to-reddish crystals with a faint aromatic odor that darken in air to a purple-red color. It is soluble in hot water, alcohol, ether, and many organic solvents. This compound is currently used for research purposes only, but in the mid-1950s it was used as an intermediate in the manufacture of dyes and as an antioxidant in the production of rubber for automobile tires, among other uses.

Asbestos is now known to cause lung cancer, and beta-naphthylamine, in one prominent case, was shown to cause bladder cancer in virtually all of the British factory workers who were exposed to it in the 1950s. However, the number of people dying because of these carcinogens is no greater than the millions of deaths attributable to aflatoxin, a naturally occurring compound produced by the common bread mold *Aspergillus oryzae*. This fungus grows on grains and peanuts when they are stored under humid tropical conditions, and the aflatoxin it produces is thought to be the cause of liver cancer in the tropics.

However, the deadliest carcinogens by far are found in cigarette smoke, and among the 40 or so that have been identified, the best studied is a compound called *benzopyrene*. This molecule, when intact, is not dangerous, but when a cigarette is smoked the benzopyrene enters the blood and travels to the liver where it is inadvertently activated. An important function of our liver is to detoxify our blood by breaking down a wide variety of compounds, from alcohol to aspirin. A special set of liver enzymes, called *mixed-function* oxidases, breaks the alcohol down and either stores or eliminates the pieces. In the case of benzopyrene, the oxidases activate the molecule in such a way that it gains the ability to bind to guanine, thus forming DNA adducts.

The binding of benzopyrene to DNA is not a problem in itself, as long as the cell is postmitotic. However, DNA adducts greatly increase the error frequency associated with DNA replication. Cells in the lung are not postmitotic but divide frequently, and if those cells contain DNA adducts, errors will be introduced into their genome with each round of the cell cycle. Making the situation even worse, other ingredients in tobacco smoke stimulate proliferation-signaling pathways, much as certain oncogenes do, forcing the cells to divide more frequently than normal. The carcinogens' combined ability to form DNA adducts and to force a cell to divide when it should not accelerates the mutation rate and onset of cancers. An accelerated mutation rate increases the risk of damaging a tumor suppressor gene or of activating an oncogene. These changes set the stage for serious trouble to come.

Lung cancer and other cancers caused by tobacco smoke kill more than 400,000 men and women every year in the United States alone and account for nearly 30 percent of annual U.S. cancer deaths. Smokers are 20 times more likely to die of cancer than nonsmokers. Worldwide, 4 million people die every year of cancers caused by tobacco smoke. In China, where two-thirds of the adult male population smokes tobacco, close to 1 million die each year of tobacco-related cancers. Lung cancer alone is so prevalent that it has obscured the incidence of all other cancers. Many people have the impression that the incidence of cancer cases has been increasing over the years, and if all cancers are simply grouped together and plotted against time, this does appear to be the case. Many believe the increased prevalence of cancer is due to pollution of our environment, the air we breathe, and the food we eat. Yet if lung cancer is subtracted from the data, we find that the incidence of other major cancers (plotted as deaths per 100,000 people), including colon, breast, and prostate cancer, has not changed since 1930. It is quite possible that the elimination of tobacco carcinogens would lower the rates for other cancers as well, since it is likely that compounds such as benzopyrene are contributing to the onset of cancers in other organs of the body. Not surprisingly, smoking tobacco is associated with an increased risk for cancers of the mouth, throat, stomach, pancreas (the deadliest of all cancers), liver, uterus, kidney, and bladder. It may also be responsible for the increased prevalence of leukemia in adults and children, the latter presumably caused by secondary smoke inhalation. Indeed, laboratory rats and mice forced to smoke the equivalent of a pack of cigarettes a day develop benzopyrene DNA adducts in virtually every tissue of the body. If we are ever able to remove tobacco carcinogens from our daily lives, it may well turn out that cancer is more a consequence of our life-style, rather than that of our protozoan ancestors.

Mechanisms of Tumor Evasion

The clinical experiments of William Coley in the 1890's demonstrating a therapeutic effect of the "*Coley Toxins*" in some patients, and the animal models of Prehn and Main in the 1950's demonstrating the existence of tumor specific antigens, established an era of active research in immunotherapy as a treatment for cancer. Several studies demonstrated that tumors arising from oncogenic viruses could induce a protective immune response during the early phases of tumor development. However, results in some animal tumor models and especially in patients with cancer, failed to demonstrate the presence of a protective immune response to the progressively growing tumor. Hersh and Oppenheim instead demonstrated that *Hodgkins disease* (HD) patients had a decreased *delayed type hypersensitivity* (DTH) response to PPD and DNBC (*di-nitrochlorobenzene*) and a diminished in vitro response to mitogen stimulation, which persisted even in patients who had achieved a complete clinical response to chemotherapy. Furthermore, Hellstrom and colleagues showed a decreased cellular immune response, but a marked increase in serum immunoglobulins in patients with melanoma. Similarly observations in patients with renal cell carcinoma, prostate and bladder cancer, lung cancer and breast cancer, suggested that tumors might impair the immune response. However the clinical relevance of these findings or the mechanisms causing them remained unclear.

A renewed enthusiasm for immunotherapy started in the 1980's with the cloning and production of pharmaceutical grade cytokines and the isolation and purification of tumor associated antigens. However the results of clinical trials in patients failed to reproduce the undisputable therapeutic benefit shown in animal models, bringing forth the need to understand how tumors escape the immune response. Various mechanisms of tumor escape have been identified ranging from the loss of HLA markers in tumor cells making them difficult to recognize by T cells, to the gradual deterioration of the immune response with the progressive growth of the tumor. Here we will discuss some of the most recent concepts on how tumor cells may escape and/or inhibit the normal function of the immune system.

Changes in Tumor Cells

Selection of Resistant Tumor Cells

The concept of "*immune surveillance*" proposed by Jones and Burnet in the 1970's suggested that the immune system was vigilant to destroy any malignant cells before they developed into a clinically relevant tumor. However, aside from the demonstration of the existence of natural killer cells there was little proof or understanding of how this mechanism worked. In the early 1990's work by Schreiber and

Table 5.1. Mechanisms of tumor evasion

Target	*Major changes*
Changes in tumor cells	Selection of tumor cells resistant to apoptosis
	Changes in the expression of HLA
	Absence of co-stimulatory molecules
Alterations in antigen presenting cells	Arrested maturation of DC
	Selective increase in DC2
Dysfunction of effector cells	Induction of regulatory T cells
	Increased apoptosis of T effector cells
	Alteration in T cell signal transduction

colleagues demonstrated that early tumor growth is comprised mostly of transformed cells that undergo apoptosis when they bind IFNγ and chemokines produced by cells of the innate immune response including natural killer cells, γδ T lymphocytes and macrophages. This effectively eliminates most of the tumor cells, however it also selects for a minority of malignant cells that have mutations or alterations that make them resistant to an immune induced apoptosis. The absence of one or more chains of the IFNγ receptor, or mutations in the tyrosine kinases associated with this receptor (Jak1, Jak2 or Stat1), prevent the triggering of the apoptosis cascade making these cells resistant to the immune surveillance mechanism. These resistant clones then develop into tumors of clinical significance unimpeded by the immune response. Therefore, the innate immune response may eliminate most transformed cells during the early stages of tumor growth, however it may also result in the selection of a resistant population of malignant cells, a process that was coined by Schreiber as cancer immunoediting. Alternatively, Khong and Restifo suggested that tumors are not rejected during early stages of tumor growth because they do not cause significant tissue damage and therefore fail to send "*danger signals*" that could activate the immune response, a concept presented by Matzinger as a means for certain normal tissues of causing immune tolerance.

Decreased HLA Antigen and Co-stimulatory Signal Expression

HLA class I antigen expression

The continued growth of tumor leads to tissue destruction and the generation of "*danger signals*," which may trigger an adaptive immune response. The activation of *tumor associated antigen* (TAA)-specific T lymphocytes occurs through the recognition of two combined signals by the T cell (i) peptides, derived from TAA, presented by self-HLA class I molecules (i.e. HLA class I antigen-TAA peptide complex) and (ii) co-stimulatory signals such as B7.1 (CD80) or B7.2 (CD86). This recognition results in the development of effector *cytotoxic T lymphocytes* (CTL) that recognize and lyse tumor cells presenting the relevant HLA class I antigen-TAA peptide complex. Therefore, tumor cells can evade hosts' immune response by being poor stimulators of T cells or being poor targets for effector CTL. Specifically, malignant cells may posses abnormalities in the expression of molecules required for effective T cell recognition, such as HLA class I antigens, costimulatory molecules and/or the TAA itself.

In the case of HLA class I antigens, a large body of evidence indicates that malignant transformation is associated with abnormalities in HLA class I antigen expression. Analysis of cell lines in long term culture, through a combination of binding and immunochemical assays, has identified distinct defects in the expression of HLA class I antigens in tumor cells. These defects do not represent artifacts of *in vitro* cell culture, since they have also been identified in surgically removed tumors by *immunohistochemical* (IHC) staining with *monoclonal antibodies* (mAb). In fact, with the exception of liver carcinoma and leukemia, IHC staining of a large number of surgically removed malignant lesions with mAb to monomorphic determinants of HLA class I antigens has identified abnormalities in the HLA class I antigen expression in 16% to 50% of all malignant lesions analyzed.

The reason(s) for differences in the frequency of HLA class I defects is (are) not known. They are likely to reflect the time length between onset of tumor and diagnosis, since a long interval gives tumor cells more chances to mutate in the genes involved in HLA class I antigen expression and allows mutated cells to over-grow cells without abnormalities in their HLA class I phenotype in the presence of T cell selective pressure, as it will be discussed later. HLA class I antigen down-regulation or loss has also been described in other tumor types. However, the number of lesions that have been analyzed is too low for one to draw definitive conclusions. These types of tumors include stomach, pancreatic, bladder, germ cell and basal cell carcinomas. It is noteworthy that HLA class I antigen loss or down-regulation does not occur in all types of malignancies. In leukemia, defects in HLA class I antigen expression in malignant cells have been only occasionally identified. This finding is not likely to reflect a lack of genetic instability in leukemic cells, since like solid tumor cells, leukemic cells harbor many genetic and/or epigenetic alterations in their DNA. Furthermore, in view of the role of immunoselection in the generation of malignant cell populations with HLA class I defects, lack of immune responses against leukemic cells is unlikely to be the mechanism. This possibility is supported by the higher frequency of HLA class I antigen abnormalities in sporadic diffuse large cell lymphoma than in immunodeficient and transplant-related lymphomas. Therefore, it is likely that the lack of defects in HLA class I antigen expression identified in leukemia reflects the time interval between the onset of leukemia and its diagnosis, which is likely to be shorter than that of solid tumors. A short time interval between the onset of leukemia and diagnosis may not allow sufficient time for cells to acquire mutations in the gene(s) involved in HLA class I antigen expression and for selective pressure to facilitate the expansion of malignant cells with HLA class I abnormalities. In the case of liver carcinoma, normal hepatocytes, which do not express or express very low HLA class I antigen levels, acquire the expression of these antigens during malignant transformation. The results obtained with liver carcinoma cell lines suggest that HLA class I antigen up-regulation may result from the induction of antigen processing machinery components by cytokines secreted by immune cells infiltrating malignant lesions.

Abnormalities in HLA class I antigen expression in malignant lesions appear to have clinical significance, since they are associated with histopathological characteristics of the lesions and/or with clinical parameters in several malignant diseases. However, depending on the tumor type, HLA class I antigen defects can be associated directly (*head and neck squamous cell* (HSCC), breast, small cell lung, prostate, bladder and cervical carcinoma and cutaneous melanoma), inversely correlated (uveal melanoma and colon carcinoma) or not associated (pulmonary adenocarcinoma, squamous cell carcinoma of the uterine cervix, cutaneous squamous cell carcinoma, large cell and large immunoblastic lymphoma and non-small cell lung carcinoma) with disease progression and/or poor clinical outcomes. The reasons for these discrepancies are not known but may reflect differences in the characteristics of the patient population, the methods of analysis and/or the system used to score HLA class I antigen expression. In addition, these findings may be attributed to differences in types of immune response elicited by tumors of different tissue or differences in routes of metastasis. An example is represented by the opposite association of HLA class I antigen down-regulation with the clinical outcome in cutaneous and uveal melanomas. HLA class I antigen down-regulation is associated with a poor prognosis in cutaneous melanoma, where

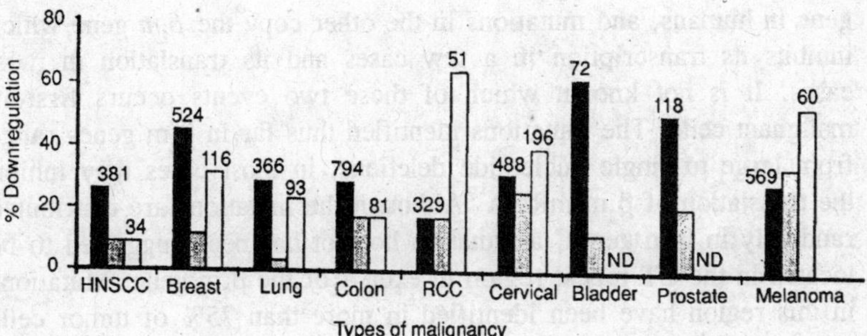

Fig. 5.1. Frequency of HLA class I antigen and TAP1 downregulation in malignant lesions of different embryological origin.

CTL are believed to control the metastatic tumor spread via the lymphatics. In contrast, HLA class I antigen down-regulation is associated with a favorable clinical outcome in uveal melanoma, where NK cells, which tend to kill tumor cells with a low HLA class I antigen expression, have been suggested to limit metastasis via the blood.

The potential role of HLA class I antigen abnormalities in the clinical course of malignant disease has stimulated the characterization of the molecular mechanisms responsible for HLA class I antigen abnormalities. Through the effort of a number of investigators, characterization of cell lines originated from malignant lesions with HLA class I abnormalities has shown that distinct molecular mechanisms underlie the abnormal HLA class I phenotypes of tumor cells. The frequency of complete HLA class I antigen loss has been found to be between about 15% in primary cutaneous melanoma lesions and 50% in primary prostate carcinoma lesions. The frequency of this phenotype varies significantly between different malignancies. As indicated above, it is likely that these differences reflect the time length between onset of tumor and diagnosis. Complete HLA class I antigen loss can be caused by defects in β_2-microglobulin (β_2m) which is required for the formation of the HLA class I heavy chain-β_2m-peptide complex and its transport to the cell membrane, epigenetic changes in the DNA or alterations in the antigen processing machinery components.

The latter play a crucial role in the assembly of functional HLA class I antigen-peptide complexes and in their expression on the cell membrane. Inactivation of the β_2m genes completely abrogates HLA class I antigen expression at the cell surface and has marked effects on peptide presentation. β_2m defects result from two events: loss of one copy of the β_2m gene at chromosome #15, which carries the β_2m

gene in humans, and mutations in the other copy the $\beta_2 m$ gene which inhibits its transcription in a few cases and its translation in most cases. It is not known which of these two events occurs first in malignant cells. The mutations identified thus far in β_2m genes range from large to single nucleotide deletions; in most cases they inhibit the translation of β_2m mRNA. Although the mutations are distributed randomly in β_2m genes, a mutation hotspot has been suggested to be located in the CT repeat region in exon 1 of the β_2m gene. Mutations in this region have been identified in more than 75% of tumor cells with total HLA class I antigen loss and have been found to parallel the mutator phenotype in tumor cells, reflecting the increased genetic instability of this region during malignant transformation of cells.

It is noteworthy, that for some tumors such as head and neck squamous cell, laryngeal, breast, colorectal, renal and bladder carcinoma, β_2m gene mutations are not responsible for complete HLA class I antigen loss. These observations suggest that genetic mutations in the β_2m gene may not be the predominant molecular mechanism underlying total HLA class I antigen loss and suggest that other mechanisms may be involved in total HLA class I antigen loss. In this regard, post-transcriptional regulation of the β_2m gene expression has been suggested as a possible mechanism for total HLA class I antigen loss. In addition, epigenetic changes that cause total HLA class I antigen loss have been observed. Hypermethylation of three HLA class I antigen loci has been observed in neoplastic cells to selectively switch off HLA class I antigen gene expression. The characteristics of these tumors are the significant reduction in or complete absence of mRNA from the heavy chain gene and normal expression of β_2m and antigen processing machinery components. DNA hypermethylation has been implicated as a major mechanism for transcriptional inactivation of HLA class I antigen genes in esophageal squamous cell carcinomas and is also responsible for the total HLA class I antigen loss in melanoma.

Selective HLA class I allospecificity loss, e.g. HLA-A2 loss, is caused by loss of the gene(s) encoding the lost HLA class I heavy chain(s) or by mutations which inhibit their transcription or translation. It is noteworthy, that selective HLA class I antigen loss results from only one mutational event in a heterozygous allelic background. This may explain why, in most malignancies, the frequency of selective HLA class I antigen losses is higher than that of total HLA class I antigen losses. As in the case of the β_2m gene, the mutations found in

HLA class I heavy chains range from large deletions to single base deletions. The mutations appear to occur randomly. Whether a mutation hotspot in the genes encoding HLA class I heavy chains exists remains to be determined.

Loss of one HLA class I haplotype, e.g. HLA-A24, -B56, -Cw7, appears to be frequently caused by loss of segments of the short arm of chromosome 6 where HLA class I genes reside, however in some instances it can be caused by the loss of specific transcription factors that specifically bind to HLA-A or HLA-B promoters. This phenotype is often identified by HLA class I genotyping and LOH analysis of chromosome 6. LOH at chromosome 6 appears to represent a frequent mechanism contributing to selective HLA haplotype loss in tumors. This finding may reflect the frequent genetic recombination events at the human *MHC* located at chromosome 6p21.3, which carries the highest density of genes among all gene loci in human chromosomes.

Total HLA class I down-regulation can be caused by multiple mechanisms. First, transcriptional activity of HLA class I heavy chain genes can be suppressed by the presence of silencer located at the distal promoter or by epigenetic mechanisms such as hypermethylation and/or altered chromatin structure of the HLA class I heavy chain gene promoters. Second, the restoration or enhancement of HLA class I antigen expression in malignant cells by IFN-γ suggests that altered regulation of non-mutated genes may play a part in defects in HLA class I antigen expression.

Lastly, the level of HLA class I antigens expressed on cells can be reduced by down-regulation or loss of antigen processing machinery components. Defects in antigen processing machinery components may effect the generation of peptides from antigens, their transport into the *endoplasmic reticulum* (ER), their loading on HLA class I antigens and/or the repertoire of peptides presented by HLA class I antigens. It is noteworthy that in the majority of cases, antigen processing machinery component loss or down-regulation can be corrected by treating cells with cytokines, e.g. IFN-γ, indicating that these abnormalities are usually caused by regulatory and not structural defects. This mechanism may explain why the frequency of down-regulation of one or multiple antigen processing machinery components in malignant lesions is high, in spite of the codominant expression of the two genes encoding each antigen processing machinery component.

An alternative, although not exclusive, mechanism is represented by the down-regulation, by IL-10, of antigen processing machinery components, which leads to reduced HLA class I antigen cell surface expression. This finding may be of clinical relevance, since a large number of human tumors secrete IL-10. Therefore, these patients, at variance with those with structural defects in HLA class I antigen-encoding genes, are likely to benefit by combining T cell-based immunotherapy with administration of IFN-γ and/or anti-IL-10 antibodies.

Information in the literature regarding antigen processing machinery component expression in various types of malignancies is scanty. Only a few components have been analyzed and only in a limited number of lesions. It is also noteworthy to point out that no information is available as to what constitutes normal or abnormal expression profiles of antigen processing machinery components in cells, since to the best of our knowledge no study has quantitated the level of antigen processing machinery component expression in normal cells of different embryological origin.

The paucity of the available information reflects the limited or lack of availability of antibodies and methodology to quantitate antigen processing machinery components. Therefore, one must exercise caution in interpreting studies that analyze antigen processing machinery component expression in malignant cells, since the phenotype of the normal counterparts is not known in many cases. Among the antigen processing machinery components, TAP1 has been most extensively investigated. TAP1 down-regulation and/or loss has been found in HNSCC, in carcinomas of the breast, small cell lung (SCLC), colon, kidney, cervix and prostate and in cutaneous melanoma with a frequency ranging from 10–84%. A few studies have investigated TAP2 expression in malignant cells and the frequency of TAP2 down-regulation tends to correlate with that of TAP1. TAP1 down-regulation or loss is likely to be caused by abnormalities in regulatory mechanisms, since in some instances they can be corrected by *in vitro* administration of cytokines, such as IFN-γ and TNF-α, and is accompanied by an increase in HLA class I antigen expression.

The increase in HLA class I antigen expression following induction of TAP1 expression is correlated with an increased susceptibility to TAA-specific CTL lysis, in most but not all cases. In addition, it is expected that the frequency of TAP down-regulation is higher than that of total HLA class I antigen losses, due to the distinct mechanisms underlying these two phenotypes. While two mutational events are required for total HLA class I antigen loss, TAP downregulation appears to be primarily due to abnormalities in regulatory mechanisms. To the best of our knowledge, structural defects in TAP1 as a result of mutations have been observed only in two human tumor cell lines.

Only recently has tapasin expression been analyzed in a few types of tumors. Abnormalities in tapasin expression can lead to reduced HLA class I antigen expression, alterations in the repertoire of peptides presented by HLA class I antigens and resistance of malignant cells to CTL. Heterogeneous and reduced levels of tapasin mRNA has been observed in HNSCC, SCLC, hepatoma, RCC, colon carcinoma, pancreatic carcinoma, neuroblastoma and cutaneous melanoma cell lines. In the majority of cases, *in vitro* incubation of cells with cytokines such as IFN-α, IFN-γ, TNF-α and IL-4 has resulted in tapasin transcriptional up-regulation. However, in the melanoma cell line COPA159 we have identified a single-base deletion at position 684 in exon 3 of the *tapasin* gene resulting in a reading frameshift of the mRNA with a subsequent introduction of a premature stop codon at positions 698–700. This cell line demonstrates reduced HLA class I antigen expression, which can be restored upon transfection with the wild-type *tapasin* allele. To a limited extent, tapasin expression has been investigated in surgically removed malignant lesions. In these studies tapasin has been found to be down-regulated in both RCC and HNSCC lesions. In the latter malignancy, this downregulation is associated with poor prognosis. If this is a cause-effect relationship, it is likely to reflect the reduced susceptibility of tumor cells to CTL-mediated lysis because of HLA class I antigen downregulation and alterations in the HLA class I antigen peptide repertoire in cells with reduced tapasin expression.

Selective downregulation of the gene products of one HLA class I locus can be caused by alterations in the transcription factors for genes encoding HLA class I heavy chains. However, there is limited information regarding selective downregulation of the gene products of one HLA class I locus, since the expression of some HLA class I allospecificities in malignant lesions has not been assessed because of the lack of appropriate probes.

The major role played by the HLA class I-TAA peptide complex in the recognition of tumor cells by CTL can be further illustrated by the association found between abnormalities in the expression and/or function of antigen processing machinery components and poor clinical course of the disease in some malignancies. This association most likely reflects the importance of these components in the generation of functional HLA class I-TAA peptide complexes. Notably, TAP1 down-regulation has been reported to associate with tumor staging and reduction in patients' survival in breast carcinoma, SCLC, cervical cancer and cutaneous melanoma. An increased frequency of TAP1 downregulation in metastatic lesions when compared to primary lesions has also been reported in breast carcinoma, cervical carcinoma and cutaneous melanoma. Most recently, the role of tapasin in the clinical course of malignant diseases has been suggested by Ogino et al. who reported that tapasin downregulation in conjunction with HLA class I antigen downregulation was associated with reduced survival in patients with maxillary sinus squamous cell carcinoma.

It remains to be determined whether this finding applies to other types of tumors. Nevertheless, all of these findings are likely to reflect the crucial role of TAP1 and tapasin in the generation of HLA class I antigen-TAA peptide complexes and suggest that alterations in the repertoire of peptides presented by HLA class I antigens may provide an alternate route of immune escape for malignant cells. This possibility highlights the need to monitor specific HLA class I antigen-TAA derived peptide complex expression in malignant lesions. To this end, we have begun to develop probes capable of recognizing allospecific HLA class I antigen-TAA derived peptide complex expression on malignant cells.

Generation of cells with HLA class I antigen defects results from mutations in the gene(s) which are involved in the expression of HLA class I antigens. It is likely that these mutations occur randomly due to increased epigenetic changes and genomic instability in the early stages of tumor development. In general the frequency of HLA class I antigen defects in metastatic lesions is higher than that in primary and premalignant lesions. It is also noteworthy to point out that especially in malignant cells isolated from patients with advanced disease the presence of multiple defects affecting different antigen processing machinery components and HLA class I subunits appears to be the rule more than the exception. Moreover, an increase frequency of HLA class I antigen loss variants have been found in recurrent metastatic lesions in patients who had experienced clinical responses following T cell-based immunotherapy.

Therefore, one important question to ask is which mechanism(s) play(s) a role in the expansion of cells with HLA class I defects in malignant lesions. In view of the continuous exposure of tumor cells to the host's immune response, one might ask whether immune selective pressure plays a major role in the expansion of cells with HLA class I antigen defects so that they become the major population in a lesion.

One can envision two possible scenarios: (i) if immune selective pressure plays a major role, then tumor cells with HLA class I defects expand because of escape from host's immune response which targets tumor cells without HLA class I antigen defects; (ii) if on the other hand, immune selective pressure does not play a role, then the expansion of tumor cells with HLA class I antigen defects is independent of the development of an immune response in the host. The available evidence derived from studies in animal model systems and in patients treated with T cell-based immunotherapy argues in favor of a major role played by immune selective pressure in the generation of malignant lesions with HLA class I antigen defects. From a practical viewpoint, the possible role played by immune selective pressure in the generation of malignant lesions with HLA class I antigen defects suggests that the use of T cell-based immunotherapy for the treatment of malignant diseases may only be successful in a limited number of cases.

HLA class I antigen downregulation may provide malignant cells with a mechanism to escape CTL recognition and destruction. This possibility has raised the question of why HLA class I antigen downregulation does not increase the sensitivity of malignant cells to NK cell-mediated cytotoxicity. The latter phenomenon has been convincingly shown in mice where MHC class I downregulation is correlated with increased target cells' susceptibility to NK cells (missing-self hypothesis). The mechanisms by which NK cells recognize and kill target cells have been poorly understood only until recently. NK cell recognition and killing mechanisms are now believed to be governed by a balance between activating and inhibitory signals received by the NK cells. These signals are generated by specific target cell ligand-NK cell receptor interactions. To date, there is evidence that the non-classical HLA class I antigens HLA-E, F, G may serve as inhibitory NK cell ligands, while the MHC class I related chain A and B (MICA and MICB) and the UL16-binding protein 1, 2 and 3 (ULBP1, ULBP2 and ULBP3) may act as activating NK cell ligands. In this regard, tumors can express stress induced ligands MICA and MICB, which inhibit NK cytotoxic function and IFN-γ production when released in soluble form.

Co-stimulatory molecule expression

To achieve activation, T cells require a minimum of two signals provided by antigen and co-stimulatory membrane proteins such as CD80 and CD86. Stimulation of T cells in the absence of co-stimulatory signals leads to anergy of T cells and eventually to T cell apoptosis.

A decreased expression of costimulatory signals CD80, CD86 and CD45 has been demonstrated in B cell malignancies, lung and colon cancer, making them not only poor stimulators of a T cell response, but also potential inducers of T cell apoptosis. In concert with these observations, in vitro experiments showed that transfection of tumor cells with the CD80 and CD86 genes, increased their immunogenicity. Although this led to the rejection of B7 transfected tumor in murine models, it did not always lead to the regression of the non-transfected malignant cells. Tumor cells can also evade recognition by T cells by decreasing the expression of tumor antigens through mechanisms that remain unclear, but appear to be independent of HLA expression. The loss of gp100, MART 1 and tyrosinase in melanoma have been associated with tumor progression and resistance to immunotherapy.

Changes in Cell Mediated Immune Response in Cancer

During the early 1980's North and colleagues developed animal models where they carefully studied T cell function during progressive tumor growth. An initial protective T cell response could be readily demonstrated during the first days after tumor implantation, followed by a rapid decline in the response with the appearance of Ly1+ suppressor T cells. This suppressor function could be transferred into naive animals and was eliminated with low doses of cyclophosphamide, re-establishing a therapeutic anti-tumor response. These findings provided an insight into a dynamic interaction between the tumor and the immune system that could be manipulated to the benefit of the host. An alternative explanation to the presence of suppressor cells came from studies on the function of cytokines produced by $CD4^+$ helper clones. Mossman and colleagues classified T helper cells according to the type of cytokines they produced and the response elicited. Th1 cells mainly produced IL2, IFNγ, and TNFα, promoting cellular responses, while Th2 cells mainly secreted IL4, IL13 and IL10, promoting antibody production. It was therefore possible that the progressive growth of tumor induced a loss of Th1 activity and an increased Th2 function, leading to a diminished cellular response and an enhanced antibody production. Most of these concepts remained as interesting research observations, but with minor relevance in the treatment of patients.

The advent of immunotherapy in the 1980's using the adoptive transfer of *tumor-infiltrating lymphocytes* (TIL) revealed to a greater extent the degree of T cell dysfunction in patients with cancer. In vitro testing of freshly isolated TIL demonstrated that these cells had a markedly decreased proliferation when stimulated with mitogens or tumor cells and had a significantly diminished clonogenic potential. This T cell dysfunction was however not limited to TIL cells, but was also seen in peripheral blood T cells or splenic T lymphocytes in tumor bearing mice. Furthermore this cellular dysfunction appeared to have a major detrimental effect on the therapeutic success of immunotherapy.

Loeffier and colleagues studying an immunotherapy model of adoptive transfer of T lymphocytes, demonstrated that T cells from mice bearing tumors for >21 days had a markedly diminished antitumor effect when used to treat tumor-bearing recipients. In contrast, T cells from mice bearing tumors for <14 days had a high therapeutic efficacy when transferred into tumor bearing recipients. In vitro tests demonstrated a diminished cytotoxic activity in the T cells from long-term tumor bearing mice, which could in part be explained by a diminished expression of the perforin gene. Sondak et al. also confirmed the diminished cytotoxic function of T cells from tumor bearing mice, which was more significant in mice bearing visceral metastases as compared to those with subcutaneous tumors. Therefore animal models not only reproduced the T cell dysfunction seen in cancer patients, but also suggested that these alterations could have an important impact on the outcome of cancer immunotherapy. These observations sparked an increased research effort to elucidate the mechanisms of tumor escape that started in the 1990's and continues today.

Major advances in understanding the fundamental mechanisms of antigen processing and presentation, costimulatory signals and T cell activation, as well as the molecular basis for T cell signal transduction, provided important tools to start exploring the intricate interactions between tumors and the immune system.

Changes in Antigen Presenting Cells

Antigen presenting cells (APC) in the form of macrophages or *dendritic cells* (DC) process and present antigens to T lymphocytes. Gabrilovich and colleagues first described a selective increase in the number of immature myeloid DC in the circulation of tumor bearing mice and cancer patients. Surgical removal of the tumor resulted in a decrease in the immature DC cells and a recovery of T cell responses. In tumor-bearing mice, the immature myeloid cells are represented by a population of Gr-1, CD11b and MHC class I positive cells. Gr-1 (+) cells do not impair T cell responses to mitogens such as Con A, but completely block T cell responses *in vitro* and *in vivo* to peptides presented by MHC class I. Therefore, immature DC preferentially inhibit CD8-mediated antigen-specific T cell responses. The increased immature DC cells appear to be result of VEGF produced by tumor cells, which arrests DC maturation by suppressing the activation of the transcription factor NFκB.

In fact, there is a high degree of association between increased serum levels of VEGF and a high numbers of immature DC in patients with gastric, lung and head and neck cancer. In addition to arresting dendritic cell maturation, tumors can also induce a selective increase in the number of DC2 cells or regulatory dendritic cells, which can induce T cell anergy. *Stromal derived factor*–1 (SDF-1) produced by ovarian carcinoma cells selectively recruits plasmacytoid dendritic cells and modulates their function. These in turn appear to preferentially activate regulatory T lymphocytes that express CD25.

Tumors may also impair the cytotoxic function of macrophages by blocking nitric oxide production. Nitric oxide is an important component of the cytotoxic mechanism displayed by macrophages, endothelial cells and neurons. Several studies have found that macrophages from patients with cancer or tumor bearing mice have a decreased production of nitric oxide when compared to normal individuals. However, these studies did not find a decreased expression of iNOS, suggesting that other mechanisms, such as the depletion of the nitric oxide substrate, arginine, may be the mechanism for the inhibition in nitric oxide production.

Induction of Regulatory T Cells

The recently described subset of regulatory T cells comprises a subset of mostly $CD4^+$, $CD25^+$ T cells, which constitute approximately 5–10% of the total $CD4^+$ cells and appear to control key aspects of tolerance to self antigens. Depletion of this T cell subset can induce an autoimmune response against endocrine organs in mice. Patients with melanoma, colon and head and neck cancer have an increased percentage of regulatory T cells ($CD4^+/CD25^+$) in their circulation. The depletion of these cells in tumor bearing mice increases the response to tumor associate antigen. However, depletion of regulatory T cells alone is not enough to treat established tumors in mice.

Apoptosis of Effector T Cells

Elimination of T cells responding to autologous antigens through the binding of *Fas ligand* (FasL) to the Fas receptor is a well-established mechanism for the induction of apoptosis and tolerance to normal tissue antigens. A high expression of FasL has been reported in tumor cells from lung carcinoma, melanoma, colon carcinoma and liver carcinoma. Therefore tumors that express Fas-ligand, or shed Fas-ligand into the serum could induce apoptosis in T cells infiltrating the site of tumor or in circulating T cells, effectively escaping the effector arm of the immune response. Several reports have recently suggested an increased percentage in apoptosis of T cells in the peripheral blood of patients with head and neck cancer. Tumor cells have also been shown to lose the expression of Fas, developing resistance to apoptosis induced by FasL expressed by effector cells of the immune system.

Changes in T Cell Signal Transduction

In the mid 1980's major advances in T cell biology provided the basis to understand the molecular events that lead to T cell activation. Among these were the elucidation of the elements that form the *T cell antigen receptor* (TCR) and the mechanisms of T cell signal transduction after antigen stimulation. Briefly two polymorphic chains, the α and β chains confer antigen specificity to the T cell and form the antigen-binding site. These are covalently linked to the CD3 complex formed by the invariant chains γδε and ζ. The latter forms homodimers ζζ (CD3ζ) or heterodimers (ζη). Two Src family members of tyrosine kinases are critical in the signal transduction of this structure, namely $p56^{lck}$ that is associated with CD4 or CD8, and $p59^{fyn}$, associated with CD3ζ. The binding of antigen to the αβ TCR complex triggers the mobilization of calcium from intracellular stores and the hydrolysis of IP3 to IP2 freeing high-energy phosphates used by kinases in the phosphorylation of several signal transduction proteins. In parallel, HLA molecules and CD80 and CD86 bind to their receptors, activating various tyrosine kinases including $p59^{fyn}$ and ZAP-70, which activate nuclear transcription factors such as NFκB that translocate into the nucleus and activate or repress various genes.

Major advances were also made in understanding the molecular changes that accompany T cell unresponsiveness or anergy. Quill and colleagues and Jenkins and Schwartz demonstrated that T cells stimulated by antigens presented on fixed *antigen presenting cells* (APC) were anergic, i.e., unresponsive to repeated antigenic stimuli and unable to produce IL2. Furthermore, stimulation of T cells with streptococcus superantigen produced a state of T cell anergy and resulted in a decreased expression of $p56^{lck}$ and $p59^{fyn}$. Anergic T cells also had several molecular changes including the inability to phosphorylate p21 Ras and a decreased ability to activate nuclear transcription factors NFκB and AP-1, important in regulating cytokine production.

In the early 1990's Mizoguchi and colleagues studying the dysfunctional T cells from long-term tumor bearing mice demonstrated a marked decrease in the expression of CD3ζ chain, $p56^{lck}$ and $p59^{fyn}$ tyrosine kinases. These changes were accompanied by a decreased tyrosine kinase phosphorylation and a diminished Ca^{++} flux. These findings provided for the first time a molecular basis to explain T cell dysfunction in cancer patients. Li and Ghosh later showed that T cells from some patients with renal cell carcinoma and from long-term tumor bearing mice were unable to translocate NFκBp65 nuclear transcription factor, resulting in a predominance of NFκBp50/50 homodimer known to act as a repressor of the IFNγ gene. In fact, cytokine production during the progressive growth of tumors in mice demonstrated a Th1 response (IL2 and IFNγ) early after tumor implantation, followed by an increased production of Th2 cytokines (IL4 and IL10) after three weeks.

Table 5.2. Most frequent T cell signal transduction abnormalities reported in cancer patients

Target	*Effect*
CD3ζ	Decreased expression
$p56^{lck}$	Decreased expression
JAK-3	Decreased expression
Calcium signaling	Decreased mobilization
NFκBp65	Inability to translocate
IL2 production	Decreased production

Results in cancer patients confirmed the initial observations in murine models. T cells and NK cells from approximately half of the patients with renal cell carcinoma, colon carcinoma, ovarian carcinoma, gastric cancer, breast cancer, prostate cancer, Hodgkins disease, acute myelocytic leukemia and other tumors showed a decreased expression of CD3ζ chain and a decreased in vitro response to antigens or mitogens. In addition, T cells from renal cell carcinoma patients also had a diminished ability to translocate NFκBp65. However, changes in signal transduction molecules were not limited to those associated with the T cell receptor. Kolenko and colleagues demonstrated that Jak-3, a tyrosine kinase associated with the γ chain, a common element to IL2, IL4, IL7 and IL15 cytokine receptors, was also decreased in T cells from renal cell carcinoma patients. Initial work in colon carcinoma and renal cell carcinoma suggested that patients with more advanced stages of the disease had a higher frequency of T cell signal transduction alterations. However, in cervical carcinoma some patients with carcinoma *in situ* already showed a diminished expression of CD3ζ, suggesting that T cell signal transduction alterations could occur early in the disease and were not an exclusive characteristic of advanced stages of cancer. Other reports have also suggested an association between the expression of CD3ζ and survival. Patients with muetastatic melanoma (Stage IV) treated with IL2 + anti-CD3 monoclonal antibody and patients with head and neck cancer that had normal levels of CD3ζ chain at the initiation of treatment had a significantly longer survival compared to those who had undetectable levels.

The expression of CD3ζ changes with treatment. Patients with non-Hodgkins lymphoma and patients with Hodgkins disease who responded to chemotherapy showed a re-expression of normal levels of ζ chain, which decreased again in patients who had a recurrence of the disease. Limited data from clinical trials in ovarian carcinoma, melanoma, renal cell carcinoma and colon carcinoma showed that patients receiving IL2 based therapies could recover CD3ζ expression. However, this did not always coincide with a full recovery of T cell function since tyrosine kinase activity was not always fully restored.

Mechanisms Leading to Alterations in T Cell Signal Transduction

Otsuji et al. and Kono et al. demonstrated in a series of elegant in vitro experiments that H_2O_2 from macrophages induced the loss of CD3ζ chain in naive T cells, a phenomenon that could be blocked by the depletion of macrophages or the addition of oxygen radical scavengers. A similar effect was seen with H_2O_2 produced by neutrophils in patients with pancreatic and breast cancer. Other macrophage products also appear to be able to alter the expression of T cell signal transduction proteins. Kolenko and colleagues showed that PGE2 in combination with substances that increase cAMP can diminish the expression of Jak-3 in naive T lymphocytes, effectively blocking signal transduction through the IL2 receptor.

A second mechanism leading to loss of CD3ζ chain was found while studying Fas-FasL induced T cell apoptosis. T cells undergoing apoptosis lose the expression of CD3ζ as one of the early changes in this process. Gangliosides expressed on the membrane of different tumors have also been shown to be powerful immunosuppressors of T cells. Uzzo et al. showed that gangliosides from renal cell carcinoma cells can suppress nuclear transcription factor NFκBp65 in T cells and induce apoptosis. Therefore the diminished expression of CD3ζ chain seen in cancer patients could in part be explained by an increased frequency of apoptotic cells in peripheral blood.

Modulation of T Cell Function and CD3ζ Expression by Amino-Acid Availability

Recent observations have demonstrated the important role of amino-acids in regulating T cell function. Among these tryptophan and arginine appear to play an important role in cancer. Dunn and colleagues demonstrated that macrophages producing Indoleamine 2, 3-dioxygenase (IDO) can deplete the essential amino-acid tryptophan and sensitizes activated T cell to apoptosis. Preliminary data in tumor bearing animals suggests that tumor cells may express IDO. The use of an IDO inhibitor, 1-methyl-tryptophan (1-MT) is currently being studied in animal models as a means reversing the inhibitory effects of this metabolic pathway.

Non-essential amino acids can also cause severe T cell dysfunction. Taheri et al. and Rodriguez and colleagues recently demonstrated that T cells cultured in the absence of arginine lose the expression of CD3ζ, have a decreased proliferation and a decreased production of IFNγ. Arginine levels can be regulated in vivo by the enzymes nitric oxide synthase (iNOS) and arginase I produced by macrophages or tumor cells.

Arginase I production in macrophages is increased by Th2 cytokines and is able to deplete the extracellular levels of arginine, causing a down-regulation of CD3ζ. In addition, cells cultured in the absence of arginine show a decreased translocation of NFκBp65 similar to these observed in T cells from cancer patients. The CD3ζ down-regulation in the absence of arginine is caused by post-transcriptional mechanisms leading to a decrease in CD3ζ mRNA stability. These recent observations have led us to postulate the following scenario for the induction of T cell dysfunction in cancer. Arginase I produced by tumor cells or macrophages depletes arginine, causing the loss of CD3ζ and inhibiting cytokine production by T cells. This results in the inability of T cells to develop an anti tumor response and may impair the efficacy of immunotherapies.

Concluding Remark

The results from in vitro immunological experiments, murine tumor models and patients with cancer clearly demonstrate that tumors have multiple mechanisms to evade the immune response. During the early stages of tumor development malignant cells can be poor stimulators, present poor targets or become resistant to the innate immune response, while at later stages, progressively growing tumors impair the adaptive immune response by blocking the maturation and function of antigen presenting cells and causing alterations in T cell signal transduction and function. Preliminary results also suggest a correlation between some of these changes and an increased metastatic potential of the tumor cells, a diminished response to immunotherapy, and poor prognosis. Carefully coordinated basic research studies and clinical immunotherapy trials will be required to fully determine the impact on the outcome of the disease and the response to treatment. However, understanding the mechanisms used by tumor cells to evade the immune system could result in new therapeutic approaches for preventing and/ or reversing these immune alterations and have the potential of improving the current results of immunotherapy trials.

6

Tumor Suppressor Gene

While oncogenes promote tumor development by increased activity or deregulation, tumor suppressor genes have to undergo loss of function for tumor development. Many hereditary cancers result from germline mutations in tumor suppressor genes that are passed on in families. In most cancers with a dominant mode of inheritance, one mutant allele of a tumor suppressor gene is inherited. When the second allele becomes as well inactivated by mutation, deletion, recombination with the mutated allele, or by epigenetic mechanisms, cancer development is initiated. In sporadic cancers, two mutations in the two alleles of the gene must occur within one cell line. Therefore, inherited cancers typically occur at earlier ages and are more often multifocal than sporadic cancers of the same type. Of note, while inheritance is dominant, tumor suppressor genes behave as recessive genes at the cellular level.

Loss of a tumor suppressor allele by deletion or recombination often becomes apparent as *loss of heterozygosity* (LOH) of polymorphic markers, e.g., microsatellites, in its vicinity. LOH analysis is a useful method to detect deletions or recombinations in tumors and can be employed to discover tumor suppressor genes in regions of the genome which consistently show LOH in one type of tumor.

Retinoblastoma has provided the paradigm for tumor suppressor genes, that also fits for several other inherited cancers. The tumor suppressor gene inactivated in retinoblastomas, *RB1*, encodes a central regulator of the cell cycle, prominently of the G1→S transition, but also aides to ensure correct mitotic segregation, affects chromatin structure and regulates apoptosis. RB1 acts by binding and controlling other proteins, prominently E2F transcriptional factors. These can activate genes required for entry into the S phase and DNA synthesis, but in certain circumstances also induce apoptosis. RB1 itself is regulated via phosphorylation by *cyclin-dependent kinases* (CDKs) which in turn are dependent on their regulatory cyclin subunits.

Multiple mechanisms are employed in human cells to regulate the cell cycle and RB1 phosphorylation, including induction and proteolysis of cyclins, phosphorylation and dephosphorylation of CDKs and induction, stabilization and proteolysis of CDK protein inhibitors. The CDK inhibitors comprise the INK4 family which specifically inhibits CDK4 and the CIP/KIP family inhibiting several CDKs. CDK inhibitors can be tumor suppressors. The most important one in this regard is CDKN2A/p16^{INK4A}, but p27^{KIP1}, p21^{CIP1}, and p57^{KIP2} are also relevant.

Alterations in cell cycle regulation in different tumors are alternatively brought about by loss of tumor suppressor gene (*RB1* or *CDKN2A*) function or by oncogene (*CCND1* or *CDK4*) activation. There are further cases, in which tumor suppressors essentially act as antagonists of oncogenes, e.g. the tumor suppressor NF1 is a GAP that limits the action of RAS proteins. Loss of tumor suppressors and activation of oncogenes therefore often have similar, albeit not fully equivalent consequences.

Whereas loss of RB1 function directly impinges on cell proliferation and differentiation, loss of tumor suppressor genes such as TP53 promotes tumor formation in a different fashion. Inactivation of TP53 compromises the ability of a cell to react to genomic damage, e.g. by ionizing radiation, as well as to hyperproliferation induced by oncogenes, or to viral infection. Therefore, loss of TP53 function permits survival and proliferation of cells accumulating mutations and thereby the emergence of a cancer. Several other tumor suppressors, e.g. BRCA1 and BRCA2, which are defective in familial breast cancers, also act primarily by protecting against genomic instability. Such '*caretakers*' can be considered as a different class of tumor suppressors from '*gatekeepers*' like RB1.

TP53, as a central regulator gene of genomic stability, may be the most frequently altered gene in human cancers. Several upstream pathways responding to different kinds of genomic instability lead to activation of TP53, mainly by post-translational regulation. In turn, TP53 acts on several downstream pathways as a transcriptional activator or repressor, and may even directly participate in DNA repair. Activated TP53 can arrest the cell cycle via induction of cell cycle inhibitors such as p21^{CIP1}, or elicit apoptosis by induction of proteins like BAX. TP53 action is limited by its induction of MDM2/HDM2 which inhibits TP53 and initiates its proteolytic degradation.

In different human cancers, TP53 is inactivated by different mechanisms. Most widely, one gene copy is inactivated by point mutations in the central DNA binding domain of the protein, whereas the other one is lost by deletion or recombination. In some tumors, HDM2 is overexpressed. The CDKN2A gene encodes not only p16^{INK4A}, but also an activator of p53, p14^{ARF1} in a different reading frame. Homozygous deletions, therefore, and certain point mutations in this gene impede the function of both TP53 and RB1.

DNA tumor viruses, e.g. the papovavirus SV40 and tumorigenic strains of human papilloma viruses, contain proteins inactivating both TP53 and RB1. This underlines the crucial role of these two proteins in the prevention of human cancer.

Tumor Suppressor Genes in Hereditary Cancers

Several recessively inherited syndromes caused by defects in DNA repair genes are associated with an increased cancer risk, often for leukemias and lymphomas. Other '*cancer syndromes*' are inherited in a dominant mode. Most of these predispose to a restricted range of cancers or even to a single tumor type, while a few are rather unselective, e.g., the rarer Li-Fraumeni and Cowden syndromes.

Typically, these syndromes show high penetrance and the life-time risk of cancer may approach 100%. As a further important characteristic, patients with familial cancers often develop cancers at a significantly lower age than in other '*sporadic*' cases. Thus, most sporadic colon or breast cancers present in patients in their sixties or seventies, but familial cases can appear already in the second or third decade of life. In addition, patients with inherited cancers may develop more than one cancer of the same type or cancers of different types. Multifocality or bilaterality is obvious in cancers of paired organs such as breast, kidney or the eyes. Patients with FAP or HPRCC can have literally thousands of individual tumors in their bowel or kidneys, respectively. A theoretical explanation for these properties of hereditary cancers was developed and later experimentally confirmed for hereditary retinoblastoma.

Retinoblastoma is a rare tumor which occurs in young children. It consists of undifferentiated or incompletely differentiated retinocyte precursors ('*retinoblasts*') forming an expanding cell mass in the back of the eye. The incidence in general is around 1:20000 live births, but in some families approximately every second child is affected on average, as expected for an autosomal dominantly inherited disease with high penetrance. Bilateral cases are extremely rare outside retinoblastoma families. Even though all patients suffering from this disease are young, on average the cancers manifest at lower age in familial cases. Retinoblastoma was recognized as such and could be treated by surgery already in the 19th century. Attentive surgeons of the time noted that patients cured of retinoblastoma tended to develop other cancers later in life, notably of the bone (*osteosarcoma*), and that their children also tended to develop the disease. Based on the assembled statistical data, in the early 1970's, a model was developed by Knudson that accounted for these observations.

The Knudson model assumes that development of retinoblastoma requires two mutations ('*hits*') within one cell to form the initial tumor cell clone. In hereditary cases, one of these hits has already occurred and is passed along in the affected families. The development of a retinoblastoma then depends on a single mutation to take place in any cell during the critical period when retinoblasts proliferate during fetal development. The probability of a mutation in a specific human gene is in the order of 10^{-6} - 10^{-7} per cell generation. So it is not unlikely for one or several mutations to occur leading to one or more retinoblastomas. If no mutation is inherited, two mutations in two cells within the same line are required. The probability for this double accident is very low and it is even more unlikely that it occurs more than once within the same person. So, in familial cases tumors are much more likely to occur at all, tend to develop more rapidly (because their expansion begins already after one hit), and they can be bilateral, whereas in children without an inherited defective allele tumors form much less frequently, on average later, and almost never in more than one place.

This theoretical model so far does not make assumptions about which genes are affected by hit 1 and hit 2. They could be two alleles of the same gene or one allele each of different genes. However, the model required that the genes behave recessively at the cellular level. Since oncogenes act in a dominant fashion, the model indicated a different sort of tumor gene undergoing inactivation in cancers. Indeed, some retinoblastomas occur in patients lacking parts of chromosome 13, with a common region of deletion within band 13q14.1. Deletions of this region were also seen in sporadic cases. Therefore, at least one of the hits in retinoblastoma formation involved loss of a gene and its function. In fact, in almost all cases of retinoblastoma the second hit also concerns the same gene and inactivates the function of its second allele. Tumor formation therefore requires inactivation of the function of this gene, which is designated a tumor suppressor gene.

The gene that is defective in the overwhelming majority of retinoblastomas is designated *RB1*. It encompasses ≈180 kb of genomic sequence, in which 27 exons code for a 4.7 kb mRNA and a 110 kDa phosphoprotein. Mutations of this gene are observed in familial as well as in sporadic retinoblastoma and osteosarcoma, but also in sporadic cases of several other cancers such as glioma, breast and bladder cancer. In familial cases of retinoblastoma, mutations in *RB1* are passed on in the germ-line. Mutations in different families comprise deletions of various sizes, ranging from cytogenetically detectable (i.e. several Mbp) to single bases, small insertions, nonsense and splice mutations and specific missense mutations which usually alter amino acids in the central portion of the protein, the '*pocket*' domain.

The second allele can be inactivated independently by deletions, insertion, or various kinds of point mutation. In a few cases, an entire chromosome 13 is lost, e.g. by mitotic nondisjunction, more frequently, large deletions obliterate sequences including 13q14.1. In some cases (only in childhood cancers), the otherwise intact second allele is not transcribed as a consequence of hypermethylation of the *RB1* promoter.

Another important mechanism involves the replacement of the intact allele by a defective copy. This can again occur by several means. In some cases, the cell contains two identical chromosomes 13, either by duplication of one remaining after loss of the other or by misdistribution of chromosomes during mitosis. In other cases, recombination between the two different chromosomes leads to replacement of larger or smaller regions of one chromosome by sequences from the other and specifically to conversion of the intact RB1 to a defective copy.

Several of the above mechanisms, specifically larger deletions and unequal recombinations or recombination followed by chromosomal loss, leave the cell not only without a functional allele of the *RB1* tumor suppressor gene, but also abolish other differences between the two chromosomal copies. So, polymorphisms in single nucleotides (SNPs) or in microsatellite sequences disappear, as heterozygous sequences become homozygous. This process is called *loss of heterozygosity* (LOH). So, LOH marks regions in a tumor genome where deletions or illegitimate recombination have taken place. Since such processes are often involved in the inactivation of tumor suppressor genes, the observation of consistent LOH in one region in a particular tumor type can be used as an indication of the presence of a tumor suppressor gene.

Many further tumor suppressors also fit the Knudson model well. Among them are *APC* in colon carcinoma, *VHL* in renal cell carcinoma, and *CDH1* in gastric carcinoma. Others follow the model at least partly. So, *BRCA1* and *BRCA2* behave according to the model in hereditary breast and ovarian cancer, but are rarely involved in sporadic cases. The converse case is more common, i.e. several tumor suppressor genes are never mutated in the germ-line, but both copies are inactivated in cancers. In other words, not all common human cancers also occur in an inherited form. It is also conceivable that mutation of one copy of a tumor suppressor gene could be sufficient to initiate the development of a cancer, albeit not as efficiently as the inactivation of both alleles. This situation is called '*haploinsufficiency*'. It is discussed for several tumor suppressors, including *PTCH* in basal cell carcinomas of the skin, *PTEN* in a variety of cancers, and *HPC1* in prostate cancer. In the case of inherited mutation in *PTCH* and *PTEN*, the case for haploinsuffiency is supported by the fact that the patients tend to have developmental abnormalities unrelated to cancer.

An entirely different situation is provided by germ-line mutations that activate oncogenes and thereby result in dominantly inherited cancers. This situation has been experimentally achieved with very high efficiency in transgenic mice, e.g. by introduction of a mutated *Ras* gene. In humans, very few inherited cancers are caused by activated oncogenes. Multiple endocrine neoplasia type 2 is caused by mutations in the *RET* proto-oncogene predisposing to cancer of several endocrine glands, notably the thyroid and adrenal glands. RET is a tyrosine receptor kinase and the inherited mutations lead to its constitutive activation. Comparable mutations in the *MET* gene, which also encodes a receptor tyrosine kinase, cause one type of papillary renal cell carcinoma. The reason why tumor suppressor gene mutations prevail in inherited human cancer is not really understood. It may partly reflect a better protection of human cells against oncogenic transformation compared to rodent cells or a pronounced sensitivity of human development to disturbances by mutated oncogenes.

RB1 and the Cell Cycle

The product of the *RB1* gene, $pp110^{RB1}$, is most of all a central regulator of the cell cycle. The RB1 protein controls the transition from the G1 to the S phase by binding to E2F1, E2F2, or E2F3 proteins and thereby repressing the promoters of genes needed for the entrance into S phase. This repression is relieved and binding to E2F alleviated when $pp110^{RB1}$ becomes hyperphosphorylated towards the end of G1. At least two successive phosphorylations are needed to inactivate RB1. Normally, the first phosphorylation is performed by a CDK4/Cyclin D holoenzyme, and is followed by further phosphorylations by the CDK2/Cyclin E holoenzyme.

Hyperphosphorylated RB1 is inactive as far as G1/S cell cycle regulation is concerned. The protein likely has also functions in the S phase, where it may be involved in chromatin organization, and during mitosis, where it may help to organize proteins for chromosome segregation. Following mitosis, RB1 is partly dephosphorylated and its hypophosphorylated state restored. In this fashion, RB1 switches between hypophosphorylated and hyper-phosphorylated states during the cell cycle.

Clearly, therefore, loss of RB1 function, at a minimum, upsets cell cycle regulation and may lead to unrestrained cell proliferation. Specifically, in the absence of RB1 immature cells such as retinoblasts may not spend sufficient time in G1 to enter a differentiated state or establish stable quiescence, i.e. G0. Worse, since RB1 may also be required for proper chromatin structure and chromosome segregation, cells may tend to become genomically instable and acquire additional alterations that favor tumor progression. At least one mechanism may protect against loss of RB1 function: Over-activity of E2F factors, particularly of E2F1, can induce apoptosis.

The mechanism of cell cycle regulation sketched so far is in fact much more complex and consists of several layers of control, even when only the G1 to S transition is considered. The activity of the CDK4 and CDK2 protein kinases depends strictly on the presence of their regulatory subunits, i.e., D-Cyclins and Cyclin E, respectively. Both fluctuate in a coordinate fashion in the course of the cell cycle. Cyclin D expression is directly dependent on stimulation by exogenous signals such as growth factors. Moreover, CDKs are only active, if they are phosphorylated in a certain pattern. Phosphorylation at one specific threonine residue by the CDK activating kinase (CAK, identical to CDK7) in conjunction with its regulatory subunit Cyclin H is activating, while phosphorylation at two different threonines is inhibitory. The phosphates at these sites are removed by CDC25 phosphatases, which also respond to external signals.

A further layer of control is provided by protein inhibitors of CDKs. There are two classes of such inhibitors, the CIP/KIP and the INK proteins. The first comprises the $p21^{CIP1}$, $p27^{KIP1}$, and $p57^{KIP2}$ proteins, the second $p15^{INK4B}$, $p16^{INK4A}$, $p18^{INK4C}$, and $p19^{INK4D}$. Their genes are now systematically designated *CDKN1A - CDKN1C* and *CDKN2A - CDKN2D*. All proteins are named according to their molecular weights. The function of the INK4 (inhibitor of kinase 4) proteins is straightforward. They compete with D-Cyclins for binding to CDK4 and block its kinase activity.

The function of the CIP/KIP proteins (CDK/kinase inhibitory proteins) is more complicated. At high concentrations, they inhibit the activity of CDKs in general, but different from INK4s they block the CDK-Cyclin holoenzymes. At moderate concentrations, they rather stimulate the assembly of CDK-Cyclin complexes. In proliferating cells, CIP/KIP proteins, in particular $p27^{KIP1}$, help to coordinate the cell cycle. Until late G1, $p27^{KIP1}$ is bound to the CDK2/Cyclin E complex delaying its activity until late G1 when CDK2 activity is required to inactivate RB1. At this point, the $p27^{KIP1}$ inhibitor is phosphorylated and rapidly degraded. On the other hand, in cells that are not supposed to proliferate, high levels of inhibitor proteins arrest the cell cycle.

The different CDK inhibitors respond to different signals that lead to cell arrest, allowing fine-tuned cellular responses to different signals. For instance, in some cell types $p15^{INK4B}$ is induced by inhibitory growth factors like TGFβ. High levels of the inhibitor protein dissociate Cyclin D/CDK4 complexes and block CDK4. They also redirect any $p21^{CIP1}$ or $p27^{KIP1}$ present towards CDK2/Cyclin E, blocking this kinase as well. By comparison, $p16^{INK4A}$ has a very slow turnover and accumulates gradually in continuously proliferating cells until its concentration becomes high enough to slow down the cell cycle or arrest it irreversibly. $p21^{CIP1}$ accumulates in a similar fashion during frequent replication, but also in response to various growth factors and to DNA damage. $p57^{KIP2}$ is expressed in a restricted range of cell types, most prominently during embryonic development where the protein appears to help establish a terminally differentiated state in specific tissues. The gene encoding $p57^{KIP2}$, *CDKN1C*, is as a rule only expressed from the maternally inherited allele, i.e. it is imprinted.

In summary, therefore, RB1 forms a node in the cell cycle regulation network which ensures that cell proliferation occurs only in response to proper sets of signals, e.g. following stimulation by growth factors via the MAPK and further signaling pathways. It is easy to imagine how this regulation network becomes disrupted by loss of function of the central RB1 protein. Alternatively to loss of RB1 function itself, other components of the regulatory network may be affected in human cancers. So, overexpression of D-Cyclins or CDK4 as a consequence of gene amplification, or mutations of CDK4 that make it unresponsive to CDK inhibitors may exert similar effects.

In addition, alterations in CDK inhibitors are found in a variety of human cancers. In a wide range of human cancers, the *CDKN2A* gene is inactivated by point mutation, promoter hypermethylation, or homozygous deletion. In fact, *CDKN2A* must also be regarded as a '*classical*' tumor suppressor gene, since both alleles are affected in such cancers, and germ-line mutations of the gene have been found in families prone to pancreatic cancer and melanoma. Of note, not all these changes may be equivalent. There is some evidence that loss of RB1 function may be the most severe defect, as one might guess intuitively.

Surprisingly, mutations or deletions of the genes encoding CDK inhibitors other than $p16^{INK4A}$ are by far not as frequent in human cancers. The *CDKN2B* gene encoding $p15^{INK4B}$ is located within 40 kb of *CDKN2A* and is often deleted together with its neighbor. However, inactivation of the gene may only be crucial in certain leukemias. Inactivation of *CDKN1C*, in accord with its more circumscribed expression, may be relevant in a tighter range of cancers. Mutations in the genes encoding $p21^{CIP1}$ and $p27^{KIP1}$ seem very rare in human cancers, but down-regulation of their expression is highly prevalent in many different cancers. It is often a good indication of tumor progression and a marker for cancers taking a more aggressive clinical course. It is neither well understood, why these genes are so rarely mutated nor which mechanisms exactly lead to down-regulation of their expression during tumor progression. In some cases, loss of $p27^{KIP1}$ may be caused by over-expression of proteins involved in its degradation at the end of G1.

TP53 as a Different Kind of Tumor Suppressor

RB1 is a tumor suppressor gene mainly because its inactivation removes an essential point of regulation of the cell cycle. Thus, its loss takes a tumor cell directly towards unrestricted proliferation and diminished dependence on extracellular signals. Of note, while RB1 inactivation favors tumor development, its actual function is not so much to suppress tumors, but to allow coordinated proliferation and differentiation during the development and maintenance of normal tissues. Accordingly, mice lacking *Rb1* are not viable and exhibit defects in the development of several tissues.

In contrast, animals can in principle live without another tumor suppressor, Tp53. However, mice lacking Tp53 succumb to tumors after a few months of life. In a rare human disease, Li-Fraumeni-syndrome, one mutant copy of the *TP53* gene is inherited. The patients develop various types of tumors in different tissues, including blood, lymphoid organs, soft tissues, the nervous system and epithelia, often early in life. In accord with the Knudson model, the tumors contain mutations inactivating the second *TP53* allele or exhibit LOH at chromosome 17p where the gene resides. The *TP53* gene is also inactivated in many different types of sporadic cancers in man. It is arguably the most frequently mutated gene in human cancer. Indeed, the main function of the TP53 protein appears the prevention of damage to the genome and of cancer, making it literally a '*tumor suppressor*'.

The approximately 20 kb *TP53* gene on chromosome 17p13.1 encodes in eleven exons a 2.2 kb mRNA, from which, as the name indicates, a 53 kDa phosphoprotein is translated. The TP53 (or simply p53) protein has a structure typical for transcriptional activators. It is composed of a central DNA binding domain, an N-terminal transactivation domain, and a C-terminal domain which contains sequences necessary for oligomerization and regulation of DNA-binding.

Indeed, TP53 can function as a transcriptional activator at several hundred genes. In many of these genes, TP53 binds as a tetramer to a symmetric specific binding sequence in the promoter region or an (often intronic) enhancer. In other genes, TP53 acts as a repressor of transcription by PolII and PolIII by binding and blocking the basal transcription factor TBP or by interacting with transcriptional repressors, e.g. SIN3A. Moreover, TP53 has several other functions that are less well characterized, such as the ability to bind to damaged DNA directly, to function as an exonuclease, to anneal nucleic acids to each other, and perhaps even to regulate protein biosynthesis at the ribosome.

Through these various functions TP53 coordinates the cellular response towards many kinds of damage to the genome, in particular, DNA double-strand breaks induced by chemical mutagens and ionizing radiation, as well as to certain kinds of cellular stress, such as guanine nucleotide imbalance, viral infection, and oncogeneinduced hyperproliferation. TP53 is also involved in the regulation of replicative senescence.

TP53 action is mostly regulated posttranslationally by phosphorylation and other modifications which alter the stability and activity of the protein. Under normal circumstances, TP53 undergoes rapid turnover in the cell, with a half-life in the 10-20 min range. For this short half-life, the MDM2/HDM2 protein is mostly responsible. It binds to the N-terminal domain of TP53 blocking its transcriptional activity and initiating its transport out of the nucleus. Furthermore, MDM2/HDM2 acts as a specific E3 ubiquitin ligase for TP53, which following oligo-ubiquitination is rapidly degraded by the proteasome.

Different pathways signal various types of damage and stress to TP53 leading to a variety of post-translational modifications. Double-strand breaks induced by ionizing radiation activate ATM and/or DNA-dependent protein kinase and extensive UV damage activates ATR which phosphorylate TP53 at Ser15 and Ser37. The checkpoint protein kinases CHK1 and CHK2, which respond to DNA damage and specifically to mitotic disturbances phosphorylate Ser20. Phosphorylation at Ser15 and Ser 20 in particular block the interaction of TP53 with MDM2/HDM2 and increase the half-life of the protein. Moreover, most phosphorylations in the N-terminal transactivation domain enhance the strength of TP53 as a transcriptional activator. In the C-terminal regulatory domain, sumolation at Lys386 helps to guide TP53 within the nucleus. Acetylation at Lys320, Lys373, and Lys382 may modulate DNA-binding, transcriptional activation, and nuclear localization. Phosphorylation at Ser392 by the double-strand RNA-dependent protein kinase PKR may activate TP53 in response to viral infections. Conversely, other phosphorylations may restrain TP53. For instance, TP53 is phosphorylated at several serines (371, 376, and 378) by PKC and at Ser315 by CDK2. Phosphorylations by p38MAPK and JNK at Ser46 and Thr81 appear to modulate the pro-apoptotic function of TP53.

Inappropriate cell proliferation, e.g. induced by oncogenic RAS, also activates TP53, mainly by an indirect mechanism. Increased proliferation is associated with increased activity of E2F factors such as E2F1. In addition to genes required for cell cycle progression, E2F1 activates the transcription of $p16^{INK4A}$ mRNA from the *CDKN2A* gene, but also a second promoter in the gene, leading to expression of a 14 kDa protein in an alternative reading frame. This protein is f therefore designated $p14^{ARF}$ ($p19^{ARF}$ in mice). It is an inhibitor of MDM2/HDM2. Therefore, '*inappropriate*' proliferation signals induce $p14^{ARF}$ which blocks MDM2/HDM2 leading to stabilization and activation of TP53. The *CDKN2A* gene is thus, in fact, a double locus with two common exons, of which exon 2 codes for both p16^{INK4A} and p14^{ARF1} in different reading frames. So, many mutations in this exon inactivate both proteins, as do homozygous deletions of *CDKN2A*. Therefore, alterations in this locus normally compromise the functions of both TP53 and RB1 indirectly.

Following its activation by one of the above pathways, TP53 induces multiple cellular responses, i.e. cell cycle arrest, DNA repair, altered secretion of growth factors (particularly of angiogenic factors), apoptosis, and, finally, its own inactivation by MDM2/HDM2. Which responses are induced in particular, appears to depend on several factors, such as the cell type, the extent of DNA damage or cellular stress, the basal and induced pattern of phosphorylation of TP53 by multiple kinases, and on competing signals. Cell cycle arrest and apoptosis occur alternatively to each other, and the fate of a cell may sometimes simply depend on which response is induced faster. Overall, several hundred genes can be activated or repressed by TP53. Therefore, the proteins act '*downstream*' of TP53 are a selection of the more established and more general mediators of TP53 action in human cells.

Arrest of the cell cycle by TP53 is mediated through rapid and strong induction of two inhibitory proteins: p21^{CIP1} and 14-3-3σ, which block the cell cycle in G1 or G2. This response appears to be common to all cell types and to follow the activation of TP53 by a variety of signals. Another common response to TP53 activation is induction of GADD45, a protein involved in DNA repair.

Induction of apoptosis by TP53 appears to proceed through different factors in different cells. Most widespread may be induction of BAX, an antagonistic homolog of BCL2, and an effector of apoptosis at mitochondria. Conversely, *BCL2* is one of the genes repressed by TP53. Several further proteins in the '*mitochondrial*' or '*intrinsic*' apoptotic pathway can be induced by activated TP53, such as p53AIP, NOXA, PUMA, and APAF1. In addition or in parallel, TP53 increases the sensitivity towards exogenous apoptotic signals, e.g. by increasing expression of the '*death receptor*' FAS. One could interprete this variety of pro-apoptotic signals as a series of back-up mechanisms evolved to ensure that apoptosis cannot be circumvented. Alternatively, this variety may allow a better choice between apoptosis and survival (with cell cycle arrest) depending on further intracellular and exogenous signals and on the cell type.

A further group of genes induced or repressed by TP53 functions in the communication with neighboring tissue, particularly with endothelial cells. For instance, TP53 induces thrombospondin (TSP1) which inhibits the proliferation of endothelial cells and thereby blocks angiogenesis.

Finally, TP53 induces a feedback mechanism to limit its own action. The *MDM2/HDM2* gene is a direct transcriptional target of TP53 and becomes relatively rapidly induced following TP53 activation. Accumulating MDM2/HDM2 blocks transcriptional activation by TP53 and causes its degradation. The efficacy of this mechanism is most dramatically illustrated by an experiment in mice. Mice lacking Tp53 are usually viable, although they die of tumors at an early age. In contrast, mice lacking Mdm2 die in utero from widespread apoptosis. Knockout of the Tp53 gene as well largely corrects this defect.

In summary, TP53 can be considered as a central node in an important network which regulates the cellular response to most kinds of genomic damage and many types of cellular stress. This explains why defects in TP53 are so widespread in human cancers. Cancers lacking functional TP53 will tolerate more DNA damage, including DNA strand breaks and aneuploidy, will condone inappropriate proliferation signals and nucleotide stress, and will less easily enter replicative senescence. Compared to cancers of the same type with wild-type TP53, cancers with mutant TP53 therefore tend to accumulate more genomic alterations and to run a higher risk of progression. The inactivation of TP53 function is brought about by several distinct mechanisms in different human cancers.

Missense Mutations Plus LOH

The most common mechanism in many different kinds of human tumors consists of missense mutations in one allele and loss of the second functional allele by deletion or recombination, which is detectable as LOH on 17p. It is likely favorable for the two changes to occur in this order, since some missense mutation in the first allele may already impede the function of TP53, with LOH completing its inactivation. In experimental models, certain mutant TP53 clearly compromise the function of unaltered ('*wild-type*') protein. They act as dominant negatives, probably by sequestering wild-type protein monomers in inactive (*tetrameric*) complexes. It is less clear, how important this effect actually is during the development of human cancers. Conceivably, the initial missense mutation might increase the probability of the loss of the second allele by compromising the ability of the cell to react to genomic damage such as illegitimate recombinations or deletions of chromosome 17p.

Most missense mutations in TP53 affect the central domain of the protein necessary for specific binding to DNA. This domain consists of a large structure made up from β-sheets stabilized by zinc ions which supports the α-helix that contacts DNA through arginine and further residues. These arginines are mutational hot-spots, but many other amino acids in the central domain can also be mutated. The exact site of the mutation also appears to depend on the carcinogen involved. Mutations in the N-terminal and C-terminal domains are found with lower frequencies and may compromise the activation and oligomerization of TP53.

Nonsense and Splice Mutations

Nonsense and splice mutations in TP53 do occur, but are less frequent. Apparently, missense mutations provide some sort of advantage, either by acting as dominant-negatives as described above, or by retaining some functions of TP53 which are advantageous to tumor cells. This issue is still under investigation.

MDM2 Overexpression

Some tumors harbor amplifications of the *HDM2/MDM2* gene. In others this gene is overexpressed by unknown mechanisms. Such overexpression likely diminishes the function of TP53. Indeed, in some cancers like sarcomas and gliomas amplifications of *HDM2* and mutations of *TP53* occur in a mutually exclusive fashion. This is a very good indication that they are indeed complementary. It should be mentioned, though, that HDM2 has functions beyond the regulation of TP53 which could be important in specific cancers (e.g. sarcomas).

Table 6.1. Mechanisms of TP53 inactivation in human cancers

Mechanism of inactivation
Missense mutations
Nonsense and splice mutations
Deletion of one allele
Overexpression of HDM2 by gene amplification or deregulation
Loss of $p14^{ARF}$ function by gene deletion, mutation or promoter hypermethylation
Loss of function of upstream activators, e.g. ATM or CHK1
Loss of function of downstream effectors, e.g. BAX
Inactivation by altered post-translational modification
Inactivation by viral oncoproteins, e.g. HPV E6

Conversely, in cancers with mutated TP53, HDM2 cannot be induced by TP53. If the mutation does not otherwise destabilize the TP53 protein, this will lead to an accumulation of the mutated protein, since HDM2 is the rate-limiting enzyme for its degradation. This is one reason, why in many cancers TP53 protein levels paradoxically are higher than in the corresponding normal tissues. Thus, in some cases, detection of increased TP53 protein levels (i.e. accumulated mutant protein) can be used for the detection of tumor cells.

Upstream Activator Inactivation

The function of TP53 is expected to be impeded by mutations in upstream pathways that provide signals for its activation. This is likely the case in ataxia telengiectasia. In this disease, activation of TP53 in response to ionizing radiation is diminished as a consequence of defects in the ATM kinase. More generally in human cancers, the loss of $p14^{ARF}$ may be important. The *CDKN2A* gene is inactivated in many different types of human cancers by deletions or point mutations, in specific cancers also by hypermethylation of its promoters. The loss of $p14^{ARF}$ would be predicted to specifically disrupt the activation of TP53 in response to inappropriate cell proliferation, e.g. as induced by oncogene activation. Of note, loss of $p14^{ARF}$ also occurs in cancers with TP53 inactivation by other mechanisms, but then, $p16^{INK4A}$ is a mutation target in the same gene. Intriguingly, loss of $p16^{INK4A}$ and RB1 appear to occur in a mutually exclusive fashion.

Cell-type Specific Down-regulation

There are a few cancers in which mutations of TP53 are extremely rare. In testicular germ cell tumors, e.g. seminomas, mutations may be very rare, because the gene is normally not very active at the stage of development from which the tumor cells arise. However, TP53 can be activated by strong signals and the presence of an intact gene is one factor responsible for the high efficacy of radiotherapy and chemotherapy in these cancers.

Inactivation by Viral Proteins

Still another mechanism is found regularly in cervical cancers and occasionally in some other cancer types. These cancers are caused by specific oncogenic strains of *human papilloma virus* (HPV). These express a protein, E6, which binds to TP53 and promotes its degradation, quite similar as HDM2. This mechanism inhibits the cellular response to the infection and active replication of the virus. If E6 expression is sustained, e.g. by activation of the viral gene through cellular enhancers, it contributes to cell immortalization and favors the accumulation of genetic alterations promoting cancer by impeding the response to DNA damage and chromosomal defects.

Indeed, other DNA viruses have developed similar mechanisms to cope with TP53 during infection. Adenoviruses, which are tumorigenic in rodents, employ the E1B protein to sequester and inhibit TP53, although the protein is not degraded. In fact, TP53 was originally discovered as a protein regularly associated with the major transforming protein of the DNA tumor virus SV40, a papovavirus infecting primates including man. This virus encodes two tumor antigens, named large-T and small-T. Large-T antigen is a multifunctional protein that regulates SV40 transcription and replication. It also binds and inactivates several host proteins, including TP53.

A second important protein sequestered and inactivated by SV40 large-T is RB1. Other DNA tumor viruses as well inactivate RB1, HPV by its E7 protein and adenoviruses by their E1A proteins. Nevertheless, adenoviruses are probably not transforming in man. However, SV40 and related papovaviruses such as BK and JC may play a role in specific human cancers. The best evidence is available for mesothelioma, where SV40 infection may synergize with exposure towards asbestos.

Classification of Tumor Suppressor Genes

The fact that DNA tumor viruses so specifically target TP53 and RB1 is another indication that these proteins are of central importance in normal cell growth as well as in cancer. They reside at nodes of networks which control cell proliferation and genomic integrity. These must be subverted or overcome for tumor growth to proceed. Many oncogenes can be arranged around one central signaling pathway (which could with some right too be called a *network*) and can be usefully classified by their biochemical function. Considered overall, tumor suppressors may exhibit a wider array of biochemical functions and act in a wider range of regulatory networks in addition to cell cycle regulation and DNA damage response.

In some of these networks, both tumor suppressors and oncogenes can be spotted and tend to be antagonists in the normal functioning of the pathway. For instance, PTEN is a negative regulator of the PI3K pathway, PTCH1 is a negative regulator of SMO in the Hedgehog pathway, APC promotes the inactivation of CTNNB1 in the WNT pathway, and NF1 mutated in familial neurofibromatosis is a tissue-specific GAP regulating RAS function. When tumor suppressors were first discovered, it was suggested to designate them as '*anti-oncogenes*'. Clearly, there is some justification for this name. However, it is misleading in so far as there is no pairwise complementarity between oncogenes and tumor suppressors. Moreover, activation of proto-oncogenes and inactivation of tumor suppressors from the same pathway typically have similar, but not identical consequences. In any case, the presence of alternatively occuring alterations in tumor suppressor genes and oncogenes suggests that it is the function of '*cancer pathways*' (or *networks*) that is crucial for cancer development, rather than that of individual genes.

Even a crude comparison between *TP53* and *RB1* suggests that there are at least two classes of tumor suppressors. Most importantly, loss of TP53 function does not directly lead to altered cell growth. Rather, it permits alterations in the cell to take place that are then directly responsible for altered growth at the cell and tissue level. One such alteration is loss of RB1 which causes altered growth and differentiation directly. Vogelstein and Kinzler have proposed to call these two kinds of tumor suppressors '*caretakers*' and '*gatekeepers*', respectively. The designation '*gatekeeper*' implies in addition that a cancer of a certain type can only arise, if the function of this particular tumor suppressor is abolished. This may indeed be true in some cases, e.g. in colorectal cancer, where the concept was developed.

Of course, further classes of tumor suppressor genes may exist. For instance, it has been proposed that some genes may be irrelevant for the growth of a primary tumor, but their loss of function would be essential for metastasis. These would then be considered '*metastasis suppressor genes*'. There is some evidence for such genes, but the concept is not as well developed as that of '*caretakers & gatekeepers*'.

So, finally, what is the precise definition of a tumor suppressor gene? The strictest definition, according to the Knudson model, would encompass all genes which lead to cancers inherited in a autosomal-dominant fashion, but behave in a recessive mode at the cellular level. Thus, one mutant, functionally inactive allele is inherited and the second one is inactivated in the ensuing tumors by point mutation, deletion, insertion, recombination, or promoter hypermethylation. Often, both alleles of these same genes are also functionally inactivated in sporadic cases of the same type. No conceptual problem arises from extending this definition to all genes that show inactivation of both alleles in many sporadic cases of a specific tumor type, if this occurs consistently or in a sizeable subgroup, and if the functional relevance for tumor development or progression can be shown.

The concept is more difficult to apply when inactivation of both alleles does not occur regularly or only one allele of a gene is consistently lost. The first case could be a random event and the second case could, e.g., be a consequence of proximity to a real tumor suppressor gene. However, haploinsufficiency is a real possibility in such cases. A gene exhibiting consistent loss of only one allele could represent a tumor suppressor, whose expression at half the normal dose is insufficient to inhibit tumor formation. Unfortunately, haploinsufficiency is very difficult to ascertain in the context of human cancers, as demonstrated by the case of NKX3.1 in prostate cancer or by the elusive tumor suppressor gene at chromosome 9q in bladder cancer. A particularly difficult case is raised by genes whose expression is consistently down-regulated in one type of cancer, but which do not show genetic alterations in structure or dosage, and not even a clear-cut epigenetic mark of stable silencing such as promoter hypermethylation. This is similar to the dilemma whether overexpressed genes are generally oncogenes. As in that case, defining the precise function of the gene and protein in question is an essential requirement for approaching this problem.

7

EPIGENETICS OF CANCER

In humans, cell differentiation does not involve changes in the base sequence or in the amount of DNA, with few exceptions. Rather, '*epigenetic*' mechanisms are employed to establish stable patterns of gene expression. In this case, '*epigenetic*' mechanisms are those which establish stably inherited patterns of gene expression in somatic cells without changes in the content or sequence of genomic DNA. Specific epigenetic mechanisms are involved in X-inactivation in female cells and for genomic imprinting, i.e. selective expression of alleles inherited from mother or father. Aberrant genomic imprinting is a cause of certain pediatric tumors, e.g. Wilms tumors. Loss of imprinting is observed in many carcinomas also of older people.

An important component of epigenetic mechanisms is DNA methylation at cytosine residues in the palindromic CpG dinucleotide sequence. In normal somatic human cells, CpG dinucleotides are mainly methylated in repetitive sequences, in the body of genes and in the regulatory regions of non-expressed genes. In contrast, relatively CpG-rich sequences overlapping the transcriptional start site of many human genes, called '*CpG-islands*', are usually devoid of methylation.

In many human tumors, some CpG-islands become aberrantly methylated. This '*hypermethylation*' as a rule is associated with silencing of the hypermethylated gene. In spite of such increases in methylation at specific sites, the overall methylcytosine content is decreased in many tumor cells, owing to partial demethylation of repetitive sequences and gene coding regions. This phenomenon is designated '*global hypomethylation*'. It may be related to chromosomal instability. Both changes are relatively straightforwardly detected and monitored, and can be used for tumor diagnostics. DNA methylation is one of several interacting mechanisms that down-regulate gene expression in an increasingly stable fashion.

The most dynamical of these mechanisms is deacetylation of histones in the nucleosomes of gene regulatory regions. Acetylation is enhanced by transcriptional activators binding to DNA and by co-activators with *histone acetylase* (HAT) activity. Conversely, deacetylation is catalyzed by histone deacetylases (HDACs) recruited by repressors or co-repressors. Methylation of histones at specific sites, prominently at the K9 of H3, by *histone methyltransferases* (HMTs) is a further step towards inactivation, while methylation at other sites, e.g. K4 of H3 stabilizes gene activation.

Modification at K9 attracts repressor proteins, e.g. HP1, but also DNA methyltransferases (DNMTs), which '*lock in*' gene silencing. DNA methylation directly inhibits the binding of some transcriptional activators and promotes the binding of repressory protein complexes which recognize methylcytosine via MBD proteins. DNMTs also interact with HDACs and HMTs, thereby reinforcing silencing. Gene activation as well as gene inactivation employ chromatin remodeling complexes which mutually interact with activators and repressors.

Aberrant gene silencing by epigenetic mechanisms in tumor cells is often, but not always accompanied by DNA hypermethylation. The underlying rules are not understood. A variety of HATs, HDACs, HMTs, and chromatin remodeling factors are implicated as oncogenes or tumor suppressors in human cancers.

Activated gene states are also propagated by epigenetic mechanisms, including specific chromatin modifications. While epigenetic mechanisms leading to inappropriate gene over-expression in human cancers are overall less well understood than those leading to gene silencing, it is clear that epigenetic mechanism contribute to the inappropriate expression of oncogenic proteins.

The concept of '*epigenetics*' can be extended to include phenomena beyond the nucleus and even beyond a single cell. It is likely that such mechanisms contribute to the establishment of stably inherited patterns of gene expression in normal tissues and in tumors. They could encompass autoregulatory loops in transcription factor networks or growth factor signal transducing pathways acting within one cell, but also stable interaction loops between different cell types, particularly mesenchymal and epithelial cells or stromal and carcinoma cells.

Mechanisms of Epigenetics Inheritance

It may seem trivial to say that cancers are caused by genetic alterations in their constituent cells, but it is not. Many properties of tumor cells are determined by their pattern of gene expression and do neither necessarily require structural alterations of gene products by mutations nor alterations in the structure of gene regulatory elements nor in gene dosage. Evidently, very different patterns of gene expression are established in normal cells of the human body and can in many cases be stably maintained during proliferation.

For instance, tissue stem cells retain their phenotype through several thousand divisions in a human life-time. Likewise, cell differentiation in humans is in general achieved without alterations in the sequence and amount of DNA. There are a few exceptions. Differentiation of B- and T-lymphocytes involves gene rearrangements with loss of small DNA segments from the immunoglobin and T-cell receptor genes, respectively. In some tissues, terminally differentiated cells are polyploid. So, theoretically, a tumor cell phenotype could be achieved by mechanisms similar to those that determine normal differentiated states. In general, mechanisms leading to a stably inherited phenotype without changes in the DNA sequence and content of a cell are designated as '*epigenetic*'. In reality, no malignant tumors in humans appear to be caused exclusively by epigenetic mechanisms. Instead, in most cancers, epigenetic alterations complement genetic alterations and in many, they appear to be essential.

The definition of what is considered as epigenetic has undergone fluctuations over the last decades. It is generally agreed that genomic imprinting and X-chromosome inactivation are prime examples. In both cases, identical DNA sequences are differentially expressed in a stably inherited fashion. One mechanism involved in fixing this differential expression is DNA methylation at cytosine residues, which is thus another exemplary epigenetic mechanism. DNA methylation is also instrumental in other instances of gene silencing and of facultative heterochromatin formation. Further mechanisms contribute, notably posttranslational modifications of histones, in particular methylation at specific lysine residues. In comparison, histone acetylation certainly regulates gene activity, but it is questionable whether this modification should be considered an epigenetic mechanism, because it is readily reversible, even without a cell division.

As DNA methylation and related epigenetic mechanisms are important for stably inherited gene silencing, other mechanisms must be responsible for stably inherited gene activation. Gene activation requires modification of chromatin in the regulatory regions of the gene and the assembly of a protein complex consisting of transcription factors binding to DNA at specific sites and co-activators. This complex interacts with basal transcription factors and RNA polymerases to initiate transcription, but also further modifies regional chromatin. It is clear that, but not entirely how active gene states are propagated through DNA replication and mitosis. Histone phosphorylation it thought to play a role. Another factor in this propagation is that cell differentiation is often achieved through transcription factor cascades which include an autoregulatory amplification step that make the process essentially irreversible. This could certainly be considered an epigenetic mechanism.

Table 7.1. Some examples of epigenetic processes in humans

Accepted	*Considered*
Genomic imprinting	Posttranscriptional histone modification, specifically histone acetylation
X-chromosome inactivation	Regulation by polycomb and trithorax proteins
Gene regulation by DNA methylation	Chromatin remodeling
Posttranscriptional histone modification, specifically histone methylation	Autoregulatory transcription factor networks
	Mutual paracrine cell-to-cell interaction networks
	Stem cell specification and maintenance

While the above mechanisms all occur essentially within the nucleus of a single cell, one could extend the concept of epigenetics to phenomena outside the nucleus and even to certain stable interactions between different cells. For instance, signals from one cell may elicit a response from another one which re-acts on the first and so on, until a stable steady-state is reached to which the system returns even after perturbations. Such signals are indeed exchanged in a homotypic or heterotypic fashion during normal tissue function and during tissue repair and adaptation. Intercellular loops are important in the regulation of tissue proliferation and differentiation and can be stably maintained throughout life. It does stretch the concept, but one could regard human embryonic development with some right as a sequence of epigenetic events. Disturbances of each of the above mechanisms contribute to human cancers.

Imprinting and X-inactivation

Most genes in humans are expressed equally strong from both alleles. About 50 genes, however, are genomically imprinted. They often occur in clusters, i.e. several imprinted genes are located within one chromosomal region. The expression of imprinted genes differs between the alleles inherited from the mother ('*maternal*') and father ('*paternal*'). Depending on the gene, expression differences between the maternal and paternal alleles may be found in every or in selected tissue, and they may be qualitative or quantitative. The most pronounced differences are found in fetal tissues and in the placenta. This observation underlies the '*battle of the sexes*' hypothesis.

According to this interpretation, genes preferentially expressed from the paternal allele promote growth of the fetus and the placenta, thereby straining the mother's resources. In contrast, genes expressed from the maternal allele tend to limit growth. This interpretation fits amazingly well with all observations. At the least, it is helpful to memorize which genes are preferentially expressed from which allele.

The best studied example of imprinted genes involves the mini-cluster consisting of *IGF2* and *H19* located near the tip of chromosome 11 at 11p15.5. They are imprinted in opposite ways. *IGF2* encodes a growth factor from the insulin family and is expressed from the paternally inherited allele. *H19* is located telomeric of *IGF2* and encodes a non-coding RNA which is expressed only from the maternal allele. It is not clear whether the H19 RNA has a function. Each gene has its own promoter, but both share the same enhancer which is located telomeric of the *H19* gene.

On the paternal allele, the enhancer interacts with the *IGF2* promoter; on the maternal allele it interacts with that of *H19*. The choice between them is imposed by a boundary element located in an intron of the *IGF2* gene. This is the '*imprinting center*' of the gene. This DNA sequence can bind the chromatin protein CTCF which prohibits the interaction between enhancer and promoter across the boundary. Binding of CTCF is sensitive to methylation of cytosines within its recognition sequence. Methylation of the boundary element on the maternal allele therefore directs the enhancer towards the *H19* promoter, diminishing expression of the *IGF2* gene. Conversely, the CTCF binding region is unmethylated on the paternal allele, allowing expression of *IGF2*.

This elegant regulatory system is disturbed in many human cancers. Most frequently, overexpression of the growth factor IGF2 is found, due to expression from every allele in the cancer cells. This corresponds to a *loss of imprinting* (sometimes abbreviated as 'LOI'). LOI can have several causes. In some pediatric cancers, notably in Wilms tumors and in germ cell cancers, imprinting may be lacking because it has never been properly set up during development.

In some cancers of adults, the maternal allele has been lost by deletion or recombination. Alternatively, imprinting may be disturbed by loss of DNA methylation at the boundary site or by altered expression of chromatin proteins involved in maintaining the boundary. In some cases, the regulation of the twin locus is so disturbed that both IGF2 and H19 become overexpressed. The issue is further complicated by differential use of promoters in the *IGF2* locus. In cancers, the P3 and P4 promoters are used preferentially, other than in normal tissues.

The *IGF2/H19* locus is certainly not the only imprinted locus deregulated in human cancers. Rather, it is best studied and due to the potency of IGF2 as a growth factor highly relevant. It is likely that LOI occurs at other imprinted loci, too, where the responsible mechanisms are at present incompletely understood.

A case in point is *CDKN1C*, which encodes the CDK inhibitor $p57^{KIP2}$. As would be expected, this growth inhibitor is expressed from the maternal allele, albeit in a tissue-specific fashion. The *CDKN1C* gene is also located on chromosome 11p15.5, centromeric of *IGF2/*H19, at a distance. Its imprinting is regulated by a different mechanism, although it again involves an '*imprinting center*', which is in this case located within an intron of the neighboring gene *KCNQ1*. Like the boundary element in the *IGF2/H19* locus, this imprinting center is differentially methylated on maternal and paternal alleles.

Intriguingly, it harbors a promoter from which another non-coding RNA is transcribed in opposite orientation to *KCNQ1*. Presently, it is not known how this leads to control of *CDKN1C* expression. However, disruption of the physical proximity between the imprinting center and *CDKN1C* by translocations leads to LOI. Such translocations are one cause of the human Beckwith-Wiedemann syndrome, which is characterized by fetal overgrowth and a propensity to childhood tumors such as nephroblastoma and hepatoblastoma. One variant of the syndrome is caused by mutations in *CDKN1C*. Moreover, $p57^{KIP2}$ is down-regulated in several carcinomas.

Mechanisms very similar to those responsible for genomic imprinting are employed in X-chromosome inactivation. As in other mammals, the second X-chromosome in human females is largely inactivated and heterochromatized, except for the small '*pseudo-autosomal*' region which is homologous to a stretch of the Y chromosome. In humans, the choice of the X-chromosome subject to inactivation is entirely random, even in extra-fetal tissues. Inactivation sets in during gastrulation due to increased expression of the non-coding (!) XIST RNA from the X-inactivation center on the chromosome destined for inactivation. This increase is initially achieved predominantly by posttranscriptional stabilization and leads to coating of the chromosome to become inactivated with XIST RNA. Chromatin is remodeled and histones are hypoacetylated and hypermethylated. Heterochromatin proteins such as HP1 bind and DNA methyltransferases methylate the promoter regions of genes, thereby fixing the inactive state. Conversely, the XIST gene becomes inactivated and methylated on the active X-chromosome of males and females. The activity states of the chromosomes are then faithfully maintained through many cell generations.

In cancer research, the present of X-inactivation has been used to investigate whether cancers are monoclonal or polyclonal based on the argument that if a cancer contains cells from only one clone, then the same X-chromosome should always be inactivated. If more than one clone was involved, expression from both should be found. Formerly, this approach used enzyme variants, e.g. the isozymes A and B of glucose-6-phosphate dehydrogenase. More recently, polymorphisms in the androgen receptor mRNA (the *AR* gene is located at Xq12) were used. In most cases, tumors were found to be monoclonal. This conclusion is a bit problematic. X-inactivation is established during gastrulation and mostly finished, when organogenesis sets in. Thus, e.g, of ≈8 cells in the foregut committed to form the liver, four each (on average) will have one or the other X-chromosome inactivated. The probability to find a liver cancer with inactivation of the same X throughout is rather high because of this fact alone. The test is also limited to cancers in females. Modern methods that follow the pattern of chromosomal alterations by microsatellite analysis yield a more reliable and more detailed picture of clonal development in human cancers.

An interesting and somewhat neglected issue is what happens to supernumerary chromosomes in aneuploid cancer cells. During development, supernumerary X-chromosomes are also inactivated. However, in some cancers they may remain active and contribute to the tumor phenotype. Conversely, germ cell cancers in males can be detected by the presence of transcriptionally active, unmethylated XIST sequences.

DNA Methylation

DNA methylation is instrumental for both imprinting and X-chromosome inactivation. In mammals, physiological methylation of DNA is restricted to the 5-position of cytosine residues, and again only to those in CpG dinucleotides. Since CG is a palindromic sequence, a CpG site can be non-methylated, hemi-methylated, i.e. in one strand only, or fully methylated, i.e. symmetrically in both strands. Except during replication, the usual state of methylated sites in human DNA is symmetrical methylation. After replication, which creates a hemimethylated site, symmetrical methylation is re-established by a maintenance DNA methyltransferase. If no re-methylation occurs, the site remains hemi-methylated and can become unmethylated in one daughter strand during the next round of replication. So, normally, removal of DNA methylation requires at least two cell cycles.

Methylation levels vary somewhat among normal tissues, with more pronounced changes during germ cell and embryonic development. In typical somatic cells, 3.5-4% of all cytosines are methylated. This is an average value, since DNA methylation is unequally distributed across the genome. Most methylcytosines are contained in repetitive sequences such as LINE and SINE retrotransposons interspersed in the genome and in CpG-rich satellites concentrated in peri- and juxta-centromeric regions. Genes and intergenic regions, too, are mostly methylated.

In contrast, regulatory regions of active genes are generally undermethylated. Specifically, in <50% of all human genes, 0.5 - 2 kb stretches around the transcriptional start site, including the basal promoter, are richer in CpG-dinucleotides than the rest of the genome, with a frequency of >0.6 found/expected in a random sequence and a higher GC content than the rest of the genome. These sequences are called '*CpG-islands*'. As a rule, they remain unmethylated throughout development and in all tissues. A prominent exception are the CpG-islands on the inactive X-chromosome which are methylated and the respective genes are silenced.

Apparently, the lack of methylation helps to mark CpG-islands as regions of potential transcription in the genome. Typically, genes with

CpG-island type promoters can be transcribed in several different cell types. DNA methylation also regulates the transcription of some other genes without CpG-islands, including some with cell-type specific expression.

CpG-islands stand out from the rest of the genome, because they contain more CpG-dinucleotides. More precisely, the rest of the genome contains less, as a consequence of cytosine loss during evolution. Hydrolytic deamination of cytosine occurs frequently, spontaneously or induced by chemicals, and yields uracil. This base is very efficiently recognized as incongruous and accordingly repaired. In contrast, methylcytosine yields methyluracil, i.e. thymine, albeit in a G-T mismatch. Such mismatches are accordingly repaired preferentially towards G-C, with the help of the protein MBD4 which recognizes the methylcytosine in the opposite strand of the CpG palindrome.

In spite of such precautionary mechanisms, over evolutionary periods, CpGs have become depleted from heavily methylated sequences by mutating to TpG (or CpA). This depletion has not affected sequences exempt from methylation and in this fashion has sculpted CpG-islands out of the genome background. In fact, the mutation rate at methylated cytosines remains higher in the present. Therefore, methylated CpGs are preferential sites of mutations not only in the human germ-line, but also in cancers.

DNA methylation patterns change substantially during development. During germ cell development, DNA is first widely demethylated and then remethylated to yield distinctive patterns in oocytes and sperm. Differential methylation at imprinted genes is also established during this period. Following fertilization, methylation again decreases across the genome, although some specific sites, e.g. in imprinted genes, are exempt from these changes. Extraembryonal tissues remain strongly demethylated, whereas in the cells of the fetus proper the genome is subjected to a wave of de-novo-methylation during gastrulation. This process largely establishes the overall level of methylation found in the DNA of somatic cells. Demethylation of genes expressed in a cell-type specific fashion then leads to the DNA methylation patterns of the various cell types. Of note, CpG-islands are in general exempt from these changes and remain unmethylated throughout development. Likewise, methylation patterns of imprinted genes follow their own rules.

These wide swings in overall methylation levels likely reflect the necessity to completely reprogram the expression of the genome, once during the development of germ cells and then again during embryonic development. A major reason why cloned embryos are often defective appears to be a failure to achieve this reprogramming properly. Very low levels of DNA methylation in germ cells may moreover signify a state of chromatin that facilitates recombination during meiosis.

Given this background, it is not unexpected that the altered state of cancer cells is often also accompanied by alterations in DNA methylation. Basically, two types of alterations can be distinguished. Both can occur in the same cell. In many cancers, overall DNA methylation levels are diminished by up to 70% compared to the corresponding normal cell type. This decrease affects mostly methylcytosine contained in repetitive sequences and is therefore termed '*global*' or '*genome-wide*' '*hypomethylation*'. In contrast, specific sites can become '*hypermethylated*'. Hypermethylation occurs, in particular, at CpG-islands which are never methylated otherwise. Like the extent of hypomethylation, that of hypermethylation differs widely between cancers, even of the same histological type. In some cancers, only individual CpG-islands become hypermethylated, whereas several hundreds are afflicted in others. Moreover, hypermethylation affects different genes in different cancers, although some genes are prone to hypermethylation in many cancer types. Alterations of DNA methylation may also affect the expression of imprinted genes.

Hypermethylation of CpG-islands is almost invariably associated with stable silencing of the affected genes. Therefore, hypermethylation is a very efficient means of gene inactivation in cancers. It is now regarded as a mechanism of tumor suppressor gene inactivation comparable to mutation and deletion. For instance, the *CDKN2A* locusis inactivated in a wide variety of human cancers. In almost every cancer type, mutation, deletion, and promoter hypermethylation are all observed as mechanisms of inactivation, although their relative contributions vary. One important difference towards mutation and deletion, however, is that hypermethylation is in principle reversible by inhibitors of DNA methylation. Of course, in cancers with hundreds of genes inactivated by hypermethylation, not each one of them is a tumor suppressor like *CDKN2A*. Rather, gene silencing via DNA methylation may reflect a '*slimming*' of gene expression.

By comparison, global hypomethylation would be expected to increase gene expression across the genome at large. There is, indeed, some evidence for hypomethylation to increase the level of '*transcriptional noise*' and to cause inappropriate expression of certain sequences, e.g. of retrotransposon sequences and of '*cancer testis antigens*', i.e. genes that are normally restricted to developing male germ cells. More importantly, perhaps, global hypomethylation is associated with enhanced chromosomal instability. The underlying mechanism are under investigation. Possibly, decreased methylation in pericentromeric repeats and interspersed repetitive sequences facilitates illegitimate recombination and chromosomal loss during mitosis.

DNA methylation patterns are set up by specific enzymes, of which DNA methyltransferases are better characterized, whereas DNA demethylases remain stubbornly elusive. In somatic cells, DNA methyltransferase 1 (DNMT1) provides the major activity. The enzyme prefers hemimethylated over unmethylated DNA by a large margin. Hemimethylated DNA originates from symmetrically methylated DNA during replication, because DNA polymerases only insert unmodified cytidines. Its preference of hemimethylated DNA makes DNMT1 an ideal enzyme to stably propagate DNA methylation states during cell proliferation. Unmethylated sites remain unmethylated, whereas methylated sites become remethylated in both daughter strands. Accordingly, DNMT1 is tightly associated with the replisome, where it binds to PCNA, and is preferentially expressed in S-phase and in proliferating cells. Establishment of methylation at previously unmethylated sites, '*de-novo-methylation*', likely requires other enzymes. The methyltransferases DNMT3A and DNMT3B may be responsible for most de-novo-methylation occurring during development.

The mechanisms leading to demethylation are more obscure. One obvious mechanism is passive. If DNA methyltransferases are kept from remethylating newly replicated DNA, successive rounds of cell proliferation will yield unmethylated DNA. During embryonic development, this mechanism is likely supplemented by active enzymatic demethylation. Which protein is responsible is a moot point. One candidate is a methylcytosine-specific glycosylase acting similar to a repair enzyme.

The known properties of DNMTs go some way to explain how changes in overall methylation could come about. They do, however, not account for patterns of methylation at specific genes and sites. Specifically, it is not clear how hyper- and hypomethylation in cancer cells are generated. It is likely that DNMTs are directed towards or prevented from certain sites and genes by interaction with other proteins. As discussed below, histone modifications and the proteins establishing and interpreting these may also direct DNMTs. Conversely, active transcription complexes appear to exclude DNMTs from promoter regions. This is apparently part of the mechanism by which CpG-islands are kept free of DNA methylation.

Cancer cells tend to over-express DNA methyltransferases. Compared to normal tissues, the expression of DNMT1 is almost always increased. However, since DNMT1 is regulated in parallel with DNA synthesis in normal cells, a large fraction of this increase may simply reflect increased proliferation. Although demonstratable in model experiments, it is questionable whether altered expression of DNMT1 as such is responsible for aberrant methylation in cancer cells. In contrast, increased expression of DNMT3A and DNMT3B observed in some cancers is certainly significant, since these enzymes are normally expressed at low levels in somatic cells. It is, however, still unclear, to which extent they are responsible for hypermethylation.

Maintenance of correct levels and patterns of DNA methylation is not only dependent on chromatin factors and DNA methyltransferases, but also on the availability of the methyl group donor *S-adenosylmethionine* (SAM). More precisely, the reactions catalyzed by DNA methyltransferases and many other methyltransferases in the cell are influenced by the ratio of the substrate and product, SAM and *S-adenosylhomocysteine* (SAH). SAM is synthesized from the essential amino acid methionine, which is recycled through several steps from SAH. The efficiency of recycling is influenced by dietary factors, prominently the supply of folic acid and vitamin B12 and varies between humans as a consequence of genetic polymorphisms in enzymes involved in folate metabolism and the '*methyl cycle*'. Deficiencies in the diet and genotype exert a synergistic effect on the DNA methylation levels in rapidly turning over cells. So, these prevalent polymorphisms may contribute to cancer predisposition and some alterations in DNA methylation observed in human cancers could be related to a synergistic effect of diet and genetic predisposition.

Chromatin Structure

While promoter methylation is a conspicuous mark of gene silencing, DNA methylation is certainly not the only mechanism involved. Many invertebrates achieve gene silencing without DNA methylation at all and even in mammals not all silenced genes become methylated. Rather, DNA methylation in general represents one of the last steps in a chain of events leading to stable gene repression and often serves to fix the state of a gene silenced by other means. It has therefore been considered a '*lock-in*' mechanism, but – to keep with the metaphor - in some cases, as during X-inactivation, the door seems already to have been locked by other mechanisms and DNA methylation acts as an additional bolt. Rather, feedback and feed-forward mechanisms tend to enforce and stabilize the active and inactive states of a gene.

The mechanisms leading to gene silencing involve histone modifications and changes in the binding of non-histone proteins to DNA. Transcriptionally active genes are characterized by acetylation of histones H3 and H4 as well as by methylation of H3 at Lys4 (K4). These changes tend to loosen the attachment of DNA to nucleosomes, allowing remodeling and the binding of transcriptional activators. Transcription activating factors recruit co-activators and exclude co-repressors. Typical co-activators exhibit themselves ***histone acetyltransferase*** (HAT) activities or attract additional proteins which acetylate and methylate histones to yield an active nucleosome structure. In this way, the active state of a gene tends to be self-reinforcing. It is not entirely clear, how this active state is propagated through S phase and mitosis. Several mechanisms are discussed. Of these, histone phosphorylation at specific sites is best characterized.

The sequence towards gene silencing starts with loss of transcriptional activator proteins and/or their replacement by repressors. These changes elicit deacetylation by histone deacetylases (HDACs). Proteins acting as transcriptional repressors recruit deacetylases and *histone methyltransferases* (HMT) with SET domains which methylate e.g. H3 at the K9 position. Some co-repressors exhibit HDAC or HMT activities themselves. A specialized class of DNA-binding repressors is constituted by polycomb proteins. Two complexes of such proteins active in man, which exhibit HMT activity.

Acetylation and deacetylation are apparently quite rapid and are readily reversible, even in a non-proliferating cell. In contrast, histone methylation is certainly not as rapidly reversible and may require replacement of a nucleosome to be removed. This would normally occur in the course of DNA replication and cell division. So, histone H3 methylations at K9 and K4 appear to constitute already a quite stable mark of gene inactivation or activation, respectively. Methylation of H3 K9 is recognized by further chromatin proteins including HP1 which is a characteristic component of heterochromatin. The same modification may also serve to direct DNMTs to the DNA on that nucleosome. In turn, DNMTs may attract HMTs and HDACs leading again to reinforcement of the chromatin state – in this case an inactive one. Moreover, the assembly of proteins at one modified nucleosome may target neighboring nucleosomes. For this reason, inactive chromatin states, as DNA methylation, tend to spread.

Methylcytosine in DNA interferes with transcription in two ways. First, some transcriptional activators cannot recognize DNA, if CpGs in their binding site are methylated. Secondly, specialized repressor proteins recognize methylated DNA. These include MeCP2, MBD2 and MBD3 which bind preferentially to methylated DNA, blocking access and also recruiting chromatin-remodeling complexes and HDACs that buttress the repressed state.

A silenced chromatin state established in this fashion amounts to facultative heterochromatin. It is normally stably inherited and not easily reversed without extensive remodeling of chromatin and demethylation of DNA which normally requires several cell cycles. Such extensive remodeling is mostly found during development. A further common consequence of heterochromatization, which may help to ensure its propagation, is a shift of replication into the later part of S phase.

The intricate and complex mechanisms involved in histone modification and chromatin remodeling are incompletely understood, even more so in humans. It is therefore likely that disturbances in these mechanisms contribute to human cancer to a much larger extent than is presently known. Alterations in DNA methylation are relatively easy to detect and have been found in a large variety of human cancers. As they represent the end of a sequence, related epigenetic mechanisms leading to aberrant gene silencing may be even more ubiquitous. An indication of the importance of these mechanisms is provided by the exquisite sensitivity of a variety of cancers to HDAC inhibitors.

Indeed, several proteins involved in chromatin modification – beyond the DNMTs – are aberrantly expressed or mutated in human cancers. HATs, HDAC, and HMTs have all been found as parts of fusion proteins in leukemias and lymphomas. Misdirection of co-repressor proteins is the crucial event, e.g., in promyelocytic leukemia. Such misdirection may, of course, also be responsible for DNA hypermethylation in carcinomas.

Overexpression of the polycomb repressor protein EZH2 has been found, e.g., in prostate and breast cancers. The polycomb protein BMI1 is also overexpressed in some cancers, prominently in acute leukemias arising from hematopoetic stem cells. Maintenance of the stem cell population in these cancers requires the BMI1 repressor. In particular, BMI1 prohibits the activation of $p16^{INK4A}$ transcription in response to the continuous proliferation of the cancer cells. Conversely, loss of repressors can also contribute to cancer development.

A prominent repressor protein is RB1 which directs deacetylation to promoters by binding to E2F factors. RB1 also elicits remodeling at E2F-dependent promoters, which could in principle make inactivation of these promoters irreversible. Compared to other pocket proteins in the RB family, such as p130 and p107, RB1 may therefore cause more persistent and in some cases irreversible inactivation of such promoters, effectively establishing replicative senescence or enforcing terminal differentiation. These relationships could explain, why loss of RB1 function represents such a large step towards cancer, and why RB1 of the three closely related pocket proteins is by far the most frequently one mutated in cancer. The precise functions and mechanisms of chromatin remodeling are only beginning to be understood. Certainly, chromatin remodeling, i.e., the reorganization of nucleosomes along a DNA sequence, is necessary when the activity state of a gene is fundamentally switched, in either direction. This mechanism could therefore be essential both in epigenetic overexpression and silencing in human cancers. The extent to which it is involved, is not known. One specific component of the SWI/SNF remodeling complex, hSNF5/INI1, which is encoded by a gene at chromosome 22q11, behaves as a tumor suppressor in rare childhood cancers of the nervous system. Apparently, in these cancers, correct differentiation fails because chromatin remodeling cannot be properly performed.

Epigenetics of Cell Differentiation

Genetic changes like the loss of RB1 function or that of a chromatin remodeling protein like hSNF5/INI1 cause cancer by obliteration of epigenetic mechanism in which these proteins are involved. It is perhaps not incidential that the cancers caused in these instances impress primarily as failures of differentiation. One could go one step further and ponder whether some cancers might be caused by purely epigenetic mechanisms and represent a specific, if aberrant form of cell differentiation. This idea is, in fact, the core of an older theory that is now obsolete as a consequence of the discovery of the multitude of genetic changes present in the great majority of human cancers. So, if any human cancers are caused purely by epigenetic mechanisms, they are rare. Most likely, they would be childhood cancers characterized by failed differentiation. Some cases of Wilms tumors may come close.

However, the theory contained an important core of truth which is still relevant and may in fact now be understudied. Cell differentiation and cancer development resemble each other in that for a large number of genes '*cell-type-specific*' patterns of expression, including strong activation as well as strict silencing must be stably established. It is plausible that the same mechanisms might be at work in both processes. These mechanisms are now partly understood for gene silencing in cancer cells. By comparison, it is hardly known how overexpression of genes in cancer cells is established by epigenetic mechanisms.

For instance, overexpression of the EGFR is an important step in the progression of many carcinomas. In some cases, this overexpression is due to gain of chromosome 7p or regional amplification at 7p12, but these alterations are not generally found in cancers with overexpression of the protein. So, overexpression is likely caused by deregulation of gene expression secondary to alterations in other genes. For instance, degradation of the EGFR requires the CBL protein which could be lacking or the protein could be stabilized as a consequence of altered phosphorylation by PKC enzymes. Still another possibility is that the *ERBB1* gene encoding the receptor is locked in an activated state by epigenetic mechanisms, comparable to the silenced state of a tumor suppressor gene established by promoter hypermethylation.

For the establishment and maintenance of an active gene state across cell division, the continuous presence of transcriptional activators is necessary. Current understanding is that transcriptional activators binding to promoter and enhancer sequences recruit co-activators to form a large protein complex, a transcriptosome, which modifies the local chromatin and guides the actual transcriptional apparatus including RNA polymerase. This local chromatin state is transmitted through mitosis in a largely unknown fashion.

In any case, the differentiation state of a cell strictly depends on the pattern of transcriptional activators expressed. Cell differentiation often involves cascades of transcription factors which successively activate each other. These cascades often involve autoregulatory loops that make the process essentially irreversible. One well-studied example is myoblast differentiation. It is initiated and carried through by muscle-specific transcription factors (MSTFs or MRFs) that belong to the basic helix-loop-helix family (bHLH) like the MYC proteins. Like these, they bind to specific DNA sequences called E-boxes. The best-known of these factors is MYOD. E-boxes are present in genes encoding the typical proteins of muscle cells, but also in the enhancers of the genes encoding the MRFs. So, activation of MRFs beyond a threshold leads to an autocatalytic cascade, in which several MRFs become expressed at increasing levels until full differentiation is achieved. The threshold may be determined by the expression of MYC factors, but also by specialized inhibitor proteins, called ID. The four small ID proteins belong to the same general class of proteins as MRFs and MYC proteins, but lack a DNA-binding domain. Rather, they heterodimerize with and block the action of cell-type specific bHLH transcription factors. Overexpression of ID proteins, sometimes as a consequence of gene amplification, is a common finding in human cancers, particularly in carcinomas.

Importantly, transcription factor cascades not only lead to expression of cell-type specific products during normal cell differentiation, but also turn off cell proliferation by interacting with cell cycle regulators. In muscle cells, cell proliferation and differentiation are mutually exclusive. MYOD not only competes with MYC, but also represses the transcription of the AP1 factors FOS and JUN in differentiated cells, while in proliferating myoblasts the reverse occurs. So this system tends to be either in one (proliferation) or the other (differentiation) state. In addition, RB1 is activated during muscle differentiation and inactivates E2F-dependent promoters required for cell proliferation, while supporting the action of MYOD.

Similar transcription factor networks are thought to act in the differentiation of other cell types. For instance, in the differentiation of hepatocytes, insulin-producing cells of the pancreas, and proximal tubule cells of the kidney, the transcriptional activators HNF4 and HNF1 may be organized in a mutually activatory autocatalytical loop stabilizing the differentiated phenotype.

In many cell types, retinoids contribute to differentiation and growth arrest. Retinoids activate one of several retinoic acid receptors, named RARα, β, or γ, which are organized in an autocatalytic cascade. The *RARB2* gene promoter contains a sequence, named a RARE (*retinoic acid responsive element*), to which retinoic acid receptors can bind and increase transcription of the gene. During differentiation induced by retinoic acid, one of the other receptors (α or γ, depending on the cell type) initiates transcription of RARβ, which amplifies its own induction. Loss of the initiating RAR or inactivation of the *RARB* gene blocks the cascade. Accordingly, a translocation linking RARα to a repressor domain blocks the differentiation of promyeloid cells in an acute leukemia. In different carcinomas, the retinoid activatory cascade is interrupted by hypermethylation of the *RARB2* promoter.

In summary, then, disruption of epigenetic mechanism leading to cell differentiation is an important component in cancer development. Conversely, cancer cells may set up their own epigenetic cascades that maintain a status of gene expression compatible with continuous tumor growth.

Epigenetics of Tissue Homeostasis

Stably inherited phenotypes can not only be achieved by mechanisms acting within one cell, but also by interactions between similar or distinct cell types. In many tissues, such interactions occur between the mesenchymal and the epithelial component. They exchange paracrine factors in the steady-state of the tissue. Upon wounding or infection, the steady-state is disturbed and the exchange intensifies leading to wound healing and immune responses.

In the skin, paracrine factors are exchanged between keratinocytes in the epidermis and fibroblasts in the dermis. Epithelial keratinocytes in the epidermis produce, a.o., the cytokine interleukin-1 (IL1), of which normally only a fraction reaches the underlying dermal tissue. Mesenchymal cells produce and secrete low amounts of the *fibroblast growth factor* 7 (FGF7), which is also called *keratinocyte growth factor* (KGF), because it stimulates the proliferation of keratinocytes and other epithelial cells. They likewise produce low amounts of GM-CSF, a factor stimulating the proliferation and maturation of myeloid cells. It acts on keratinocytes, too, promoting their proliferation, but more strongly their differentiation. Upon damage to the epidermis, IL1 is released and binds to its receptor on fibroblasts. This activates the JNK and p38 MAPK pathways and leads to an increased activity of JUN transcriptional activators at the promoters of the *FGF7* and 7 *GM-CSF* genes. Increased secretion of FGF7 and GM-CSF stimulates proliferation and differentiation of the keratinocyte compartment, until it is healed and the IL1 concentration returns to normal levels. This is, of course, a simplified description, as many more factors are involved. Moreover, during wound healing a substantial reorganization of the extracellular matrix takes place which is performed, e.g., by proteases secreted from fibroblasts and invading immune cells in response to IL1 and GM-CSF. Immune cells are attracted by cytokines, chemokines and other factors from the activated fibroblasts. Another level of regulation is required to limit the ensuing inflammation.

The crucial argument in this example is that normal tissues use mutual paracrine interactions to achieve tissue homeostasis and to react appropriately to its disturbances. This could certainly be considered an epigenetic mechanism. Importantly, this type of interaction also takes place in cancers between tumor cells and the tumor stroma. However, in cancers, these interactions are grossly disturbed and do not lead back to a steady-state, but to a continued expansion of the tumor mass. Disturbances of paracrine interactions are also crucially involved in the co-carcinogenic effect of HIV.

A case in point is angiogenesis, an essential process in many cancers, that can be activated by genetic or epigenetic mechanisms. Some cancers carry mutations which lead to the constitutive production of pro-angiogenic growth factors such as VEGF or bFGF (FGF2) that stimulate branching of capillaries and proliferation of endothelial cells. In benign tumors and malignant renal cell carcinomas arising in the Von-Hippel-Lindau syndrome, this constitutive production is due to mutations in a regulator of the cellular response to hypoxia. As a consequence, HIF (*hypoxia-induced factor*) transcription factors are overactive and enhance the production of pro-angiogenic growth factors. So, in this case, a specific genetic change is responsible for increased angiogenesis.

Other cancers do not carry according genetic defects. Instead, when the tumor mass has exceeded the size that allows sufficient supply of oxygen by diffusion, tumor cells become hypoxic. This elicits a normal physiological response, viz. induction of HIF transcription factors leading to the production of angiogenic growth factors. These stimulate angiogenesis. Accordingly, the supply of oxygen (and other nutrients) improves allowing further expansion of the tumor to the point where oxygen becomes limiting again leading to further induction of HIF, angiogenic growth factors and continued angiogenesis. This epigenetic vicious circle is often exacerbated by genetic defects in the cancer cell, e.g. TP53 mutations that diminish the production of anti-angiogenic factors.

It is important to realize that by such paracrine interactions the tumor cells change the character of the normal cells with which they interact. While these cells need not become genetically altered (although this has been occasionally reported), they are persisently activated, which can alter their properties considerably. Experimentally, it can be demonstrated that stromal cells from malignant tumors acquire an '*epigenetic memory*', i.e., their activated state tends to persist even if the actual cancer cells are removed. This is plausible, if one considers the role of epigenetics in cell differentiation. Interactions between tumor cells and neighboring normal stromal cells are particularly important during metastasis. Setting up stable interactions is crucial for the survival and eventual expansion of metastatic cells. This presupposes a selection for those cancer cells which fit into the target tissue and their successful adaptation to the local environment. For instance, metastatic prostate cancer cells adapt so well to the microenvironment in the bone by interacting with local osteoblasts and osteoclasts that they have been termed '*osteomimetic*'. As in normal tissues, these mutual interactions are to a great deal mediated by exchange of paracrine growth factors, and to some extent by direct cell-to-cell interactions.

A final example of epigenetic mechanisms relevant to both normal tissues and cancer concerns stem cells. Stem cells are defined as cells with unlimited proliferation potential, the ability to generate differentiated derivatives, and the ability to do this by asymmetric division generating another stem cell and a more differentiated daughter cell. Stem cells which can give yield to any cell-type (in principle) are called *pluripotent*. In a healthy adult human, two types of stem cells are present: those of the germ-line and tissue stem cells. Tissue stem cells are probably not pluripotent. Rather, they can give rise to a limited number of diverse cell types. They are therefore also labeled as '*tissue precursor*' cells and as '*multi-* or *oligopotent*'. As the DNA of stem cells does not differ from that in (most) somatic cells, they must be defined by epigenetic mechanisms. In fact, both intercellular and intracellular mechanisms are involved.

Intracellular mechanisms include the expression of hTERT and of active telomerase, which allows the escape from replicative senescence. The other mechanism inducing replicative senescence upon continued cell proliferation, viz. induction of CDK inhibitors is likewise repressed. Specifically, accumulation of $p16^{INK4A}$ appears to be prevented by a polycomb repressor complex with BMI1 as its crucial component. It is not precisely clear, how pluripotency is maintained. In germ cells, expression of specific transcription factors appears to be involved. For instance, the transcriptional activator OCT3/4, now systematically called POUF5, is expressed in the germ line and in the early embryo. Its expression is lost, when pluripotent cells in the epiblast become committed to specific tissues. It is also strongly expressed in germ cell cancers and is necessary for their continuous proliferation. Germ cells and perhaps tissue precursor cells also have patterns of DNA methylation different from those typical for somatic cells. These are accordingly reflected in germ cell cancers. In germ cells as in germ cell cancers, moreover, expression levels of both RB1 and TP53 may be relatively low. This may prohibit a commitment to specific pathways of differentiation as well as replicative senescence.

In the testes and ovaries, respectively, primordial germ cells reside in an environment that allows their maintenance and organized differentiation towards mature oocytes and spermatozoa. Oogenesis is almost completed after the fetal period, whereas spermatogenesis continues throughout life and the stem cells remain present in the epithelia of the seminiferous tubules of the testes. There, they divide assymetrically to give rise to spermatozoa after several differentiation steps including meisosis. The location within the testicular epithelia is on one hand crucial for the survival of these cells, as they tend to undergo apoptosis outside this environment. On the other hand, primordial stem cells can principally develop into tumors when placed into the wrong environment. This is exemplified by experimental teratocarcinomas in specific mouse strains, which appear to arise by purely epigenetic mechanisms. However, germ cell tumors in humans do show chromosomal aberrations. In contrast, normal primordial germ cells contain the same amount and the same sequence of DNA as somatic cells. Thus, the mechanisms that make them immortal and pluripotent are purely epigenetic. The tubules of the testes are an example of a stem cell '*niche*'. This niche is actively maintained not so much by the germ cells themselves, but by the surrounding testicular tissue. Cells in this tissue provide, e.g., SCF (*stem cell factor*), a ligand for the receptor tyrosine kinase KIT.

Tissue stem (precursor) cells are less obvious and in humans they are only beginning to become characterized. Like primordial germ cells, however, they do not differ in DNA amount or sequence from their differentiated progeny. Instead, their state appears to be determined by their location in particular niches within a tissue, e.g. near the basis of crypts in the intestine or near the root of hair bulbs in the skin. Maintenance of their state appears to be achieved partly by growth factors produced by the surrounding mesenchyme. WNT factors in the intestine and WNT factors as well as SHH in the skin are thought to be essential. Less is known about the intracellular mechanisms which maintain their stem cell character. Very likely, telomerase expression is involved and may be stimulated via MYC through WNT or SHH-dependent pathways.

In contrast to primordial germ cells or cells of the epiblast, tissue-stem cells may not be pluripotent. Rather, they may be committed to a limited spectrum of differentiation fates, which may, however, involve quite different types of cells. For instance, stem cells of the large intestine are precursors of enterocytes, enteroendocrine, Paneth and goblet cells, which exhibit quite different functions. Moreover, if transplanted into a different environment, tissue stem cells may show a great deal of plasticity. Thus, bone marrow stem cells can not only give rise to many different types of blood cells and of the immune system, but even to some kinds of epithelial cells such as hepatocytes or to endothelial cells. Again, these different differentiation potentials must be imposed by epigenetic mechanisms that are at present insufficiently understood.

Clearly, most cancers likewise develop some kind of stem cell phenotype, by different mechanisms. In a number of cancers pathways involved in the maintenance of tissue stem cells are activated by mutations in components of these pathways or by autocrine mechanisms. This mechanism is likely responsible for the precursor cell phenotype of colorectal cancers and basal cell carcinoma of the skin. *Chronic myelocytic leukemia* (CML) is also clearly a stem cell disease caused by overactivity of '*cancer pathways*'.

Other cancers also resemble stem cells in possessing apparently unlimited proliferation potential, and most express telomerase. In some cancers, there is even evidence for a subpopulation which gives rise to a larger fraction of more differentiated tumor cells. However, it appears that in many cancers the stem cell properties are acquired secondarily. So, cancers do not necessarily develop directly from stem cells, although some certainly do. Others may develop from cells at a more differentiated stage that resume the phenotype of their precursor cell. Still others may acquire only selected aspects of a stem cell phenotype, such as telomerase expression. While the stem cell properties of cancers are often caused by genetic aberrations, a stem cell phenotype can be established by purely epigenetic mechanisms and this could well important in some cancers.

8

Gene Expression in Cancer

The principle of cDNA microarray hybridization takes advantage of the property of DNA to form duplex structures between two complementary strands. In this technique, the cDNA probes, which are arrayed onto a glass slide and represent the sequence of known genes or *expressed sequence tags* (ESTs), interrogate fluorescently labeled cDNA targets synthesized from extracted mRNA. In two-color microarray experiments, the differentially labeled cDNA targets (e.g., from tumor and normal tissue) hybridize to their respective cDNA probe sequences tethered to the slide. After imaging the microarray slide for signal intensities in each color channel, the relative expression ratio for each arrayed gene can be determined. In contrast to traditional gene-by-gene expression monitoring (such as Northerns), the cDNA microarray technique is limited only by the number of genes printed on the slide and, therefore; allows the analysis of gene expression on a truly genomewide scale.

In 1994, Drmanac et al., who used radioactive targets hybridized onto filter-immobilized *polymerase chain reaction* (PCR)-amplified cDNA probes, described gene expression monitoring using microarrays. In 1995, Schena et al. first described the hybridization of two-color fluorescently labeled targets to cDNA microarrays printed on glass. The two-color detection scheme has the advantage over radioactively labeled targets by allowing rapid and simultaneous differential expression analysis of two biologic samples, with one color used as a reference for normalization purposes. The reference allows for compensation of target-to-target and slide-to-slide variations in intensity owing to DNA concentrations and hybridization efficiencies, and thereby permits comparisons among multiple biologic samples across many experiments.

With more than 2,800,000 human EST sequences available at the latest UniGene build 137, representing 50–90% of all human genes, it is now possible to uncover the gene expression profiles of human cancers, querying the expression of thousands of genes in a single experiment. Global gene expression of different types of cancer may allow the development of expression profiles unique for a cancer and may lead to the development of rapid diagnostic assays. It may also identify secreted and membrane proteins that can be used for early diagnosis and for monitoring therapy. Gene expression profiles can also be correlated with clinical data to help predict biologic behavior and may allow us to direct therapy. In addition, this information may be useful in dissecting out the pathways involved in therapy failure, or malignant transformation with oncogenic transcription factors, and may ultimately provide novel therapeutic targets. Interest in microarray technology has risen in the pharmaceutical industry for new cancer drug discovery and for monitoring the effects of novel therapeutic agents. The list of potential uses of this technique is endless and is not limited to cancer research.

The following protocols are meant to be a general guide to setting up a microarray facility; other kits, reagents, and protocols may be substituted where necessary.

MATERIALS

All materials may be stored at room temperature unless otherwise noted.

cDNA Microarray Production

Clone production

1. Luria-Bertani (LB) broth.
2. Superbroth.
3. 96-Well round-bottomed plates.
4. ThinSeal Plate Sealers.
5. 96-Well Culture Blocks.
6. Airpore Tape Sheets.
7. Carbenicillin.
8. Ampicillin.
9. 96-Pin inoculation stamp.
10. 100% Ethanol.

Isolation of plasmid DNA

1. 96-well Alkaline Lysis Miniprep Kit. Store all buffers at 4°C.
2. 1 *M* Tris-HCl, pH 8.0.
3. 0.5 *M* EDTA, pH 8.0.
4. 100% Ethanol.

PCR amplification of clones

1. Cycleplate thin-walled PCR plate.
2. Cycleseal PCR Plate Sealer.
3. MJ Research (DNA Engine Tetrad) PTC-225 Peltier Thermal Cyclers.
4. 10X PCR Buffer (4°C).
5. Ampli Taq Polymerase (–20°C).
6. dNTPs (100 m*M* stocks) (–20°C).
7. Diethylpyrocarbonate (DEPC)-treated H_2O.
8. AEK M13 forward (F) and reverse (R) primers, a custom oligo (–20°C):
   (a) AEK M13F: 5'-GTTGTAAAACGACGGCCAGTG-3' (stock concentration of 1 m*M*).
   (b) AEK M13R: 5'-CACACAGGAAACAGCTATG-3' (stock concentration of 1 m*M*).

Quantification of PCR product

1. FluoReporter Blue Fluorometric dsDNA Kit (4°C).
2. Microfluor 2 White 96-well U-bottomed plates.
3. Lambda *Hin*dIII fragments (–20°C).
4. Perkin-Elmer Luminescence Spectrometer LS50B.

Purification of PCR product

1. 96-Well V-bottom plates.
2. Cyclefoil plate sealers.
3. Super T21 Centrifuge.
4. 1575 ImmunoWash.
5. 100% Ethanol and 70% ethanol.
6. 3 *M* Sodium acetate buffered to pH 6.0.
7. 3X Saline sodium citrate (SSC): 20X SSC stock: 3 *M* NaCl, 0.3 *M* sodium citrate. Dilute accordingly.
8. Quart-size heat-sealable bags.
9. Electric sealer.

Poly-L-Lysine pretreatment of glass slides

1. Gold Seal slides: These slides have consistently low intrinsic fluorescence.
2. 50-Slide stainless steel slide racks and glass tanks.
3. Sodium hydroxide (pellets).
4. 100% Ethanol: The source alcohol should be examined in a fluorometer to ensure that it has very low levels of contaminating fluorescent organic compounds.
5. 0.1% (w/v) Poly-L-lysine.
6. Tissue culture phosphate-buffered saline: 8 g/L of sodium chloride, 0.2 g/L of potassium chloride, 1.44 g/L of sodium phosphate dibasic anhydrous, 0.24 g/L of potassium phosphate monobasic.
7. 25-Slide plastic slide racks and plastic tanks with lids.

Blocking slides after printing with succinic anhydride

1. 1-Methyl-2-pyrrolidinone.
2. Succinic anhydride.
3. 1 *M* Sodium borate, pH 8.0. Adjust pH of boric acid with sodium hydroxide.
4. Stratagene UV Stratalinker 2400.
5. 30-Slide stainless steel slide rack.
6. 30-Slide glass submersion tanks.
7. 100% Ethanol.
8. Glass beakers (500-mL) and stir bars.
9. Large glass dish (14-in. casserole).
10. Large round Pyrex dishes (8-in. diameter).
11. Plastic slide box.

RNA Extraction and Target Production

RNA extraction

1. Virsonic 100 with microprobe (conical titanium probe, 1.8-mm-diameter tip).
2. RNeasy Midi Kit.
3. TRIzol (4°C).
4. Microcon-30.
5. β-Mercaptoethanol.
6. DEPC H_2O.
7. Chloroform.
8. Isopropanol.

9. 50 m*M* Sodium hydroxide.
10. 70% Ethanol.

Direct labeling of cDNA with fluorescent dyes

1. 10X Low T dNTPs nucleotide mix (–20°C): 25 μL each of dGTP, dATP, and dCTP for a 0.5 m*M* final (1/10) concentration; 10 μL of dTTP for a 0.2 m*M* (1/10) concentration; and 415 μL of DEPC H_2O for a total volume of 500 μL (100 m*M* dNTPs).
2. FluoroLink Cy3-dUTP 1 m*M* (photosensitive) (–20°C).
3. FluoroLink Cy5-dUTP 1 m*M* (photosensitive) (–20°C).
4. SuperScript II reverse transcriptase (RT) enzyme, 5X First Strand Buffer, 0.1 *M* dithiothreitol (DTT) (–20°C).
5. Anchored oligo-dT (d-20T-d[AGC]) (1 μg/μL) primer (–20°C).
6. Rnase Inhibitor RNAsin (–20°C).
7. DEPC H_2O.

Target purification

1. 0.5 *M* EDTA, pH 8.0.
2. 1 *M*Tris-HCl, pH 7.5.
3. 1 *M* Sodium hydroxide.

Microarray Assembly

1. Poly dA (10 mg/mL) (–20°C).
2. Yeast tRNA (4 mg/mL) (–20°C).
3. Human Cot-1 DNA (concentrated to 10 mg/mL) (–20°C).
4. 50X Denhardt's (–20°C).
5. 10% Sodium dodecyl sulfate (SDS).
6. Slide hybridization chamber.
7. 20X SSC: 3 *M* NaCl, 0.3 *M* sodium citrate.

Posthybridization Slide Washes

1. Glass Coplin staining jars.
2. 25-Slide plastic slide racks.
3. Wash Solution #1: 0.1% SDS + 0.5X SSC in ddH_2O (filtered).
4. Wash Solution #2: 0.01% SDS + 0.5X SSC in ddH_2O (filtered).
5. Wash Solution #3: 0.06X SSC in ddH_2O (filtered).

Methods

cDNA Microarray Production

The choice of which genes or ESTs to print are user specified. For human cancer profiling, we are currently using the "22K" human gene set comprising 22,320 human UniGene clones available from the IMAGE consortium and distributed by Research Genetics. Within the set are approx 4000 clones corresponding to known genes; the rest are unknown genes or ESTs. Currently, arrays of up to 15,000 probes are printed. The probe DNA is made from the IMAGE clones, which are arrayed in 96-well format and are used as template for PCR amplification.

Currently, prefabricated high-density microarrays can be purchased from a number of sources such as TeleChem. Companies such as Incyte offer microarray hybridization and analysis services to investigators who provide the RNA. The Affymetrix GeneChips are high-density arrays of oligonucleotide probes synthesized simultaneously on a large glass wafer by photolithography. Protocols for RNA preparation and microarray hybridization for these commercial solutions vary considerably.

Clone production

Pregrowth of clones to ensure maximum plasmid production

1. In sterile 96-well round-bottomed plates, add 100 μL of LB broth/well with 100 μg/mL of carbenicillin.
2. Thaw frozen 96-well library plates containing source bacterial cultures and spin briefly for 2 min at 200 rcf to remove condensation and droplets from the sealer.
3. Sterilize the 96-pin inoculation stamp between samples using 100% ethanol, and flame the pins using appropriate safety precautions.
4. After briefly allowing the inoculation block to cool, dip the pins in the library plate, and then inoculate the equivalent LB plate ensuring correct orientation. Sterilize the inoculation pins as in step 3.
5. Reseal the library plates with plate sealers (ThinSeal). Store the library plates at –70°C.
6. Incubate the growth plates in a humidified oven overnight at 37°C.

Inoculation of deep-well culture blocks

1. Add 1 mL of Superbroth, containing 100 μg/mL of carbenicillin, to each well of the 96-well culture blocks using an eight-channel pipettor.
2. Using the 96-pin inoculation stamp, inoculate the 96-well culture blocks.
3. Cover (Airpore sheets) and place the blocks in a 37°C shaker incubator (200 rpm) for 24 h.

Isolation of plasmid DNA

1. Isolate plasmid DNA from the cultures using the miniprep kit according to the manufacturer's protocol.
2. Resuspend the plasmid DNA in 200 μL of T. low E. (10 m*M* Tris-HCl, 0.1 m*M* EDTA).
3. Store the DNA at –20°C and use as template for PCR amplification.

PCR amplification of clones

The isolated DNA is used as a template for PCR amplification with vector primers (AEK-M13) using a 96-well format, typically 12 plates at a time.

1. Make a PCR reaction mix by combining the components.
2. Using a multichannel pipet, transfer 99 μL of the master mix to each well of the PCR plates (Cycleplates).
3. Using a multichannel pipet, transfer 1 μL of appropriate template DNA in each well taking care to retain the plates orientation and order.
4. Cover the plates with sealers (Cycleseal) and place in a thermo-cycling device.
5. Amplify the templates using the following cycle conditions:
   (a) Step 1. 96°C for 30 s.
   (b) Step 2. 94°C for 30 s.
   (c) Step 3. 55°C for 30 s.
   (d) Step 4. 72°C for 150 s.
   (e) Step 5. Repeat steps 2–4, 24 times.
   (f) Step 6. 72°C for 5 min.

Quantification of PCR product

1. Analyze 2 μL of each PCR product by electrophoresis on a 2% TAE agarose gel containing 0.5 μg/mL of ethidium bromide. We obtain a digital image of the gel under UV illumination and analyze the electrophoresis products to ensure that a single band of distinct size is produced for each sample. The intensity of the band gives an estimate of the relative amount of product.
2. Quantify the PCR products using fluorometric quantitation. Expected yield is ~100 μg/mL.

Purification of PCR product purification

1. Prepare an ethanol/acetate precipitation mix (150 m*M* sodium acetate, pH 6.0, in ethanol). Add 200 mL of the precipitation mix to each well of a V-bottomed 96-well plate.

Table 8.1. Components for PCR reaction mix

Reagent	*Stock*	*Final*	*Volume per 1000 reactions (mL)*
PCR buffer	10 X	1 X	10
dATP	100 m*M*	0.2 m*M*	0.2
dTTP	100 m*M*	0.2 m*M*	0.2
dGTP	100 m*M*	0.2 m*M*	0.2
dCTP	100 m*M*	0.2 m*M*	0.2
AEK M13F	1000 μ*M*	0.5 μ*M*	0.05
AEK M13R	1000 μ*M*	0.5 μ*M*	0.05
Ampli Taq Polymerase	5 U/μL	0.05 U/μL	1
DEPC H_2O			87.1

2. Using a multichannel pipettor, transfer the remaining (approx 97 mL) PCR products to their corresponding wells containing the precipitation mix.
3. Place the plates in the –80°C for 1 h, or overnight at –20°C, to precipitate the DNA.
4. Allow the plates to thaw (to reduce brittleness and melt any ice), and spin in a high-speed swinging-holder centrifuge (Sorvall Super T21). We typically spin stacks of three plates at 1600 rcf for 1 h.
5. After centrifugation, remove the supernatant from plates, and dispense a 70% ethanol wash, 150 mL/well, using a plate-processing station such as the Bio-Rad 1575 ImmunoWash.
6. Centrifuge the plates as in step 4 at 1600 rcf for 1 h, and remove the supernatant. In a dust-free area, allow the plates to dry overnight without lids and covered with clean paper towels.
7. Resuspend the PCR products in 40 μL of 3X SSC. Seal the plates with foil sealer making sure that all wells are tightly sealed. Place the plates in an airtight heatsealed bag with a moistened paper towel, and place in a 65°C oven for 2 h.
8. Remove the cooled plates and store at –20°C.

Poly-L-Lysine Pretreatment of Glass Slides

Treatment of slides with a coat of poly-L-lysine allows the target DNA to adhere to the surface and minimize loss during hybridization.

1. Place new Gold Seal microscope slides into a stainless steel 50-slide rack.
2. Prepare cleaning solution in a large glass beaker (500 mL is required per 50-slide glass tank): 400 mL of ddH_2O, 100 g of

NaOH, of 600 mL of 95% ethanol. Dissolve NaOH in water, and then add ethanol. Stir until the solution is clear. If the solution does not clear, add H_2O until it does.

3. Dispense the cleaning solution into 50-slide glass tanks. Submerge the rack in the cleaning solution and shake for 2 h on an orbital shaker.
4. Remove the slides and rinse with fresh ddH_2O for 2–5 min. Repeat the wash four times, each time using fresh ddH_2O.
5. Move the clean slides to 25-slide plastic racks.
6. Prepare the poly-L-lysine solution as follows (for two boxes of 25 slides each): 35 mL of poly-L-lysine (0.1% [w/v]), 35 mL of tissue culture PBS, 280 mL of ddH_2O.
7. Dispense the poly-L-lysine solution into plastic 25-slide containers. Submerge the rack in poly-L-lysine solution, cover with a lid, and shake for 1 h.
8. Rinse once in ddH_2O for 1 min.
9. Centrifuge the rack in a low-speed swinging-holder centrifuge to remove free liquid.
10. Immediately transfer to a clean slide box.
11. Allow the slides to age for 2 wk before printing.

Microarray slide printing

The next stage is printing of DNA probes on the coated glass slides. The printing process refers to the robot-driven sequential transfer of individual purified PCR-amplified fragments from a 96-well micro-titer tray to exact, pre-defined locations on glass slides. Several arrayers are available from commercial companies: Affymetrix 417 Arrayer, Cartesian Technologies, Beecher Instruments, Genomic Solutions, BioRobotics. It is also possible to build you own arrayer for approx US $25,000, and arrayers have been built in several academic settings.

The Cancer Genetics Branch custom-built arrayers, using "*quill*"-type pens, print sequentially up to 16 spots at once on each of 48 or 96 slides, wash and dry the print pens before picking up the next set of cDNAs, and repeat until a complete 96-well plate of probe DNA has been printed. At this time, 96-well plates must be manually changed; however, an autoloading mechanism is in development. Each pen collects approx 200–500 nL and deposits between 2 and 3 nL (0.2–0.5 ng) of PCR product.

After printing is complete, identifying marks are etched along the top of each slide (print number and slide number) with a diamond scriber and the slides are placed in plastic slide box (use simple plastic slide boxes with no paper or cork to shed particles).

Blocking slides after printing with succinic anhydride

To reduce nonspecific binding of strongly negatively charged target on microarray slides, the positively charged amine groups on poly-L-lysine-coated slides are passivated by reaction with succinic anhydride. We routinely process 48 slides at a time.

1. Age the slides for 1 wk at room temperature after printing.
2. Place the slides in a glass casserole dish and cover with plastic wrap. UV-crosslink printed cDNA with a dose of 450 mJ of UV energy.
3. Place the slides in stainless steel 30-slide racks, and place the racks in clean glass tanks. Prepare the passivation reaction (for one tank) in a dedicated, dry 500-mL beaker: 6 g of succinic anhydride, 325 mL of 1-methyl-2-pyrrolidinone, 25 mL of 1 *M* sodium borate, pH 6.0. When succinic anhydride has completely dissolved, add 25 mL of 1 *M* sodium borate buffer while mixing, and quickly pour onto the slides.
4. Shake the slides for 20–30 min on an orbital shaker—some precipitation will occur. While blocking, boil ddH_2O in a clean Pyrex dish using a hot plate, so that it will be ready after the reaction.
5. Remove the slide holder from the passivation reaction, and dunk immediately in boiling ddH_2O to denature the DNA. Turn off the heat source and let stand for 2 min in the nearly boiling ddH_2O bath. Remove the slide holder, and dunk in a fresh glass tank with 100% ethanol to dehydrate the slides.
6. After 3–5 min in ethanol, remove the slides and centrifuge dry in a low-speed swinging-holder centrifuge.
7. Place the dry slides in a clean slide box.

RNA Extraction and Target Production

RNAs isolated from the cells or tissue one wishes to analyze are used as the template for synthesis of fluorescently labeled cDNA targets. For cell lines, RNA first extracted using a Qiagen RNeasy kit followed by a further round of purification using TRIzol yields excellent results. The amount of total RNA in each channel required for a microarray experiment varies from 50 to 200 μg, with the precise amount varying with the size of the array and fluorescent nucleotide used.

Considerable thought should be given to what reference cell line or tissue to use for your microarray experiments. The reference should be abundant and offer at least a minimal intensity for all genes printed on your array (if a gene has no intensity in the reference channel, then ratios and other statistical calculations cannot be computed because the denominator cannot be zero).

RNA extraction

1. For the RNeasy kit, follow the manufacturer's guidelines. At the final elution stage, elute with two successive aliquots of 150 μL of RNase-free water.
2. Determine the concentration of your RNA in 50 m*M* NaOH. At this time it may be convenient to aliquot out appropriate quantities (55–220 μg) of your RNA before beginning the second round of purification.
3. Extract the eluted RNA a second time by adding 1 mL of TRIzol/0.3 mL of eluent, vortexing, and following manufacturer guidelines for RNA extraction. You may leave the precipitated RNA in isopropanol at –80°C for later use.
4. If the RNA is to be used immediately, wash the RNA pellet twice with 70% ethanol, remove the ethanol, and dry the pellet.
5. Resuspend the dried RNA pellet (50–200 μg) in 400 μL of RNase-free H_2O. Take 1 μL for final RNA concentration measurement, and make sure the total amount of RNA for labeling with Cy3 is 80–100 μg, and 150–200 μg for Cy5.
6. Transfer the RNA to a Microcon-30 and centrifuge at 14,000 rcf for 7–12 min to concentrate the RNA. Concentrate the RNA to <14 μL .
7. Elute the RNA and bring to a final volume of 14 μL with DEPC H_2O.

Direct labeling of cDNA using fluorescent dyes

The labeling of complex probes is accomplished by direct incorporation of fluorescent nucleotides during an RT reaction. Currently, the factors of labeling efficiency, fluorescent yield, spectral separation, and nonspecific binding make the Cy3/Cy5 pair the most useful for our detection system. Although a number of conjugated fluorophores are available (dCTP, dUTP, amino-allyl dUTP RT coupled to mono-functional dyes), we have found that Amersham Pharmacia dUTP-conjugated Cy3/Cy5 yields consistent results. Other labeling systems are being tested.

1. Preanneal RNA with anchored oligo-dT (d-20T-d[AGC]) (1 μg/μL) primer: 14 μL of RNA, 3 μL of anchored oligo-dT primer. Incubate in a thermocycler at 70°C for 5 min and cool to 42°C.
2. Mix the RT labeling reaction: 4 μL of Cy3 *or* Cy5-dUTP (1 m*M*), 8 μL of 5X First-Strand Buffer, 4 μL of 10X low T dNTP mix, 4 μL of 0.1 *M* DTT, 1 μL of Rnase Inhibitor RNAsin, 2 μL of SSII RT.
3. Add RT labeling mix to the preannealed RNA.
4. Incubate at 42°C for 30–60 min.
5. Add 2 μL of SII RT enzyme, incubate at 42°C for another 30–60 min, and cool to room temperature.

Target purification

The labeled target reaction must be purified to remove unincorporated nucleotides.

1. To stop the labeling reaction, add 5 μL of 0.5 *M* EDTA, pH 8.0, and mix well.
2. To hydrolyze the RNA, add 10 μL of 1 *M* sodium hydroxide and mix well. Incubate at 65°C for 20–30 min, then cool to room temperature.
3. Add 25 μL of 1 *M* Tris-HCl, pH 7.5, to neutralize the NaOH.
4. Purify each labeled color individually for the first purification. In Microcon-30 spin columns, add labeled target and bring up to a total volume of 400 μL with DEPC H_2O. Spin the column at 16,000 rcf for about 8 to 9 min to a volume of approx 50 μL.
5. Recover each target. For the second purification, pool the Cy3- and Cy5-labeled targets for an experiment in a new Microcon-30 column, and bring up to a total volume of 400 μL of H_2O.
6. Concentrate the combined targets to a 25-μL final volume for hybridization.

Hybridization

Hybridization volumes may vary depending on array size. The following is based on a 20 × 40 mm array. Adjust volumes proportionally and use appropriate sized cover slips for smaller/larger arrays.

Microarray assembly

1. Make the hybridization mixture containing competitor DNA (to reduce nonspecific binding and background): 25 μL of pooled Cy5/Cy3 labeled targets, 1.5 μL of poly dA (10 mg/mL), 1.5 μL of

yeast tRNA (4 mg/mL), 1.5 μL of human Cot-1 DNA (10 mg/mL), 1.5 μL of 50X Denhardts, 5 μL of 20X SSC.

2. Denature at 98°C for 2 min and cool on wet ice for 10 s.
3. Add 0.8 μL of 10% SDS.
4. Pipet hybridization targets up and down several times until well mixed, and place the mixture on a microarray under a 24 × 50 mm glass coverslip.
5. Place the microarray slide in a hybridization chamber with 15–20 μL of 3X SSC to maintain humidity within the chamber.
6. Incubate the microarray hybridization chamber in a 65°C water bath for 12–18 h.

Posthybridization slide washes

After hybridization, the hybridization solution and any unbound target must be removed from the surface of the slide to reduce background.

1. Remove the microarray hybridization chamber from the water bath.
2. Dispense wash solutions into Coplin staining jars. Open the hybridization chamber and immediately place the slide in Wash #1 until the coverslip slips off. Once the coverslip comes off, agitate gently for 2 min.
3. Transfer the slide to Wash #2 and agitate gently for 2 min.
4. Transfer the slide to Wash #3 and agitate gently for 2 min.
5. Place the slide in a plastic 25-slide rack and spin in a centrifuge equipped with a swinging carrier (horizontal) that can hold the slide holder. Spin immediately.
6. Scan the slide as soon as possible.

Image Acquisition

Target fluorescence intensities at the immobilized probes can be measured using a variety of commercially available scanners. The following is a brief list scanners and contact information:

1. *Affymetrix*: 418 Array Scanner—Scanning laser digital imaging epifluorescence microscope; 5320 nm (350 mW) and 6350 nm (350 mW) lasers with 3-min scan time per slide.
2. *Agilent*: Under development.
3. *Axon*: GenePix 4000—532-nm (20-mW) and 635-nm (15-mW) lasers with 10-μm pixel resolution and 5-min scan time per slide.
4. *Beecher Instruments*: Scanner—laser confocal, two simultaneous photomultiplier tube channels, three lasers: 488 nm at 75 mW,

532 nm at 100 mW, 633 nm at 35 mW with 10- to 100-μm pixel resolution.

5. *Genomic Solutions*: GeneTAC LS IV and GeneTAC 2000—Charge-coupled device camera with high-energy xenon light source; can scan up to four fluors per slide.
6. *GSI Lumonics*: ScanArray LITE, ScanArray 4000, ScanArray 5000—Scanning confocal laser GHeNe 543 nm (Cy3) and RHeNe 632 nm (Cy5).
7. *Molecular Dynamics*: Array Scanner—Confocal optics, nine-element lens; HeNe and NdYag lasers; scanning time per slide: 5 min for single color, 11 min for two color.
8. *Packard Instruments*: BioChip Imager—Epifluorescence confocal scanning laser system. 543 nm (Cy3) and 633 nm (Cy5) HeNe lasers with 50-, 20-, or 10-μm pixel resolution.

The scanners used by our laboratory are Beecher Instruments or Agilent custom-built dual-laser confocal microscopes that generate two-color simultaneous digital scans saved to an IBM PC. Intensity data are integrated in 10- to 15-μm square pixels and recorded at 16 bits.

Image Analysis and Normalization

The two image files generated by the scanner are analyzed using software tools developed by Chen et al. for the ScanAlytics IPLab image-processing package. These software tools can be used with any image file format to extract raw target intensity information as well as to compute background-corrected intensities and expression ratios, *confidence intervals* (CI), and to allow for data integration of all clone information. As each probe is roboticly printed to a predefined position, the scanned images are overlaid with a grid that divides the images into segments, each containing a target spot.

All clone information, including gene name, clone identification number, chromosome and radiation hybrid–mapped location, and source microplate position, is attached to each segment by this process. Each of the images is assigned a pseudo-color (e.g., Cy5 = red and Cy3 = green). The probe spot is identified within each segment, and the target fluorescent intensity is calculated for each color by averaging the intensities of every pixel inside the detected spot region. The local background intensity around each spot in each color is also measured within each segment. For every spot in each color channel, the final target intensity values are derived by subtracting the local background intensity from the average fluorescent intensity.

Next, a normalization constant is determined to compensate for differential efficiencies of labeling and detection of Cy3 and Cy5. The process involves calculating the average intensity, in both color channels, for a set of internal controls consisting of 88 housekeeping genes. These genes are preselected and have been verified on numerous hybridizations as being stable for most experiments (red:green ratio = 1.0). The normalization constant is then derived and used to calculate a calibrated red:green ratio for each cDNA spot within the image. In addition the ratio variance of the 88 control genes is used to calculate 99% CIs in which the ratios are statistically no different from 1. The output of the analysis is in the form of a pseudo-colored image of the entire array. Individual spots can be highlighted using the mouse cursor, and information including gene name, clone identity, intensity values, intensity ratios, normalization constant, and user-defined CIs can be obtained. A spreadsheet of expression ratio data for each spot is generated.

Sensitivity and specificity

It is estimated that that the sensitivity of this method allows the detection of mRNA species comprising 1:10,000 of the mass of poly (A)+. Comparisons among the microarray experiments with Northern hybridizations have confirmed this technique to be reliable. Our experience to date has indicated the high consistency of microarray data for determining ratio changes; however, there is some variation in the exact value of the ratios obtained by these two methods. In some instances, the ratio obtained by microarray analysis underestimates that obtained by Northern analysis. Possible causes for this under-estimation include reaching a probe intensity saturation limit at the highest intensities under our current detection system. Additionally, the largest ratio changes frequently have one of the measurements near the lower limit of detection, and at these levels the effects of background and nonspecific binding are more apparent, causing variance at the higher ratio measurements. Other causes of discrepancy may be owing to nonlinear binding characteristics of target to probe. Currently, we can detect up to 300-fold ratio changes with accuracy.

Data Mining and Statistical Analysis

All data from each experiment can be downloaded into a relational database such as FileMaker Pro (Claris) and further parsed for comparing data across experiments as well as for extracting data from individual array hybridizations. It is obvious that large-scale, high-throughput experimental methods require information processing coupled to a variety of analysis tools. Software tools such as ArrayDB can also be used to integrate information from many Internet sources, such as NCBI Entrez, UniGene, and KEGG databases, with experimental gene expression data. Hierarchical clustering of biologic samples and genes is a commonly applied mathematical strategy to organize gene expression data. Algorithms such as multidimensional scaling are proving to be an informative way to visualize expression profiles. More complex data analysis systems are currently being devised for complex clustering of data.

PRECAUTIONS

1. There currently exists in the literature a confusing interchangeable nomenclature system for referring to hybridization partners termed probes and targets. For the purpose of this chapter we refer to the tethered DNA (of known identity) on the microarray slide as the probe, and the fluorescently labeled cDNA (synthesized from unknown mRNA messages) as the hybridization targets.
2. Use extreme care to avoid cross-contamination. Cross-contamination will be evident when PCR products are gel electrophoresed and present multiple bands. Contaminated clones will require restreaking and sequencing.
3. It is recommended that a slight excess of PCR reaction mix than what is actually required be made.
4. Take care to remove air bubbles and ensure proper mixing of the reaction mix.
5. We use the FluoReporter Blue Fluorometric dsDNA kit, Dynex Microfluor plates, lambda *Hin*dIII fragments for standards, and a Perkin-Elmer Luminescence Spectrometer LS50B.
6. Ensure proper mixing of the PCR solution with the precipitation mix. Failure to do so will decrease the concentration of DNA yield.
7. Use rubber pads between the stacked plates to prevent cracking and breakage.
8. Heat and cool the plates slowly to prevent condensation on the sealer and upper rim of the well.
9. It is important to wear powder-free gloves at all times and avoid contact with detergents or other compounds that may cause background fluorescence.
10. It is important to remove all traces of cleaning solution. Failure to do so will hinder poly-L-lysine coating the reaction and will

adversely affect microarray results (low-intensity spots, high background).

11. Aged slides will be very hydrophobic (water drops leave no trail when they move across the surface).
12. A new slide should be marked for use as a template to line up the coverslip when putting together the microarray experiment, because the printed spots will not be visible after the slide-blocking procedure.
13. The reaction solution must be prepared in completely dry containers. All glassware, stir bars, and graduated cylinders should be dedicated to slide blocking and should not be cleaned with detergents, which can adversely affect this reaction.
14. A number of groups have found that rapid or slow hydration of the DNA on the slide after printing followed by a quick-drying step improves DNA distribution or signal strength. This has not been observed for materials prepared by our procedure, so it is routinely omitted.
15. When water is added, the anhydride will begin to rapidly decompose, so add the mix to the slides very quickly. It is helpful to dispense the sodium borate buffer from a prealiquoted 50-mL conical tube.
16. Cover the dish with aluminum foil to reduce evaporation and simultaneously boil ddH_2O in a microwave to replenish evaporative loss.
17. High-quality RNA is crucial to the success of a microarray experiment. It is also possible to use 2–4 μg of poly(A)-purified mRNA in the target synthesis reaction. Smaller quantities of RNA may be used in conjunction with RNA amplification techniques, which are currently under development.
18. Cell lines should be harvested under consistent conditions and lysed rapidly. It is recommended that you sonicate the very viscous lysate with several 5-s bursts to disrupt the genomic DNA before applying to the RNeasy column. We use the microprobe (conical titanium probe 1.8-mm-diameter tip) at a setting of 5, dissipated power approx 5–10 W. When extracting RNA from tissue add the frozen sample directly to the TRIzol without thawing with immediate homogenization.
19. Factor in an approx 10% loss of RNA from each TRIzol purification round.

20. Overdrying may make resuspension of RNA difficult and may adversely affect results.
21. Do not concentrate to dryness, because the sample may be lost or difficult to recover. Proper volume is when the filter is partially dry on visual inspection.
22. The flowthrough may be saved at this step for high-performance liquid chromotography recovery of unincorporated fluorophores.
23. Appropriate competitor DNA should be used for microarrays of clones from other organisms, such as mouse.
24. For the best results, apply pooled targets to the center of the coverslip, and then, using the template slide as a guide, place the inverted microarray slide from above.
25. Use paper towels and vacuum suction to completely dry the outer surface of the chamber.
26. Take care that the coverslip does not scratch the microarray surface.

9

Cancer Therapies

The versatility, adaptability, and extreme cleverness of cancer cells have made it very difficult for scientists to develop methods to either contain or eradicate this disease. Treatment is complicated by the exact nature of the cancer cells, the tissue they arose from, and the tissue or tissues they end up colonizing. Many cancers, such as those affecting the colon or liver, remain tucked away in the darker recesses of the body, where they are hard to detect and even harder to treat. Other cancers, such as melanoma or retinoblastoma, are at or near the surface of the body, and thus are more accessible to observation and treatment. All cancer therapies try to target characteristics that are peculiar to cancer cells so as not to damage normal cells. This could be a mutated protein, a peculiar behavior pattern, such as an increased rate of cell division, or an elevated demand for oxygen to support the cancer cell's high metabolic activity.

Angiogenesis Blockers

All cells, whether they are cancerous or not, need to be vascularized in order to receive the oxygen and nutrients required to support metabolic activity. Blood vessels also carry away metabolic waste products, such as carbon dioxide, which is expelled from the body by the lungs, and urea, expelled by the kidneys. The circulatory system, consisting of an extensive collection of arteries, veins, and capillaries, provides these essential services. Installing this system requires the formation of new blood vessels, a process that is called angiogenesis.

Angiogenesis is, of course, extremely important during embryogenesis, when the circulatory system is being formed, and during growth to adulthood. Vascularization during development is so efficient that virtually every cell in the body is less than 100 μm away from the nearest capillary. *Angiogenesis* also has many important roles to play during adulthood, such as wound healing, formation of the *corpus luteum* after ovulation, formation of new endometrium after menstruation, and remodeling the vasculature of skeletal muscle after long periods of exercise.

There are many factors involved in the formation of blood vessels, but the best understood are a tyrosine kinase called *vascular endothelial growth factor* (VEGF) and a gene regulatory protein called *hypoxia-inducible factor* 1 (HIF-1). A shortage of oxygen in any cell of the body activates HIF-1, which, in turn, stimulates production and secretion of VEGF. The VEGF protein induces proliferation of endothelial cells (cells that make up blood vessels) that sprout from the nearest capillary and, following the VEGF concentration gradient, grow towards the hypoxic cells. Once the cells are vascularized and begin receiving an adequate oxygen supply, HIF-1 is inactivated and production of VEGF drops off, thus terminating angiogenesis.

Tumors, like normal tissue, cannot grow to more than a millimeter or two in diameter without being vascularized. Consequently, angiogenesis is a prime target for cancer therapy. Clinical trials are currently in progress to test angiogenesis inhibitors on cancers of the breast, prostate, brain, pancreas, lung, stomach, ovary, and cervix, as well as leukemia and lymphomas. So far the studies have had limited success. Endostatin, a widely studied drug that is toxic to endothelial cells, showed great promise in preliminary studies. It is safe to administer, but it has failed to demonstrate antitumor effects. An extract from the Asian fruit *Gleditsia sinensis* (GSE) has been shown to be an effective blocker of VEGF transcription but has yet to progress beyond the basic research stage. Another compound, extracted from green tea, called GTE is known to be a powerful blocker of endothelial cell proliferation but, like GSE, it is still at the preclinical stage of development. The most successful angiogenesis blocker tested so far is an anti-VEGF antibody called *bevacizumab*. This drug is being tested in phase I clinical trials, but it will be several years before this drug or any of the other known angiogenesis blockers are approved for routine medical use.

Biotherapies

Cancer therapies that exploit the body's immune system are known as *biotherapies* or *immunotherapies*. The use of an antibody to deactivate

VEGF is an example of a biotherapy. Biotherapy exploits the properties of the adaptive immune system, which involves the *white blood cells* (WBCs) called *T lymphocytes* and *B lymphocytes*. B lymphocytes produce antibodies tailored for microbe antigens. T lymphocytes, or T cells, are activated by other white blood cells, called *monocytes*, in a way that alerts the T cell to specific invader antigens. The T cell uses this information to hunt down and destroy those invaders. T cells enlist the aid of other lymphocytes by secreting small signaling molecules called *cytokines*. A special kind of T cell, called a *natural killer* (NK) lymphocyte, is activated by the release of cytokines but focuses its attention on attacking and killing infected cells rather than the invading microbe. The immune system also attacks cancer cells because they usually contain mutated proteins, displayed on the cell surface, that are treated as being of foreign origin. Biotherapies exploit the strategies of the immune system by employing cytokines, bone marrow stimulants, and monoclonal antibodies.

Cytokines

The first successful biotherapy came with the isolation of a cytokine known as *interferon*, which stimulates NK cells and seems to have a direct effect on some cancer cells by slowing their growth rate and stimulating more normal behavior. The U.S. *Food and Drug Administration* (FDA) has approved the use of interferon to treat kidney cancers, lymphoma, and Kaposi's sarcoma. Other cytokines, called *interleukins*, have been used to specifically boost the response of T lymphocytes. There are more than 30 known interleukins, but the most promising so far is interleukin-2 (IL-2), which has been approved for the treatment of kidney carcinomas and melanoma. In addition, clinical trials are under way to test the effectiveness of IL-2 as a treatment for cancers of the colon, ovaries, lung, brain, breast, prostate, and bone marrow (leukemia).

Bone Marrow Stimulants

Biological therapies sometimes take a more generalized approach to treating cancer. One such effort involves the use of *colony-stimulating factor* (CSF) to stimulate cell growth in the bone marrow. Its presence increases the number of WBCs, thus augmenting the immune response, but it also increases the number of *red blood cells* (RBCs) to improve the overall health and vitality of the patient. RBCs contain the oxygen-carrying pigment hemoglobin and have the very important job of delivering oxygen to all of the cells. Thus, CSF helps ensure that all cells are receiving an adequate supply of oxygen and that the patient does not become *anemic*. This is an important consideration since the patient may also be receiving chemotherapy or radiotherapy, both of which can damage the bone marrow, leading to an increased incidence of secondary infections and anemia. Administration of CSF can help counteract this effect and, indeed, makes it possible for a patient to tolerate levels of chemotherapy or radiotherapy that would not be possible otherwise.

Monoclonal Antibodies

The final form of biotherapy, currently being practiced, involves the use of *monoclonal antibodies* (MAbs). A single type of B cell, grown in culture, produces these antibodies, which are specific for a single antigen. All the cells in the culture originate from a single founder cell that produces the desired antibody. The cells are thus clones of the original cell, so the antibody they make is said to be monoclonal. MAbs are produced by injecting a single kind of human cancer cell into mice to stimulate the production of antibodies. The mouse cells producing the antibodies are isolated and fused with a culture of immortalized human cells to produce a hybridoma. The hybridomas are also an immortalized cell line, and thus can produce a very large quantity of the antibody. Production of MAbs maximizes the specificity of the antibody to ensure that it will not react with or damage antigens on normal cells. MAbs can be designed to attack cancer cells directly, or they can be linked to cytotoxic substances that destroy the cancer cell after it encounters the MAb.

Rituxin and *Herceptin* are two MAbs that have been approved by the FDA as cancer treatments. Rituxin is used to treat Hodgkin's lymphoma, and Herceptin is used to treat breast cancer. Clinical trials are under way to test a large number of MAbs for the treatment of cancers.

Bone Marrow Transplants

Transplanting *bone marrow* (BM) is a common method for treating *leukemia* and *lymphoma*. It is also required when radiotherapy is used to treat other forms of cancer, because this therapy often destroys or damages the patient's bone marrow. There are three types of BM transplants, each defined in terms of the donor tissue: *autogeneic transplants*, in which patients receive their own BM; *syngeneic transplants*, in which patients receive BM from an identical twin; and *allogeneic transplants*, in which patients receive BM from unrelated individuals. Autogeneic transplants are most commonly used when chemotherapy or radiotherapy has damaged the patient's bone marrow. Patients suffering from leukemia or lymphoma generally receive syngeneic or allogeneic transplants. Syngeneic transplants are preferred, in order to avoid immune rejection. However, very few patients have identical twins; consequently, the great majority of BM transplants are *allogeneic*. Allogeneic transplants will be attacked by the immune system, giving rise to a condition known as *graft-versus-host disease* (GVHD), making it necessary for these patients to take immuno-suppressant drugs for the remainder of their lives.

The immune system's decision to accept or reject a given tissue is based on the exact nature of the glycocalyx, the molecular forest covering the surface of each cell in the grafted tissue. The glycocalyx consists of millions of different kinds of glycoproteins that protrude from the cell surface. Immunologists call these glycoproteins cell-surface antigens. Members of the immune system, particularly T lymphocytes, can tell if a cell is foreign or not by examining these glycoproteins. Immunologists have identified many of these glycoproteins and use this information to match donated BM to prospective patients. Given that there are so many different kinds of antigens it may seem like an impossible task. However, some glycoproteins seem to be more important than others, when it comes to invoking GVHD, so immuno-logists have obtained good results by matching just five or six strong antigens. Matching BM for a few antigens still leaves many that are unmatched, and consequently the grafted tissue will be rejected over time. However, a partial match can still reduce the amount of immuno-suppressants the patient must take over a lifetime while improving the long-term survival of the transplanted tissue.

CHEMOTHERAPY

Certain drugs may be used to kill or inhibit the growth of cancer cells. The nature of a drug varies depending on the type of cancer, its location in the body, the effect it has on normal body functions, and the overall health of the patient. In general, cancer drugs damage DNA, block the synthesis of DNA and RNA, or damage the mitotic spindle. Cancer drugs can also interfere with normal physiology by blocking steroid hormone receptors that stimulate cancer cell growth.

Drugs that Target DNA

These agents chemically damage DNA and RNA, leading to a disruption of replication (*DNA synthesis*) or transcription (*RNA synthesis*). In some cases these drugs lead to the production of defective messenger RNA that is incapable of coding for protein. Examples of this type of drug are cisplatin, doxorubicin, and etoposide.

Drugs that Block DNA and RNA Synthesis

These drugs work by blocking the formation of ribonucleotides or deoxyribonucleotides, essential building blocks for RNA and DNA. Without nucleotides, the cell cannot replicate, cannot repair its DNA, and is incapable of synthesizing new proteins. Examples of these drugs are methotrexate, mercaptopurine, and fluorouracil.

Drugs that Damage the Mitotic Spindle

The mitotic spindle is a collection of microtubules that serve to carry the chromosomes to opposite poles of a dividing cell. Disruption of the spindle is an effective way of blocking cell division. Drugs in this class include Vinblastine, Vincristine, and Taxol.

Drugs that Block Hormone Receptors

Breast cancer may be caused by the lifelong exposure of breast cells to the growth-stimulating effects of the female steroid hormone, estrogen. Under normal circumstances, the effects of estrogen are essential for the growth of breast cells leading to the production of milk after a woman gives birth. However, if a tumor appears in the breast, a reasonable strategy is to neutralize the stimulatory effects of estrogen, in the hope that it will arrest the growth of the cancer. A plant extract called *tamoxifen* has been shown to be an estrogen antagonist; that is, it binds to the estrogen receptor, thus blocking the hormone's normal functions. For men, counterpart to this strategy involves the use of anti-androgen drugs, specifically to block testosterone receptors, to treat prostate cancer. A drug used for this purpose is called *bicalutamide*.

Chemotherapy may be administered daily, weekly, or monthly but generally occurs in cycles that include long rest periods, giving the body a chance to recover. Normally the drugs are administered intravenously (IV) although some may be taken as a pill or, in the case of surface cancers such as melanoma, applied directly to the skin. Patients requiring many IV treatments are fitted with a catheter, a soft flexible tube that is inserted into a large vein, thus avoiding the necessity of daily injections.

Drugs used in chemotherapy are designed to target cancer cells, but they often damage or kill normal cells as well. Death of normal cells leads to a variety of side effects, some of them quite severe. Cancer drugs target actively dividing cells; consequently, any normal tissue consisting of proliferating cells will also be affected, most notably the bone marrow, digestive tract, testes, ovaries, and hair follicles. Some drugs may also affect postmitotic cells in the heart, kidney, bladder, lungs, and nervous system. In some cases, these tissues may be permanently damaged. Given the range of tissues affected, it is not surprising that chemotherapy involving the first three categories described above is associated with a large number of side effects: fatigue, nausea and vomiting, pain, hair loss, anemia, secondary infections, and poor blood clotting.

Fatigue

Feeling tired, with a complete lack of energy, is the most common symptom reported by cancer patients. This is partly due to the stress of hospitalization and the lack of sleep this may entail, but it is mainly the result of low blood counts and poor appetite brought on by the cancer drugs.

Nausea and vomiting

This side effect is due almost entirely to the death of epithelial cells lining the digestive tract. These are actively dividing cells that are very sensitive to chemotherapy. Anticancer drugs are designed to minimize this side effect, but residual discomfort may be minimized with anti-nausea treatments.

Pain

Chemotherapy sometimes damages neurons in the peripheral nervous system, leading to burning, numbness, and tingling or shooting pain, usually in the finger or toes. Some cancer drugs can also cause mouth sores, headaches, muscle pain, and stomach pain associated with nausea and vomiting. These pains are usually no more severe than those accompanying a flu, and are treated with common painkillers such as aspirin or acetaminophen.

Hair loss

Hair follicles, like intestinal epithelium, are actively dividing cells that are killed by chemotherapy. The death of these cells is responsible for the loss of hair, not only on the head, but also over the entire body. The hair grows back when chemotherapy is discontinued, but sometimes the new hair is a different color, or it has a different texture.

Anemia

Chemotherapy greatly reduces the bone marrow's ability to make *red blood cells* (RBCs); consequently, the amount of oxygen reaching the cells is reduced. A decrease in the RBC count leads to a condition known as anemia, the symptoms of which include shortness of breath, dizziness, and a feeling of being tired and weak. In severe cases, anemia can be treated with a blood transfusion, or with a growth factor called *erythropoietin* that stimulates the formation of RBCs.

Infection

In addition to reducing production of RBCs, chemotherapy also reduces the production of *white blood cells* (WBCs), the cells of the immune system. Consequently, the patient becomes more susceptible to infections and must take precautions, such as staying away from people who have a cold or flu, and avoiding sharp objects that might cut the skin, such as sewing needles and razors. Treating the patient with colony-stimulating factor, a type of hormone that promotes the growth and differentiation of white blood cells, offsets the reduction in the WBC count.

Blood clotting problems

In addition to RBC and WBC, the bone marrow produces a third kind of blood cell, called *platelets*, which are needed for the blood to clot properly. In the absence of external cuts, low platelet counts can lead to excessive bruising, red spots under the skin, blood in the urine, bleeding nose and gums, and headaches.

CRYOSURGERY

Freezing cancer cells or tumors with liquid nitrogen (–196°C) is called *cryosurgery*. For external tumors of the skin, liquid nitrogen is applied with a very fine spray gun. For internal locations, surgeons use an instrument called a *cryoprobe* that is placed in contact with the tumor. Ultrasound imaging is sometimes used to monitor the placement of the probe and freezing of the tissue. The treatment generally involves three freeze-thaw cycles to ensure destruction of the cancer cells.

Cryosurgery is used to treat skin, prostate, lung, and cervical cancers. Research is in progress to test the effectiveness of this treatment on other types of cancers, such as cancers of bone, brain, spine, and windpipe. This procedure offers several advantages over other forms of treatment. It is less invasive than ordinary surgery, requiring only a small incision in the skin for insertion of the cryoprobe and imaging tube. Treatment is highly localized, with minimal damage to surrounding tissue, and can be repeated many times. The main disadvantage of this procedure is that it can be used only on tumors confined to a small area. In addition, cancer cells that have separated from the main tumor mass will be missed. Consequently, cryosurgery is often used in conjunction with chemotherapy or radiotherapy.

Cryosurgery does have some side effects, but they are much less severe than those associated with other forms of therapy. Used on liver cancers, the procedure will sometimes damage the bile ducts or major blood vessels, leading to hemorrhage (extensive bleeding) or infection. Cryosurgery of the prostate gland can damage the urinary tract and local nerves, leading to sexual impotence and incontinence (lack of control over urine flow), although these side effects are often temporary.

Gene Therapy

Since cancer is a disease of the genes it can, in theory, be treated by either repairing the defective gene or by introducing a normal copy of the gene into the affected tissue. This procedure, known as *gene therapy*, was pioneered in the 1990s to treat genetic deficiencies of the immune system. Since that time, more than 600 gene therapy trials have been launched in the United States alone, of which 60 percent are designed to treat various types of cancer.

Introducing a gene into a cell is a complex and often dangerous business that depends on the natural ability of viruses to infect cells. Some RNA viruses, called *retroviruses*, have the added ability to incorporate their genome into cellular chromosomes. Scientists have developed methods for adding a human gene to the retroviral genome, so that when the retrovirus infects a cell and inserts its genome into a chromosome, it has, in effect, delivered and installed the therapeutic gene. To be sure, there are many wrinkles in this procedure, and much work is needed to ensure the virus does not damage the cell or the patient, and that the therapeutic gene is expressed at levels sufficient to cure the cancer.

Most of the gene therapy trials aimed at treating cancer introduce a normal copy of the tumor suppressor gene *p53*. *p53* codes for a protein (P53) that blocks cell division in abnormal cells and can, if necessary, force defective cells to commit suicide. The *p53* gene is abnormal in more than half of all cancers and is thus a prime target for therapy. Currently, *p53*-gene therapy clinical trials are under way to treat cancers of the ovaries, breast, prostate, head and neck, liver and bone marrow (*leukemia*). Other genes, specific for breast cancer (BRCA1 and BRCA2), melanoma (CDKN2, or cyclin-dependent kinase

N2), and colon cancer (MSH1 and MSH2) are also the subject of gene therapy trials.

Side effects associated with gene therapy are invariably due either to immune attack on the cells that become infected with the vector (the virus carrying the therapeutic gene) or to complications resulting from insertional mutagenesis, whereby the vector damages a cellular gene when it inserts itself into a chromosome. In the former case, the immune response can be so extreme as to lead to multiorgan failure and subsequent death of the patient. In the latter case, insertional mutagenesis can produce additional cancers.

Laser Therapy

Some cancers may be treated with high-intensity light—a laser—that shrinks or destroys localized tumors. This treatment is often required to treat cancers that are resistant to chemotherapy or radiotherapy. Three types of lasers are currently in use: *carbon dioxide* (CO_2), *neodymium aluminum garnet* (NAG), and *argon*. The CO_2 laser, being of medium intensity, is best suited for treating skin cancers and other superficial tumors. The NAG laser is of high intensity and can penetrate deeper into tissue than light from other lasers can. The light can be carried through optical fibers to organs and tissue deep within the body. The argon laser has the lowest intensity and is used to treat the most superficial skin lesions. It is also used in photodynamic therapy.

CO_2 and NAG lasers are used routinely to treat cancers of the vocal cords, skin, lung, vagina, and colon. The side effects associated with this form of cancer therapy are the same as those for cryosurgery.

Photodynamic Therapy

Treatment using the argon laser, in conjunction with photosensitizing agents to destroy cancer cells and tumors, is called *photodynamic therapy*. The photosensitizing agent is injected into the bloodstream and absorbed by cells throughout the body. The agents are designed to remain in cancer cells longer than in normal cells. When the treated cancer cells are exposed to the argon laser light, the agent absorbs the light energy, causing it to release oxygen-free radicals that kill the cells. The timing of the therapy is important. It must be given after the agent has left normal cells but when it is still present in cancer cells. In 1998 the FDA approved the use of an agent called porfimer sodium (Photofrin) for the treatment of lung cancer. Several clinical trials are also under way to test the effectiveness of Photofrin on cancers of the bladder, brain, larynx, and oral cavity.

The side effects associated with this therapy can be severe. Photofrin makes the skin and eyes sensitive to light for six weeks or more after treatment. Patients have to avoid sunlight and bright indoor light. Moderate exposure to daylight can result in red, swollen and blistered skin. Other temporary side effects include coughing, difficulty swallowing, abdominal pain, painful breathing and shortness of breath. Photodynamic therapy was invented by Dr. Julia Levi, professor of microbiology at the University of British Columbia.

RADIOTHERAPY

The use of ionizing radiation to destroy cancer cells and tumors is known as *radiation therapy*, X-ray therapy, irradiation, or simply radiotherapy. This therapy relies on high-energy electromagnetic beams or subatomic particles to damage the DNA in cancer cells so that the cell is incapable of dividing and quickly dies. The main goal is to kill the cancer cells while leaving the normal cells intact. This can be achieved in some cases by focusing the beam of radiation on specific parts of the body or, if possible, directly on the cancerous tumor. Thus radiotherapy has the potential for greater precision than chemotherapy and produces fewer side effects.

Most patients receive external radiotherapy, in which a machine directs the high-energy radiation at the site of the tumor. The most common type of radiation machine is called a linear accelerator. This machine heats a radioactive substance, such as cobalt-60, causing it to liberate high-energy rays. Accelerators can produce X-rays and gamma rays (from cobalt), as well as protons and neutrons. Internal radiotherapy is also possible, in which a radioactive material is sealed inside a holder that is implanted near or within a tumor. This procedure is sometimes used after a tumor has been removed surgically. The implant is placed in the tumor bed (the area previously occupied by the tumor) to kill any residual cancer cells.

For most types of cancer, radiotherapy is given five days a week for six or seven weeks. The total dose of radiation depends on the size of the tumor, but normally, to minimize damage to surrounding tissue many small doses of daily radiation are preferred to fewer larger doses. This strategy is augmented by the recent development of computer-based radiotherapy, which allows precise mapping of the tumor and surrounding tissue so that multiple beams can be shaped to the contour of the treatment area. This type of radiotherapy is used extensively to treat prostate cancer, lung cancer, and certain brain tumors. Radiotherapy is also used to treat cancers of the skin, tongue, breast, uterus and bone marrow. Side effects are as broad as those described for chemotherapy, although less severe.

STEM CELL THERAPY

Stem cells are progenitor cells, capable of differentiating into many different cell types that reside in various parts of the body. These cells are used to restore bone marrow in patients who have received chemotherapy, or radiotherapy, for a variety of cancers, but are most commonly used to treat leukemia and lymphomas. In the latter case, the patient's cancerous bone marrow or lymph glands are destroyed with radiotherapy and then reconstituted using stem cells.

Stem cell therapy is similar to the use of bone marrow transplants but has three major advantages: First, the cells are easily isolated from peripheral blood or from umbilical cord blood; second, stem cells are less likely to invoke *graft-versus-host disease* (GVHD), particularly those from umbilical cord blood, thus most patients do not require immunosuppressants; third, because of reduced risk of GVHD, the donor tissue can be allogeneic and there is no need for tissue matching.

The patient receives the stem cells through a venous catheter placed in a large vein in the neck or chest area. The cells travel to the bone marrow, where they produce new white blood cells, red blood cells, and platelets in a process called *engraftment*. Reconstitution of the bone marrow takes several weeks, although full recovery of the immune system can take a year or more. The most severe side effect associated with this therapy is the risk of serious infections developing during the period of bone marrow reconstitution. Other side effects such as nausea, vomiting, and hair loss are due to the radiotherapy.

CLINICAL TRIALS

The fight against cancer is waged on three fronts simultaneously: in research laboratories, where scientists are trying to learn more about cancer cells, in the hospitals where patients are treated with the various therapies described previously, and in clinical trials where new procedures, or modifications to preexisting methods, are tested for their effectiveness. Several hundred such trials are under way worldwide. We begin with a brief introduction to the organization of clinical trials as they are conducted in North America and Europe.

Four Phases

Clinical trials are conducted in four phases and are always preceded by research conducted on experimental animals such as mice, rats, or monkeys. The format for preclinical research is informal; it is conducted in a variety of research labs around the world, with the results being published in scientific journals. Formal approval from a governmental regulatory body is not required.

Phase I clinical trial

Pending the outcome of the preclinical research, investigators may apply for permission to try the experiments on human subjects. Applications in the United States are made to the *Food and Drug Administration* (FDA), the *National Institutes of Health* (NIH), and the *Recombinant DNA Advisory Committee* (RAC). RAC was set up by NIH to monitor any research, including clinical trials, dealing with cloning, recombinant DNA, or gene therapy. Phase I trials are conducted on a small number of adult volunteers, usually two to 20, who have given informed consent. That is, the investigators explain the procedure, the possible outcomes, and especially, the dangers associated with the procedure before the subjects sign a consent form. The purpose of the Phase I trial is to determine the overall effect the treatment has on humans. A treatment that works well in monkeys or mice may not work at all on humans. Similarly, a treatment that appears safe in lab animals may be toxic, even deadly, when given to humans. Since most clinical trials are testing a new drug of some kind, the first priority is to determine a safe dosage for humans. Consequently, subjects in the Phase I trial are given a range of doses, all of which, even the high dose, are less than the highest dose given to experimental animals. If the results from the Phase I trial are promising, the investigators may apply for permission to proceed to Phase II.

Phase II clinical trial

Having established the general protocol, or procedure, the investigators now try to replicate the encouraging results from Phase I, but with a much larger number of subjects (100–300). Only with a large number of subjects is it possible to prove the treatment has an effect. In addition, dangerous side effects may have been missed in Phase I because of a small sample size. The results from Phase II will determine how safe the procedure is and whether it works or not. If the statistics show that treatment is effective and toxicity is low, the investigators may apply for permission to proceed to Phase III.

Phase III clinical trial

Based on Phase II results the procedure may look very promising, but before it can be used as a routine treatment it must be tested on thousands of patients at a variety of research centers. This is the expensive part of bringing a new drug or therapy to market, costing millions, sometimes billions, of dollars. It is for this reason that Phase III clinical trials invariably have the financial backing of large pharmaceutical or biotechnology companies. If the results of the Phase II trial are confirmed in Phase III, the FDA will approve the use of the drug for routine treatment. The use of the drug or treatment now passes into an informal Phase IV trial.

Phase IV clinical trial

Even though the treatment has gained formal approval, its performance is monitored for very-long-term effects, sometimes stretching on for 10 to 20 years. In this way, the FDA retains the power to recall the drug long after it has become a part of standard medical procedure. It can happen that in the long term, the drug costs more than an alternative, in which case, health insurance providers may refuse to cover the cost of the treatment.

Breast Cancer

Tumor detection

Three recent trials assessed the value of *magnetic resonance imaging* (MRI) in screening women for breast cancer. These studies examined whether MRI might be a more effective screening tool than mammo-graphy. The results were presented at the annual meeting of the American Society of Clinical Oncology (ASCO), held in Chicago on June 2, 2003. Effectiveness was measured in two ways: *Sensitivity* (how well the procedure detects a cancer when one is present), and *specificity* (how well the procedure avoids false positives, or a result suggesting a tumor is present when there is none). If screening suggested the presence of cancer, a biopsy was performed to confirm or deny the finding.

In the first study, which ran from November 1999 to August 2002, researchers in the Netherlands evaluated 1,911 high-risk women at several centers throughout the country. The women received a *clinical breast exam* (CBE) twice yearly, a yearly mammography, and a yearly MRI. Researchers evaluated each woman's mammography results independently of her MRI results, so if one imaging system suggested the presence of cancer the evaluator would not be biased towards expecting to see signs of cancer from the other system. Each woman in the study was followed for about two years. During this time, investigators found invasive breast cancers or noninvasive tumors (ductal carcinoma in situ) in 40 of the women. Forty-six percent of the tumors were small (1 centimeter or less) and 77 percent were confined to the breast. While the clinical breast exam detected 16 percent of the tumors and mammography found 36 percent, MRI sensitivity was found to be 71 percent. MRI sensitivity was even more pronounced in cases of invasive cancer (spread beyond the layer of tissue in which it developed), with 20 percent found by CBE, 26 percent by mammography, and 83 percent by MRI. Although more sensitive, MRI was less specific than the other two methods, leading to a greater number of false positives. Twelve percent of the time, MRI suggested that there was a cancer when there was none, compared to 5 percent for mammography and 3 percent for CBE.

In a second trial, conducted at the University of Bonn in 1998 and involving 462 women, researchers have found that MRI offers a sensitivity of 96 percent, compared to 25 percent for CBE and 43 percent for mammography. Moreover, in contrast to the Dutch study, this trial found that MRI actually resulted in fewer cases of false positives than the other forms of screening, leading the German researchers to suggest that MRI should replace mammography as a screening tool for high-risk women.

In a third study, which did not directly compare MRI with other forms of breast cancer screening, researchers at the Memorial Sloan-Kettering Cancer Center in New York reviewed medical and radiology reports for 54 women with BRCA mutations who had 115 MRI exams between 1998 and 2002. They found that MRI was 100 percent sensitive for correctly detecting breast cancer (finding a tumor when there was one), but only 83 percent specific. That is, 17 percent of MRI's results were false positives. The investigators concluded that MRI sensitivity is encouraging, but that the high false-positive rate limits its use as a routine practice.

Investigators from all of the trials agree that while MRI looks very promising, further research will be needed to reduce the number of false positives before it can be recommended as a routine procedure.

Tamoxifen treatment for breast cancer

A study published in the February 19, 2003, issue of the *Journal of the National Cancer Institute* concluded that women at high risk for breast cancer who took the *drug tamoxifen* (a compound that blocks the cell-stimulatory effects of estrogen) were less likely to be diagnosed with benign (noncancerous) breast conditions than women who took a placebo. The study participants, enrolled in the Breast Cancer Prevention

Trial at the Cancer Research Network in Plantation, Florida, took tamoxifen for five years.

The researchers found that the risk of developing benign tumors was reduced by 28 percent for women in the tamoxifen group. In addition, women treated with tamoxifen had 29 percent fewer biopsies than women who received a placebo. The reduction in biopsies was seen predominantly in premenopausal women. The results suggest that tamoxifen inhibits the formation of early breast abnormalities, such as hyperplasia, that could develop into metastatic or invasive cancer.

Chemotherapy

Dr. Sandra Swain, chief of the National Cancer Institute's Cancer Therapeutics Branch, recently concluded a study evaluating the side effects of doxorubicin (Adriamycin), widely used in cancer chemotherapy. Doxorubicin is a highly effective anticancer drug but it is suspected of increasing patients' risk of *congestive heart failure* (CHF). In CHF the heart has trouble beating normally because of damage to the heart muscle. To evaluate the risk of CHF from treatment with doxorubicin, Swain and her colleagues looked back at the medical records of 630 patients who received a placebo instead of dexrazoxane (a drug that blocks doxorubicin side effects) in three trials conducted in the 1990s. Patients were followed up to find out whether they had experienced CHF at any time, either while they were enrolled in the study or later.

A total of 32 of the 630 patients (5 percent) had doxorubicin-related CHF. In 11 cases the CHF occurred while the patient was enrolled in the trial; in the other cases, it occurred later. Ten of 172 patients (6 percent) aged over 65 experienced the problem, compared with 22 of 458 patients (5 percent) aged under 65. It was estimated that the percentage of patients with doxorubicin-related CHF rose with increasing doses of the drug. At a dose of 550 mg/m^2, they estimated that 26 percent of patients would experience this adverse event. The estimate rose to 48 percent at a dose of 700 mg/m^2. A total of 149 patients (24 percent) experienced a "*cardiac event*" (either CHF or a test result indicating that the heart is pumping less blood than normal) while enrolled in the study. Swain and her colleagues estimated that, at a dose of 550 mg/m^2, 65 percent of patients would have a cardiac event. Dr. Swain recommends that all patients with metastatic breast cancer who receive more than 300 mg/m^2 of doxorubicin also receive dexrazoxane to minimize the risk of heart problems. However, the use of dexrazoxane is only approved for breast cancer patients with disease that has spread, and only after they have received a cumulative dose of doxorubicin of 300 mg/m^2.

Colon Cancer

A study conducted at the University of North Carolina, Chapel Hill, and at the Norris Cotton Cancer Center in Lebanon, New Hampshire, has shown that taking aspirin every day for as little as three years reduces the occurrence of colorectal polyps by 19 percent to 35 percent. The results were published on March 5, 2003, in the *New England Journal of Medicine*. These data confirm numerous earlier observational studies suggesting that people who regularly take aspirin have lower rates of colorectal adenomas. Adenomas are abnormal growths (polyps) that precede the development of most colorectal cancers.

Previous studies have shown that people who regularly take aspirin to treat conditions such as arthritis have lower rates of colorectal polyps, colorectal cancer, and colorectal cancer deaths. Based on these results, as well as on animal models and laboratory data, the *National Cancer Institute* (NCI) supported the current trial, in which people were randomly assigned to aspirin or a placebo and followed for a several years. The study suggests that daily aspirin may be an appropriate supplement to regular surveillance procedures in individuals who are at risk of developing colon cancer. The trial participants were adults with either a previous colorectal adenoma or previous early-stage cancer successfully treated with surgery.

Lung Cancer

Non-small-cell lung cancer (NSCLC) accounts for about 80 percent of all lung cancer cases. The average five-year survival rate is about 50 percent for patients whose NSCLC is found early and treated with surgery before it has spread to other organs. In advanced-stage disease, chemotherapy offers modest improvements in median survival, although overall survival is poor.

Docetaxel, a drug that inhibits mitosis, is the current standard treatment for NSCLC that recurs after chemotherapy. In previous studies, docetaxel improved survival compared with other chemotherapy drugs or observation, but was found to cause severe side effects, such as fever and infections. Other studies have suggested that the experimental drug pemetrexed might be an effective alternative to docetaxel. Pemetrexed is an enzyme inhibitor that interferes with the body's production of vitamin B (folic acid), which is essential for normal cell growth.

In the current study, which ran from March 2001 to February 2002 at Indiana University in Indianapolis, 571 patients with recurrent NSCLC were given docetaxel or pemetrexed in a phase III clinical trial. As of May 2003 the survival rate of the patients was about the same whether they were treated with pemetrexed (8.3 months) or docetaxel (7.9 months). Patients in both treatment groups had about a 30 percent chance of surviving for one year. Survival was no different between the two groups of patients, but those treated with pemetrexed were less likely to suffer from fever and infections caused by low levels of white blood cells. They were also less likely to be hospitalized for fever or other side effects or to need treatment to stimulate production of white blood cells. In addition, patients treated with pemetrexed suffered less hair loss and less numbness in the arms and legs.

Melanoma

Scientists at the *National Cancer Institute* (NCI) have found a new method for modifying the immune system of cancer patients to induce cancer regression. By inhibiting a molecule associated with T lymphocytes called *cytotoxic T lymphocyte-associated antigen* 4 (CTLA-4), the immune system is able to attack some patients' tumors. CTLA-4 was inhibited with an antibody leading to tumor shrinkage in patients with metastatic melanoma. In addition to the tumor shrinkage, the treatment also induced evidence of autoimmunity, that is, signs that the immune system was attacking not only tumors, but normal tissue as well. However, treatment with steroids completely eliminated all symptoms of autoimmunity that occurred in the trial.

The 14 patients in the study received an antibody that blocks CTLA-4 activity, plus a cancer vaccine made up of a small segment of a protein found on the surface of melanoma cells. The hope is that the vaccine will stimulate the immune system to attack cancer cells, but in previous clinical trials, this type of vaccine alone did not cause melanoma tumors to shrink. Researchers speculated that CTLA-4's inhibition of T cell activity might be in part responsible for this lack of an effective immune response. Blocking CTLA-4 did indeed improve the response to treatment. In two of the patients in the study, all tumors, which included significant metastases in the lung and brain, disappeared completely. A partial response, defined as a 30 percent to 100 percent decrease in tumor size, was seen in one additional patient. In another two patients, some tumors decreased in size, but other tumors continued to grow. Six patients, including all of those whose tumors regressed, experienced significant autoimmune effects in normal tissues in response to the treatment. The enhanced activity of immune cells in these patients led to symptoms including skin rashes, inflammation of the colon, and hepatitis. With treatment, all of these symptoms were resolved.

Metastasis

When a tumor spreads to the vertebrae, the spinal cord can be compressed and can cause some patients to lose mobility or bladder control. Researchers wondered whether surgery to remove the tumor in addition to radiation would benefit cancer patients by alleviating the pressure and stabilizing the spine. Spinal cord compression occurs in 10 to 20 percent of all cancer patients, especially lung, prostate, and breast cancer patients.

A randomized phase III study of 101 patients compared the advantages of surgery combined with radiation as opposed to radiation alone in relieving spinal cord compression. In this NCI-funded study, as much tumor as possible was removed from the spinal columns of 50 patients, who were then treated with radiation. Fifty-one patients received radiation only. Patients who received surgery in addition to radiation for their spinal compression showed a marked improvement in their ability to walk as compared to patients receiving radiation only. Surgically treated patients also maintained continence for a much longer period. Sixteen patients in each group entered the study unable to walk. Nine patients treated with surgery and radiation regained the ability to walk (56 percent), compared to only three receiving radiation alone (19 percent). The study was stopped early due to the overwhelming benefits of surgery combined with radiation.

10

METASTASIS

The spread of solid cancers beyond the confinements of their tissue compartment into other parts of the same tissue and successively into neighboring tissues (*invasion*) and distant organs (*metastasis*) is the defining property of malignancy. Invasion and metastasis are decisive for the clinical course of most cancers. Invasion and metastasis are complex processes, particularly in carcinomas, since normals epithelia are strongly adherent and are confined by a basement membrane. Before or during invasion, carcinomas activate their surrounding connective tissue, eliciting inflammation and angiogenesis. Actual invasion by carcinoma cells involves decreased cell adhesion and increased motility as well as destruction of the basement membrane and remodeling of the extracellular matrix. Metastasis, in addition, requires cancer cells to enter blood or lymph vessels, to survive there, to extravasate, reattach, and proliferate in a different tissue. Furthermore, during invasion and metastasis, cancer cells need to evade cytotoxic cells of the immune system such as *cytotoxic T-cells* (CTL) and *natural killer* (NK) cells.

Invasion and metastasis require an extensive reorganization of carcinoma cells, particularly of their cytoskeleton and their surface. Likely, this reorganization involves coordinated changes of gene expression and cell structure that impress as '*programs*' for invasion or metastasis. These '*programs*' are predominantly secondary consequences of mutations in oncogenes or tumor suppressor genes, but are aided by specific mutations, e.g. in cell adhesion molecules.

Changes in cell surface molecules accompany altered cell-cell and cell-matrix interactions during invasion and metastasis. Molecules mediating homotypic interactions such as E-cadherin and connexins are down-regulated or mutated. Expression patterns of proteins mediating interactions with the extracellular matrix, such as integrins, are changed. Various other proteins on the cell surface including adhesion molecule, antigenic glycoproteins, and recognition proteins for immune cells are expressed at altered levels, alternatively spliced or processed or mutated.

Successful invasion depends crucially on interactions with non-tumor '*stromal*' cells, i.e. tissue mesenchymal, endothelial and inflammatory cells, which also display changes in gene expression and behavior. The emergence of '*activated stroma*' may distinguish highly malignant carcinomas.

The destruction of the basement membrane and other extracellular matrix components in connective tissues surrounding a carcinoma is predominantly accomplished by proteases secreted from tumor and stromal cells, notably metalloproteinases and plasmin. Various members of the *matrix metalloproteinase* (MMP) family are over-expressed in tumor tissues and their inhibitors (TIMP) are often down-regulated. Proteases also activate latent growth factors from their storage sites in the extracellular matrix that act on carcinoma and stromal cells.

Angiogenesis is a prerequisite for the progression of many solid tumors. Migration and proliferation of endothelial cells which form new blood capillaries and lymph vessels is stimulated by several factors secreted by tumor cells and reactive stroma, such as VEGFs, PDGF, and certain FGFs. Recent evidence indicates that the changes in gene expression during tumor invasion are contingent on an overall activation of protein synthesis in tumor as well as stromal cells evident as an increase in expression of translation initiation factors and phosphorylation of translational proteins.

Paracrine interactions between tumor and stromal cells are copious in carcinomas. At least during early progression stages, carcinoma cells may still depend to a large extent on growth factors from the stroma for their survival and proliferation. In turn, carcinoma cells stimulate production of growth factors from the stroma acting on carcinoma cells, stromal, immune and endothelial cells. Moreover, tumor cells secrete factors like TGFβ which stimulate proliferation of connective tissue cells, but inhibit lymphocytes.

Interactions with stromal cells are probably even more crucial in the establishment of metastases. While tissues with microcapillary systems, such as liver, lung, and bone, are obviously preferred targets for metastases for mechanical reasons, the actual pattern of metastases does not only depend on mechanical and anatomical factors. Rather, to survive and expand, metastatic tumor cells need to set up mutual interactions with stromal cells in the target tissue. This is the molecular basis of the '*seed-and-soil*' hypothesis.

Primary tumors and metastasizing tumor cells are potential targets of the immune system. Multiple mechanisms limit its ability to eliminate tumor cells. They comprise production of inhibitory cytokines, down-regulation of recognition molecules and of death receptors used by cytotoxic immune cells and even active counterattack by expression of death receptor ligands.

Invasion and Metastasis as Multistep Processes

Even more than tumor expansion as such, the extent of local invasion and distant metastasis determine the clinical outcome of cancers, especially in solid cancers like carcinomas. Invasion and metastasis can be regarded as multistep processes, where invasion towards a certain stage constitutes a prerequisite for metastasis. Each step requires and selects for certain properties of the tumor cells. Therefore, overall, metastasis may be a very inefficient process. While details vary, invasion and metastasis of a carcinoma in general can be roughly described by the following sequence of steps:

1. While the carcinoma proliferates and extends laterally and vertically within the epithelium, the tumor cells become less adherent to each other and to adjacent normal epithelial cells.
2. The underlying stroma becomes activated and inflammation may occur. The basement membrane which separates the epithelium from the underlying mesenchymal connective tissue is partly or completely destroyed.
3. The tumor continues its growth into the connective tissue. This is one of the more variable steps. Some carcinomas continue to grow as solid, coherent masses compressing the neighboring connective tissue or develop processes that spread into it, breaking up the *extracellular matrix* (ECM). From other carcinomas, small groups of cells or single cells split off and migrate into the underlying tissue, sometimes in an '*indian file*' pattern and sometimes as adherent clusters. These migrations, even by single tumors cells, involve remodeling of the ECM.
4. In fact, the invasion of stroma by tumor cells is not as one-sided as it may appear. It is accompanied by altered gene activity in stromal cells, with some changes promoting and others inhibiting

invasion. The type of stromal reaction may be one of the most important factors determining the ability of a tumor to metastasize. Often, cells of the immune system are attracted, by signals emanating from the stroma and from tumor cells. This can result in pronounced inflammation. Like the stromal reaction, the effect of inflammation is ambiguous; it may impede or promote invasion.

5. A critical step in invasion is reached when the growing or migrating tumor cells encounter blood or lymph vessels and invade them. Like the previous steps, this can occur by a tumor mass growing through the vessel wall into the lumen or by single tumor cells squeezing through the vessel lining. By this '*intravasation*' step tumor cells gain access to the circulation and can reach distal organs by '*lymphogenic*' or '*hematogenic*' routes. Gaining access to blood and lymph vessels is also not necessarily a one-directional process. Since many tumors induce angiogenesis, capillaries sprout from blood and lymph vessels into the direction of the tumor mass. Since these are often leakier than normal vessels, they may offer easier access to the circulation.
6. Independent of whether metastasis occurs, invasion may continue into further layers of the organ from which the carcinoma arises, through a tissue capsule, into surrounding adipose tissue and into neighboring organs. An important spreading route for some cancers, e.g. of the kidney, liver, ovary and pancreas, is through the lumen of the retroperitoneum or the peritoneum ('*transcoelomic metastasis*').
7. When tumor cells have entered into lymph vessels, they are transported to the filtering system of the local lymph nodes, where some may survive and start lymph node metastases. Cells from these metastases may eventually penetrate towards the main lymph vessels and eventually enter the blood by this route. Tumor cells or debris and signal molecules from tumor and stromal cells transported to the lymph nodes influence the immune reaction towards the primary tumor.
8. Tumor cells having entered into blood vessels can theoretically spread to any part of the body. However, they are larger than normal blood cells and are not well adapted for survival in a moving liquid. Survival in the blood to reach distant tissues may be limiting for metastasis.
9. To form metastases, carcinoma cells must exit from the circulation by '*extravasation*'. Most often, this appears to take place in organs

with microcapillary systems, such as the liver, the lung, the kidney, and bone. Because of their size, carcinoma cells (and certainly cell clusters) get stuck in capillaries. This is not sufficient, however, to establish micrometastases.

10. In the new tissue environment, carcinoma cells have to reattach to the matrix, survive, sometimes for extended periods, and eventually start to expand into micrometastases, which again can lie dormant for many years. After all the complicated previous steps, it may be surprising to learn that this step is by many considered the most critical, i.e. least efficient step in metastasis formation.
11. The final step in metastasis is the expansion of micrometastases to actively growing tumors. This requires establishment of a sufficient nutrient supply and interaction with a different type of stroma, often including once more induction of angiogenesis and further local invasion.

Although invasion and metastasis are such important processes in the course of cancer progression, they are incompletely understood. This is largely owed to their complexity, since at almost every step complex interactions between different cell types and extracellular tissue components are involved. In addition, the early steps of metastasis in humans can rarely be observed. Moreover, metastases specimens are not regularly available for investigation, particularly from carcinomas, since they are rarely treated by surgery. Therefore, much of our knowledge on this matter is inferred from experimental animal models, which are by themselves complex enough. At this stage, therefore, many individual factors involved in invasion and metastasis have been identified and selected interactions have been pinpointed. However, there are considerable deficits in understanding the relative importance of this factors and how they interact with each other.

One particular important issue is what drives the overall process of invasion and metastasis. Two alternative ideas are entertained. One hypothesis maintains that tumor cells acquire one property after another as they proceed through the steps outlined above. At each step (or at least at many), the best adapted tumor cells are selected from the numerous variants created by inherent genomic instability. The alternative hypothesis holds that the '*invasion* and *metastasis*' program is an inherent property of certain cancers that is expressed very early on in their development. This second hypothesis would predict that primary cancers are more similar to their metastases than to each other in their genetic alterations and gene expression patterns, and that primary cancers which metastasize show more similar alterations to one another than to those that do not. This has indeed been observed in some investigations using expression profiling methods, e.g. in breast cancers. Current opinion therefore leans towards the second hypothesis. Interestingly, and perhaps not unexpectedly, the most striking differences between metastatic and non-metastatic cancers were found in the gene expression pattern of the stromal rather than the tumor cells. The distinction between these two hypotheses is important for cancer diagnosis. The prognosis of a cancer can only be determined from a sample from the primary site, if the ability to metastasize successfully is reflected in molecular parameters of the primary tumor. It would be difficult, if the primary cancer was a mixture of cells with different abilities to metastasize and/or if this ability developed gradually.

Genes and Proteins Involved in Cell-to-Cell and Cell-matrix Adhesion

Epithelial cells adhere to each other and interact with each other through several types of contacts. Morphologically distinct and functionally important contacts include adherens junctions, gap junctions, and tight junctions (occluding junctions).

Occluding junctions seal epithelia and define the apical and lateral membrane compartments of an epithelial cell. Therefore, their loss in a carcinoma cell is associated with the loss of cell polarity.

Adherens junctions are arranged in a belt-like configuration (hence '*belt desmosomes*') between adjacent epithelial and are intracellularly connected to actin filaments. The proteins actually mediating homotypic interactions between adjacent epithelial cells are cadherins, of which E-Cadherin is a typical representative. Interaction between E-Cadherin molecules is Ca^{2+}-dependent. On the cytoplasmic surface of the cell membrane, E-Cadherin is linked to actin filaments by α-Catenin and β-Catenin. Down-regulation or mutation of E-Cadherin is frequent in human cancers and often occurs during tumor progression. In some invasive tumors, E-Cadherin is replaced by other members of the family with adhesion properties more suitable for a migrating cell, e.g. N-Cadherin. This is labelled a '*cadherin switch*'.

Spot desmosomes are connected to cytokeratin filaments in the epithelial cell by desmoplakin and plakoglobins. The actual contact between cells is again made by specialized cadherins.

Gap junctions also contribute to adhesion between cells, but primarily are communication channels that connect cells of the same type in epithelia or in other tissues, e.g. the nervous system. They allow the passage of small molecular weight molecules (≈1000 Da), in particular of cations such as Ca^{2+} and K^{+}, but also of other small signaling molecules such as cyclic AMP. Gap junctions are formed from one connexon in each partner cell, which consists of six connexin molecules. Different connexins are expressed in a tissue-specific fashion accounting for the specificity of the interaction. Gap junctions are temporarily closed, when cells separate from their neighbors for division. Closure is regulated by phosphorylation of connexins. Gap junctions are also sensitive to high Ca^{2+} levels and accordingly shut when cells become apoptotic or necrotic. In cancers, gap junctions become as a rule inactive during tumor progression and tissue-specific connexin expression is down-regulated.

In addition to adhering to each other, at least the basal cells in an epithelium are attached to the basement membrane. This contact is made through integrins which bind fibronectin and laminin in the extracellular matrix. On the cytoplasmatic side they are attached to actin filaments via α-actinin, vinculin and talin. Integrins are heterodimers consisting of each one α and β subunit. There are >17α - and >8β subunits in humans. A typical integrin of an epithelial basal cell is $\alpha_2\beta_1$. A specific integrin, $\alpha_6\beta_4$, is a constituent of hemidesmosomes. These also attach epithelial cells to the basement membrane matrix, but are attached to the cytokeratin cytoskeleton on the cytoplasmatic face. The composition of integrins is cell-type specific, and changes in migratory cells. For instance, cells of the hematopoetic lineage down-regulate their expression of $\alpha_4\beta_1$ integrin, when they have become differentiated and leave the bone marrow. Tumor cells often express different integrins than their normal counterparts. Down-regulation of integrins accounts, e.g., for the failure of chronic myelogenous leukemia cells to remain in the bone marrow sufficiently long for complete differentiation. In carcinomas, too, changes in integrin composition may be essential for invasion and metastasis, with some integrins favorable and others inhibitory for invasion.

Cell-to-cell adhesion and cell-matrix adhesion elicit signals within the cell, e.g. integrins through protein kinases like FAK, ILK, and SRC family tyrosine kinases that influence several pathways regulating cell growth and survival. In epithelial cells, lack of attachment tends to cause anoikis, a specific kind of apoptosis. Alterations in signaling as a consequence of altered adhesion in carcinoma cells must therefore be compensated. This may be the reason, why altered SRC expression is a common finding in cancers. Importantly, the ability to migrate is not simply acquired by loss of adhesive properties. Instead, cell migration requires a dynamic pattern of adhesion contacts that may overall be more complex than in a cell residing in a tissue.

A single cell migrating through a tissue needs to adhere to the extracellular matrix to just the right extent, i.e. sufficiently tightly to pull itself through the tissue, but not so tightly as to become unable to extricate itself. Moreover, if a net movement is to be achieved, attachments need to be established at a leading edge and be broken at a trailing edge by well-localized proteolysis, and cytoskeletal contractions must be coordinated. Localized activation of proteases at certain points on the cell surface is therefore a prerequisite for migration in a tissue. Some normal and tumor cells also move by a more amoeboid mode with less attachment and less activity of the actin cytoskeleton.

In fact, carcinoma cells more often migrate as cell clusters or cell files, or even expand like cell sheets during fetal development. These modes of migration nevertheless require reorganization of cell-to-cell adhesion and the cytoskeleton compared to cells in a resting epithelium. For instance, they may be accompanied by changes in the integrin isotypes and in the type of cadherin present. Some carcinomas also undergo a morphological change to a more mesenchymal phenotype, called an '*epithelial-mesenchymal transition*' (sometimes abbreviated as EMT). This allows them to invade and migrate as single cells, which is otherwise more typical of hematological and soft tissue cancers. However, cell-to-cell and cell-matrix adhesion remain dynamic in tumor tissues, as a rule, and the EMT can be reversible.

The course of E-Cadherin expression in the course of prostate cancer development illustrates the dynamic nature of changes in cell adhesion in cancers. E-Cadherin becomes down-regulated during invasion of prostate cancer cells into the stromal tissue compartiment, but is re-expressed in many metastases. A modulation of gene expression in this fashion is obviously more efficiently achieved by epigenetic than by genetic alterations. So, the promotor of the *CDH1* gene encoding E-Cadherin is hypermethylated in some carcinomas in a highly variable fashion that is associated with a variable expression of the protein.

In contrast, cancers with a diffuse-type growth pattern down-regulate specific cell adhesion molecules irreversibly. Again, E-Cadherin can serve as an example. Diffuse-type gastric cancer is characterized by highly invasive small groups of loosely adherent undifferentiated tumor cells. In this cancer type, E-Cadherin is regularly inactivated by mutation and deletion of the gene. In fact, germ-line mutations in *CDH1* are responsible for rare familial cases of this cancer.

Mutations in E-Cadherin are among the few genetic changes that specifically alter cell adhesion molecules in carcinoma cells. A much wider range of changes on the surface of tumor cells are achieved by epigenetic mechanisms. These include aberrant methylation of genes like *CDH1* and others associated with more or less strong down-regulation of expression. In other cases, up-regulation, altered splicing, or altered processing of cytoskeletal and membrane proteins are observed. Often, these changes in invasive tumor cells give the impression of a coordinated switch in gene and protein expression towards an '*invasion program*' rather than that of an accumulation of alterations in individual genes selected to yield an invasive phenotype.

Nevertheless, some among the myriad changes at the cell surface of cancer cells may be more important than others and may be decisive for invasion and metastasis. In particular, down-regulation of specific genes appears to be required for metastasis in certain cancers, although these genes do not influence the growth of primary tumors. Such genes have been designated '*metastasis suppressor genes*'. Most of them encode cell surface proteins, but some of them are protein kinases relaying signals from the cell surface, e.g. MEKK4.

For instance, KAI1 is a cell adhesion molecule encoded by a gene located on chromosome 11p12. Although this chromosomal region is subject to LOH in different carcinomas, the gene is never mutated or affected by promoter hypermethylation. Nevertheless, expression of KAI1 is down-regulated in many aggressive carcinomas.

Another gene in this category is CD9, which encodes a cell surface protein that sequesters EGF-like growth factors. Decreased expression of CD9 or KAI1 in primary tumors indicates a higher likelihood for the presence of metastases.

A more complex case is CD44. Like all proteins with the CD designation, it was first discovered as a lymphocyte surface antigen, but is expressed on many different cell types. It recognizes and binds to hyaluronic acid. In this fashion, it may function as an adhesion receptor directing lymphocytes to specific tissues. The *CD44* gene is spliced in several alternative ways. As a consequence, altered expression in carcinomas may take the form of outright down-regulation with promoter hypermethylation or that of expression of CD44 variants that could contribute to the '*targeting*' of metastatic cells.

Genes and Proteins involved in Extracellular Matrix Remodeling during Tumor Invasion

The structure of the extracellular matrix is generated by a backbone of fibrillar proteins and proteoglycans. This matrix is in a dynamic state. Structural proteins are synthesized by fibroblasts and other cells embedded in connective tissue. These same cells, together with cells of the immune system and from blood vessels, are responsible for the turnover of the extracellular material. Turnover and remodeling of the ECM are enhanced during inflammation and wound repair, as they are during tumor invasion. In fact, essentially the same mechanisms and enzymes are involved in each situtation.

The key enzymes among the many involved in ECM remodeling are proteases, and among these the *plasminogen activator* (PA) protease cascade and the *matrix metalloproteinases* (MMPs). These proteases degrade components of the basement membrane as well as proteins and proteoglycans of connective tissue extracellular matrix. They process other proteases and enzymes as well as growth factors and they liberate '*latent*' growth factors from their storage sites in the extracellular matrix. These growth factors then act on several different cell types, including or inhibiting proliferation or eliciting apoptosis in some cases. Among the factors that are activated in this fashion are FGFs (*fibroblast growth factors*), HGF (*hepatocyte growth factor*), and TGFβs. Obviously, proteins on cell surfaces can also be substrates.

The end result of the plasminogen activator cascade is localized activation of plasmin near the surface of specific cells. The inactive precursor of plasmin, plasminogen, is synthesized and secreted mainly in the liver and is present throughout the body. It is specifically cleaved to an active protease by plasminogen activator, abbreviated uPA (for '*urokinase-type plasminogen activator*'). The activity of uPA is localized to cell surfaces by its binding to a specific membrane receptor, uPAR ('*urokinase receptor*'). The uPAR in turn is localized on the cell surface by dynamic interaction with specific integrins. Thus, cell-type dependent expression of the uPAR is one mechanism of directing plasmin activity to a specific location. Plasmin activity is further localized by a dynamic association of the uPAR with integrins on the cell surface.

Conversely, the expression of *plasminogen activator inhibitor* 1 (PAI-1) prevents the cleavage of plasminogen and thus excludes plasmin from the environment of cells that express it. Furthermore, the protein protease inhibitor α_2-antiplasmin limits the activity of plasmin in the extracellular fluid in general. Plasmin is best known for its ability to digest fibrin, but it is also capable of digesting a range of ECM proteins as well as of cleaving and activating latent growth factors, pro-MMPs, and pro-uPA.

An even wider range of substrates can be digested by *matrix metalloproteinases* (MMPs). There are at least 23 members of the MMP family in man. Between them, they are able to degrade every protein in the extracellular matrix, although each MMP displays preferences for certain substrates. All MMPs have a similar basic structure with a Zn^{2+} ion essential for catalytic activity. Accordingly, compounds that complex Zn^{2+}, such as hydroxycarbamates or tetracyclines, are inhibitors, although often not specific for one member of the family. More specific inhibitors have been designed and have been tested in clinical trials.

As usual for proteases, MMPs are synthesized as proproteases ('*zymogens*'), and since most of them are secreted, they contain initially a signal peptide. The membrane-type MMPs differ from all others by containing a transmembrane domain at their C-terminal end. This locates them to the cell surface. Since pro-MMPs, mostly MMP-2, are among their substrates, they contribute to precisely localized protease activity, as would be required at the edges of a migrating cell or the growth cone of a tumor mass.

The MMPs are not only regulated at the level of activation from pro-enzymes, but also substantially at the transcriptional level. Their basal expression is cell type dependent and various factors induce their expression. These (depending again on the cell-type) include interleukins and growth factors of the EGF, FGF and TGFβ families, as well as stress and adhesion signals. Intracellularly, these factors act through one of the ERK, JNK, or p38 MAPK cascades which increase transcription by activating AP-1 factors at a conserved binding site in the gene promoters.

As for plasmin, specific as well as general protease inhibitors limit the activities of MMPs. MMPs are confined to local activity by ubiquitous protease inhibitors in blood and extracellular fluids, mainly α_2-macroglobulin and α_1-antiprotease. Moreover, they are restricted as well as directed by specific inhibitors, the *tissue inhibitors of metalloproteinases* ('TIMPs'). There are four members of this family, TIMP-1 through TIMP-4. They bind to the substrate-binding site of the MMPs, but cannot be cleaved by their catalytic centres. TIMPs also block the activation of pro- MMPs. The TIMP inhibitors are produced by a broader range of cell types than the proteases, and at least

TIMP-2 is often constitutively expressed. However, the expression of most TIMPs is additionally regulated at the transcriptional level. In general, the same factors that induce MMPs are involved, but additional cytokines such as TNFα as well as glucocorticoids and retinoids are active, at least in the regulation of TIMP-1.

It would be too simplistic to state that the activity of MMPs in a tissue depends on the relative levels of MMPs and TIMPs, for two reasons. (1) TIMPs exert a number of (not too well defined) effects on cells beyond inhibiting MMPs. TIMP-3, in particular, appears to act as a pro-apoptotic factor. It is accordingly down-regulated in many tumor cells, usually by promoter hypermethylation. (2) While antagonism between TIMPs and MMPs is the rule, there are clearly exceptions. One of the better defined ones is that TIMP-2 is a cofactor in the activation of MMP2 by membrane-type MMPs. This example illustrates the likely role of TIMPs in physiological tissue remodeling. MMPs are produced by specific cell types, but TIMPs by most others. This means that MMP activity is limited to specific sites within a tissue 'around' cells that perform the remodeling, while other cells remain protected. In fact, even the MMP activity 'around' an actively remodeling cell may not be homogeneously distributed, as particularly evident during cell migration.

The changes in protease and protease inhibitor expression taking place during tumor invasion must be considered on this background. In many human cancers, protease expression and activity are increased during tumor progression and invasion. Typically, mRNA and protein levels of several proteases are enhanced, e.g. of MMP-2, MMP-7, MMP-9, and MMP-14 as well as of uPA. Conversely, TIMPs tend to be down-regulated, most consistently TIMP-3. Enhanced expression of MMPs and of uPA/plasmin are almost generally associated with a worse outcome, i.e. primary tumors with increased expression are more likely to have metastasized than those with low expression.

The relationship between TIMP expression and tumor behavior is not as consistent. Whereas TIMP-3 down-regulation is often found in more aggressive cancers, decreased expression of the other inhibitors is not always predictive of a particular clinical course, and in some cancers the relationship is inverse. For instance, increased expression of TIMP-1 may indicate a worse prognosis in breast cancer. The explanation for this apparent paradox may lie in the question where precisely the proteases and the inhibitors are expressed. In many carcinomas, the increased expression of MMPs is found in the stromal part of the tumor. While tumor cells largely stain negative for many MMP mRNAs and proteins, often expressing only MMP-7, the stromal cells, fibroblasts and particularly invading macrophages and monocytes, express a full range of active proteases. Conceivably, in this situation, the expression of TIMPs may actually protect the carcinoma cells. This type of distribution of protease expression between carcinoma and stromal cells appears to be most pronounced in adenocarcinomas and other cancers arising from glandular structures, whereas other carcinomas, e.g. from squamous epithelia, express a wider range of MMPs themselves.

Thus, tissue remodeling during tumor invasion is far from a one-sided affair and in most cases requires an active contribution by the tumor stroma. This may be part of the explanation why an '*active stroma*' gene expression '*signature*' in expression profiling studies correlates with the presence of metastases.

Angiogenesis

As tumors exceed a minimum size, nutrients such as glucose and amino acids as well as oxygen can no longer reach their center by diffusion. Conversely, end products of metabolism such as lactate, ammonia and bicarbonate cannot diffuse out easily. In fact, this minimum size may be no more than a few cell layers in diameter, in the order of 70 μm. Beyond this size, primary tumors as well as metastases must lie dormant, disperse, or acquire a vasculature. During the progression of many tumors, the development of a vascular supply is a critical step designated as the '*angiogenic switch*'. In primary tumors, this switch often takes place during or as a prelude to invasion. In metastases, it may often mark the crucial transition from micro-metastases to actively growing tumors.

Most malignant tumors develop a vasculature by angiogenesis, i.e. the sprouting and proliferation of local capillaries. In some cases angiogenesis is supplemented by vasculogenesis, the de-novo-formation of blood vessels from hemangioblasts which are recruited from hematopoetic stem cell precursors. In other cases, tumors grow along existing blood vessels. In a few tumor types characterized by high cell plasticity, such as some melanomas and prostate cancers, cancer cells trans-differentiate into endothelial cells, forming '*tunnel-like*' structures themselves or contribute endothelial cells to capillaries formed by angiogenesis.

Like many other individual events during tumor invasion, angiogenesis is not restricted to malignant tumors, but also takes place during inflammation and wound healing. Angiogenesis is also a normal process in the cyclically growing tissues of females, most of all in the endometrium, and during tissue hypertrophy, e.g. in muscle. However, like tissue remodeling during tumor invasion, tumor angiogenesis is a less orderly and often deregulated process. It often results in relatively incomplete, leaky capillaries which allow tumor growth at the periphery with continued undernutrition and hypoxia towards the tumor center, to the extent of necrosis.

Angiogenesis starts by extension of normal capillaries which thereby become leaky and allow plasma proteins like fibrinogen to escape into the perivascular space. This contributes to the laying down of a matrix which is used by perivascular cells ('*pericytes*') to migrate into the tissue. Concomitantly, the basement membrane surrounding the vessel is degraded, a.o. by MMPs from activated endothelial cells and stroma. Endothelial cells then proliferate and the capillaries ramify extending into the surrounding tissue towards or into the tumor mass. While the proliferation of endothelial cells is transient during normal angiogenesis, it often remains permanent during tumor angiogenesis. Moreover, during normal angiogenesis, the newly emerging capillaries eventually become covered by pericytes and a vascular basement membrane once more, but this part of angiogenesis is not usually completed during tumor angiogenesis. Tumor capillaries also show irregular shapes and irregular orientations.

The irregular growth, shape and function of tumor capillaries compared to normal capillaries are likely consequences of the differences in which normal and tumor angiogenesis are regulated. Regulation of angiogenesis is achieved by a network of factors, some of which are pro-angiogenic and some anti-angiogenic. Their interplay is often depicted as a balance, which the predominance of one or the other sort of factors tilts towards or against angiogenesis. However, it needs to be considered that angiogenesis (like cell migration) is a spatially ordered process. In order to achieve proper angiogenesis, these factors must act in a spatially ordered fashion. So both the overall balance and the local balance are relevant. Some of the pro-angiogenic and anti-angiogenic factors are produced in a localized fashion. For instance, among the pro-angiogenic factors are FGFs, e.g. bFGF (FGF2), which are deposited in the ECM and liberated by proteases such as MMP-2 and plasmin. Conversely, several break-down products of matrix collagens generated by MMPs and other proteases, such as endostatin and arrestin, are among the most potent inhibitors of angiogenesis and limit its extent in normal circumstances. The disorganization of tumor tissue and tumor stroma may therefore constitute one factor causing the disturbances in tumor capillaries.

Table 10.1. Some important pro-angiogenic and anti-angiogenic factors

Pro-angiogenic	*Anti-angiogenic*
VEGFA, VEGFB-D	Thrombospondin (TSP1)
PDGF	Angiostatin (plasminogen fragment)
FGFs, particularly FGF2 and FGF1	Arrestin (collagen IV fragment)
Angiopoetins ANG1, ANG2	Canstatin (collagen IV fragment)
IL8	Endostatin (collagen XVIII fragment)
	Tumstatin (collagen IV fragment)

A second difference between normal and tumor angiogenesis concerns the growth factors involved. It is thought that most tumors do not provide a similar 'balanced' assortment of growth factors for stimulation of angiogenesis as found in normal tissues. Tumors secrete to various degrees FGFs, EGF-like factors, and PDGF, as well as the angiopoetins ANG-1 and ANG-2 and cytokines like IL8 that stimulate capillary sprouting and endothelial cell proliferation, or they stimulate the production (synthesis and release) of such factors from stromal cells. Inflammatory cells, in particular, secrete prostaglandins which promote angiogenesis. This is associated with an increase in the prostaglandin biosynthetic enzyme *cyclooxygenase* 2 (COX2).

However, the main factor eliciting angiogenesis in tumors is VEGF (*vascular endothelial growth factor*), which is over-expressed in many human cancers. So, in cancers the angiogenic growth factor '*cocktail*' may be biased towards VEGF, and assorted other factors like FGF1 and FGF2. In fact, there are several related VEGF genes, VEGFA through VEGFD. The VEGFC and VEGFD proteins are thought to be mainly responsible for induction of lymphangiogenesis by tumors. The VEGFA gene is translated into several different proteins, from alternatively spliced mRNAs. VEGFA proteins increase capillary permeability and endothelial cell proliferation, mainly through the VEGFR2 receptor tyrosine kinase expressed by endothelial cells. Some tumor cells also express VEGFR1 or VEGFR2, so VEGFs can additionally act as autocrine factors.

Enhanced expression of VEGFA in tumors can be a consequence of several genetic and epigenetic events. Some activated oncogenes, e.g. of the RAS family, induce VEGF expression. Conversely, TP53 down-regulates VEGFA and several other pro-angiogenic factors, at least under some circumstances, and also increases the expression of anti-angiogenic factors. Among the genes regularly induced by activated TP53 is *TSP1* which encodes thrombospondin 1, one of the most potent inhibitors of angiogenesis. So, several of the most consistent changes in human cancers, such as RAS mutations and TP53 loss of function would be expected to augment VEGFA expression and angiogenesis.

In normal cells, VEGFA expression is controlled by the oxygen partial pressure. Hypoxia leads to increased stability of specific transcriptional activators, designated *hypoxia inducible factors* (HIF). The accumulating HIF1α or HIF2β factors (which depends on the cell type) combine with a cofactor, ARNT (HIFβ), and activate the transcription of a set of genes that contain a specific binding element in their basal promoters. One of the most responsive genes is VEGFA. Constitutive activation of HIF factors by an inherited defect in their regulation is the cause of Von-Hippel-Lindau disease which predisposes to renal cell carcinoma and other, less malignant tumors. However, in many other cancers HIF activity is also elevated, typically as a consequence of hypoxia, and VEGFA is induced as a consequence.

As angiogenesis is such a crucial step in the expansion of many cancers and of their metastases, it may constitute an excellent target for therapy. This idea is particularly attractive, as the proliferating cells in angiogenesis are largely normal endothelial cells, which lack genomic instability. It is therefore less likely that they develop resistance to the treatment than actual cancer cells. Several inhibitors of angiogenesis have been used or are currently investigated in clinical trials, including physiological protein inhibitors of angiogenesis like endostatin and angiostatin, antibodies to VEGFA or VEGF receptors, and chemical inhibitors of the VEGFR, PDGFR, and FGFR tyrosine kinases.

Interactions of Invasive Tumors with the Immune System

As carcinomas spread beyond their compartment barrier provided by the basement membrane, they encounter cells of the immune system. These are attracted by chemokines and other signals emananating from the tumor stroma and from the tumor cells themselves. As a consequence, different types of immune cells, including macrophages, granulocytes, and various types of lymphocytes are found in the activated stroma of human carcinomas and even in between compact carcinoma masses. While the immune response to the tumor may indeed limit its growth, it is evidently overcome in advanced cancers, and in many cases its effect may even be ambiguous.

This is so because the presence of immune cells in tumor stroma and the tumor mass as such does not necessarily indicate an active response against the cancer cells, even though ample evidence indicates that immune responses against cancers are regularly initiated. In cancer patients, B-lymphocytes as well as T-lymphocytes are usually found that are directed against antigens present on the tumor cells. For instance, many patients with advanced stage cancers carry antibodies against mutated TP53 protein. Likewise, *cytotoxic T-cells* (CTL) and *natural killer* (NK) cells can be isolated from patients which specifically kill their tumor cells in vitro.

It is generally assumed that a cellular immune response, as opposed to a humoral response, is required for the successful rejection of a tumor. Tumor cell killing can be performed by cytotoxic T-cells directed against antigens presented by the MHC (*major histocompatibility complex*) and recognizing co-stimulatory molecules on the tumor cell surface. Cells that lack MHC expression or are marked by antibodies are, conversely, targets for NK cells. However, in vivo, these cytotoxic cells are often not successful in eliminating the cancer cells. While the reasons for this are not fully understood, several factors are known to be involved.

Table 10.2. Mechanisms limiting the immune response to cancers

Mechanism
Accessibility of the tumor mass to immune effector cells
Antigen presentation and cytokine secretion by professional antigen-presenting cells
Antigen presentation by tumor cells
Anergy of cytotoxic T-cells
Recognition of tumor cells
Efficiency of cell killing
Counterattack of tumor against immune cells

Accessibility

Compact tumor masses may not be well accessible to immune cells. In this regard, the insufficiency of its vascular system may work in favor of the cancer. In stroma-rich cancers, the stroma may provide a buffer against the immune response.

Presentation by Professional Cells

Tumor antigens are present on many cancers, but to be recognized by the immune system they need to be presented, best by '*professional*' antigen-presenting cells, e.g. dendritic cells. These do not seem to function optimally in many cancers.

Presentation by the Tumor Cells

Cancer cells may down-regulate proteins required for the processing and presentation of antigenic peptides, e.g. proteasomal proteins, the TAP transporter, or frequently the MHC itself.

Activation of T-cells

This may one of the most ubiquitous mechanisms, as many tumor cells, including cancer and stromal cells, secrete cytokines which limit the activity of cytotoxic T-cells. Conversely, cytokines activating T-cells such as IL2 may be lacking or be sequestered in the tumor milieu. Many advanced carcinomas, e.g., are themselves unresponsive to TGFβ, but secrete high amounts of the factor, which are liberated from the extracellular matrix and processed towards its active form by proteases in the activated stroma. TGFβ stimulates proliferation of stromal cells and the production of matrix proteins, but also inhibits the activation and proliferation of T-cells. This contributes to the characteristic '*anergy*' of T-cells isolated from actual tumor tissues.

Recognition of Cancer Cells

Down-regulation of MHC expression at the tumor cell surface diminishes recognition by cytotoxic T-cells. Cells with down-regulated MHC should be preferred targets for NK cells, but tumor cells might also downregulate receptors for NK cells like MICA and MICB, while retaining inhibitory KIR receptors.

Efficiency of Cell Killing

Cancer cells become resistant to the mechanisms by which T-cells kill, which is usually some form of apoptosis. For instance, many tumor cells down-regulate the FAS (CD95) death receptor which is activated by the FAS ligand expressed on the surface of cytotoxic T-cells, or express a soluble form that diverts the immune cells. Post-receptor defects like FLIP overexpression or Caspase 8 mutations may contribute, as might overactivity of the anti-apoptotic PI3K and NFκB pathways.

Counterattack

Tumor cells may not only contribute to anergy of T-cells, but even actively destroy them. For instance, some cancer cells secrete the FAS/CD95 ligand themselves and mount a counterattack towards the immune cells.

While the immune response towards the actual tumor cells is often blunted by these and further mechanisms, the presence of immune cells in the tumor and its stroma may contribute considerably to the destruction of the tissue. For instance, proteases secreted by macrophages and granulocytes destroy extracellular matrix, cytokines secreted by immune cells stimulate the proliferation of stromal and tumor cells as well as angiogenesis, and reactive oxygen species produced by macrophages may contribute to mutagenesis. The COX2 enzyme is thought to play a dual role in this regard, by producing prostaglandins and reactive oxygen at the same time.

The immune response is directed towards a tumor by several signals. Among the more important ones are chemokines. Chemokines are 8 - 20 kDa peptides, of which there are >50 in man. They are produced, e.g., by activated macrophages and granulocytes to attract further immune cells towards a site of infection or other tissue damage. It is therefore not surprising that chemokines are produced and secreted by stromal cells in many cancers. More surprisingly upon first thought is that cancer cells themselves also often produce chemokines, e.g., CXCL12. This chemokine activates a specific receptor, CXCR4, on the surface of immune cells, but also of hematopoetic and endothelial precursors. The receptor is also expressed on some cancer cells. So, production of CXCL12 may have several consequences, which in effect can favor cancer growth. (1) Attraction of immune cells may lead to tissue destruction favoring invasion and metastasis. (2) The factor may promote growth and survival of cancer cells expressing the CXCR4 receptor. (3) CXCL12 may promote the recruitment of precursor cells for vasculogenesis. (4) Activation of CXCR4 leads to strongly increased production of TNFα which itself may exhibit another array of effects.

Thus, like other normal physiological processes that are '*coopted*' during tumor invasion, the immune response towards tumor cells is distorted and often seems to be diverted towards promoting cancer spread instead of achieving its destruction.

Importance of Tumor-stroma Interactions

In the course of cancer invasion, therefore, several normal cell types, fibroblasts, endothelial cells, and immune cells are influenced by the actual cancer cells and in effect contribute to growth and spread of the tumor. It is now thought that the activation of stroma is in many cases rate-limiting for tumor invasion.

Similar interactions may be repeated during the establishment of metastases. However, there is one crucial difference in that during invasion cancer cells interact with essentially the same cells as their normal counterparts. Thus, interactions between tumor and local stroma may resemble those during normal tissue homeostasis and particular those during wound repair, although they are deregulated and distorted. However, during metastasis, cancer cells enter a novel environment. To expand into secondary tumors they need to activate this new environment, e.g., to provide nutrients and growth factors. The ability to achieve this interaction depends on both the cancer cells and their new environment. Such interactions may determine the sites of metastases more than anatomical relationships.

For instance, mammary cancers and prostate cancers have a propensity for metastasis to bone which appears to be determined by their ability to set up paracrine interactions with osteoclasts or osteoblasts in this tissue. Like many other aspects of metastasis, the precise relationships are not understood and are the subject of current investigations. Most studies are based on the hypothesis that metastasis is determined by an adequate interaction between tumor cells and target tissue. This is the current version of the '*seed-and-soil*' hypothesis which was proposed by Paget already in the 19th century.

One unexpected example of interactions between metastatic cancer cells and their target tissue concerns chemokines. Unlike their normal counterparts, carcinoma cells express receptors for chemokines, which typically become induced during a hypoxic phase of cancer development. Breast cancers tend to express the CXCR4 receptor for CXCL12. Its ligand is normally mainly found in lymph nodes, lung, liver, and bone, which are the preferred sites of metastasis for this cancer. Melanomas, in comparison, often express the CCR10 receptor. Its ligand CCL27 is predominantly expressed in skin. So, the unusual propensity of melanomas to metastasize to skin may not only be due to a '*natural*' affinity of melanocytes, but also to this relationship. Clearly, though, the presence of chemokines is only one factor of several preparing the '*soil*' for metastases.

Another subject of current investigation is the behavior of stroma during local tumor growth. As described above, tumor stroma is no longer regarded as a a passive medium invaded by the tumor, but as an active contributor to the success of tumor invasion. If so, genetic and epigenetic alterations in stromal cells might contribute to cancer growth, in addition to alterations in the actual carcinoma cells. Indeed, cultured senescent fibroblasts, as they may occur in tissue of older persons, secrete growth factors to which carcinoma cells, but not normal epithelial cells, respond. In similar experiments, fibroblasts from activated tumor stroma have been found to stimulate the proliferation of early carcinoma cells. In breast carcinomas, mutations of *PTEN* and *TP53* have been reported to occur in either stroma or carcinoma cells, in a mutually exclusive fashion. Such findings point towards a kind of vicious circle, in which mutations in the carcinoma drive alterations in the stroma that again promote the progression of the carcinoma, etc.

Yet another complication in this context is tumor '*mimicry*'. As carcinomas progress, they often lose markers of differentiation, including the cytokeratins typical of epithelial cells as well as cadherins, and cells change morphology. Some carcinoma cells, in vivo as in culture, assume a spindle-like shape which is quite similar to that of a typical mesenchymal fibroblast in the tumor stroma. This change, sometimes called EMT, is particularly frequent in cells that have lost expression of E-Cadherin and other epithelial adhesion proteins. By their morphology alone and even by staining for cytokeratins and other epithelial markers, these cells are difficult to identify as being derived from the cancer. Moreover, some tumors present with a stem-cell phenotype and can differentiate into several different cell types. This property is typical of certain '*embryonic*' tumors like teratocarcinomas and Wilms tumors. Nevertheless, '*mimicry*' of other cell types has been documented for a much wider range of cancers. So, tumor cells may appear as fibroblastoid components of stroma, as endothelial cells in tumor capillaries, or as osteoblast-like cells in bone metastases. This means that some cancers may not fully depend on recruitment of active stroma for invasion or metastasis, but generate it themselves by trans-differentiation '*mimicry*'.

11

MUTATIONAL ANALYSIS OF CANCER

DETECTION OF POINT MUTATIONS IN TUMOR DNA

In recent years, we have seen a dramatic improvement in our ability to detect nucleotide changes in tumor DNA using a number of techniques for mutation detection that have become routine instruments in many laboratories. The choice of a suitable method or methods of mutation analysis is governed by many factors, including the costs, experimental sensitivity, expected mutation pattern in the target sequence and its functional consequences, as well as staff expertise, personal experience, and preference. The primary selection criterion for such a method is the ability of a technique to search for the presence of unknown mutations in the analyzed regions (scanning methods) as opposed to looking for known mutations already characterized at the nucleotide level. Scanning procedures represent a cost-effective alternative to nucleotide sequencing, but usually at a price of an inferior detection rate. The former group of techniques includes procedures based on conformation polymorphism changes, denaturing gradient gel electrophoresis, constant denaturant capillary electrophoresis, and mismatch repair and RNase cleavage methods. The latter group, exemplified by techniques using sequence-specific oligonucleotides, oligonucleotide liagation assay, and ligase chain reaction, is less frequently used for analyzing molecular changes in tumor samples. A wise choice of most appropriate procedures is a crucial step for the identification of molecular changes underlying cancer development and for the correct interpretation of mutation screening.

Single-Strand Conformation Polymorphism Analysis

Single-strand conformation analysis (SSCP) is one of the simplest scanning techniques for detecting unknown mutations. Sequence variants usually exhibit differences in mobility of single-stranded fragments under nondenaturing electrophoretic conditions. Mobility shifts of DNA fragments result from mutation-induced changes of the tertiary structure of DNA. The term *polymerase chain reaction* (PCR)-SSCP refers to a PCR-amplified product analyzed by SSCP.

SSCP is particularly useful when searching for small deletions or insertions and single-base mutations and polymorphisms. Note that large insertions or deletions on the order of kilobases encompassing the amplified region are likely to go undetected.

Materials

Polymerase Chain Reaction

1. Template: high-molecular DNA or cDNA extracted from tumor/ normal cells.
2. *Taq* polymerase.
3. PCR buffer.
4. dNTPs.
5. Tested oligonucleotide primers.
6. Double-distilled H_2O.
7. α-^{32}P-dCTP or α-^{33}P-dCTP for isotopic detection.
8. Suitable restriction endonucleases, if the fragment size is too large for sensitive detection.
9. Formamide buffer: 95% formamide, 0.05% bromophenol blue, 0.05% xylene cyanol, 50 m*M* NaOH.
10. Thermal cycler.

Gel Electrophoresis

1. Gel electrophoresis apparatus.
2. Power pack.
3. Gel plates.
4. Combs.
5. Plastic film.
6. Filter papers.
7. Optional: temperature control of gel plates (water jacket, fans).
8. Acrylamide/bisacrylamide
9. Ammonium sulfate.

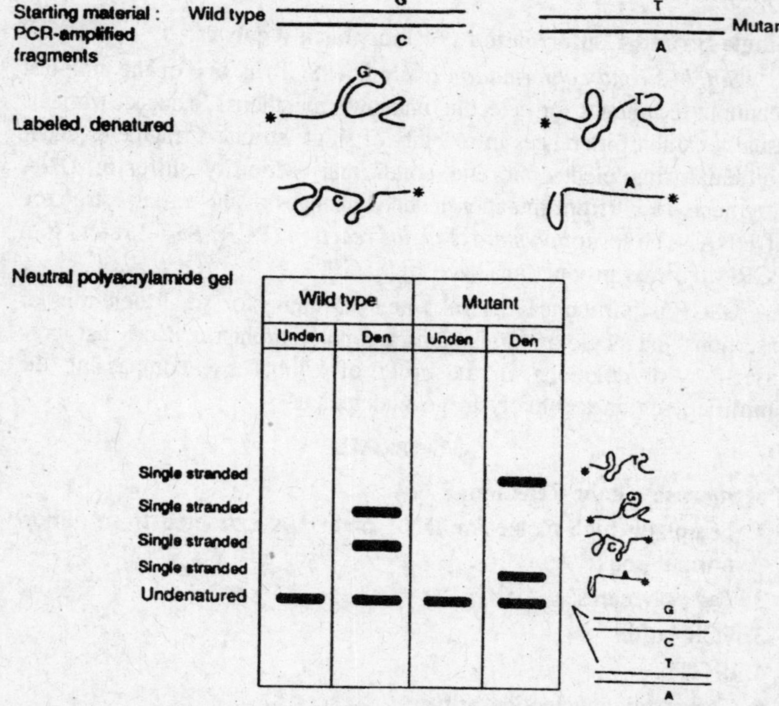

Fig. 11.1. The principle of single strand conformation polymorphism analysis.

10. TEMED.
11. Glycerol.
12. 10X Tris-borate EDTA (TBE) buffer: 0.9 *M* Tris-borate, 20 m*M* EDTA.
13. For isotopic detection of labeled fragments: Kodak X-OMAT films, X-ray cassettes, developer.

Methods

Polymerase Chain Reaction

PCR usually involves the incorporation of a label, either directly into the product or via an isotopically or nonisotopically labeled oligonucleotide primer. Alternatively, DNA fragments can be labeled after electrophoresis (e.g., by silver staining). The PCR should be tested using an agarose gel before running SSCP gels to determine whether the product is clean. PCR products with spurious bands should be avoided. A meticulous computer-assisted oligonucleotide primer design will pay off here.

A typical 100-μL PCR setup for direct isotopic labeling includes 10 μL of 10X PCR buffer (containing 1.5 m*M* $MgCl_2$), 5 μL of dNTP (2.5 m*M* stock solution), 5 μL of primer mix (final concentration 0.1–1 μ*M*), 5 × 5 μL of DNA (10–100 mg/μL), 0.5 μL of *Taq* polymerase (5 U/μL), approx 0.1–0.5 μL of α-^{32}P or α-^{33}P-dCTP (10 mCi/mL, 3000 Ci/mmol), and ddH_2O up to 100 μL. This amount is for at least five separate PCR reactions. A 20-μL reaction contains 5 μL of the template, which is convenient for dispensing multiple samples. The concentration of the labeled dNTPs depends on the sequence composition of the amplicon. After adding the enzyme-containing mixture to the template, thermal cycling should commence as soon as possible.

When using multiple samples, the amount of each template in the reaction tube should be the same. The usual amount of DNA per reaction is 50–100 ng. If the efficiency of PCR is markedly different from sample to sample (e.g., owing to the presence of enzyme inhibitors following DNA extraction from paraffin-embedded tissue), the template concentration should be further adjusted. However, loading different amounts of differentially labeled PCR products may result in altered mobilities of DNA fragments, and this may lead to difficulties in the interpretation of SSCP patterns. Different signal intensities from different samples are generally associated with a suboptimal detection rate, and every effort should be made to normalize the signal to allow the accurate evaluation of fragment mobility.

After completing the PCR, a restriction endonuclease digestion may help achieve a suitable fragment size for SSCP if the initial amplicon is too large. However, this extra step may be costly when analyzing multiple samples, and a subsequent complex SSCP pattern may be difficult to interpret.

Before running the electrophoresis, a formamide buffer is added in excess. No mixing is necessary before denaturing samples on a PCR cycler and loading onto an SSCP gel.

Gel Electrophoresis

1. Assemble glass plates for the gel.
2. In a beaker, mix the following components for a 100-mL gel solution: 5 mL of 10X TBE, 12 mL of 40% acrylamide/bisacrylamide (crosslinking 2.5%), 5 mL of glycerol, 1 mL of 10% ammonium persulfate, and ddH2O up to 100 mL.
3. Add 50 μL of TEMED and immediately pour into the gel plate assembly. Insert the comb and leave for at least 1.5 h to polymerize.

4. Remove the comb, clean the plates, assemble the gel, and fill the tank reservoir with 0.5X TBE. Check that there are no air bubbles in the gel, that the wells are undamaged, and that there is no leakage between the wells. Loading bromophenol dye to suspected wells is helpful for identifying leakages.
5. Denature the PCR products at 95°C for 5 min and load the wells. If the gel is run at room temperature, the applied power should not lead to an increased temperature of the plates. A thermometer attached to the plate is useful for monitoring the electrophoresis.
6. After completing the electrophoresis, transfer the gel to a sheet of filter paper, cover with Saran Wrap, and dry using a gel dryer. Expose the dried gel to an X-ray film for a few hours to overnight. Several exposures may be required for the correct reading of the autoradiogram.

Sensitivity of PCR-SSCP

The sensitivity of the PCR-SSCP method has been subject to controversy. Although the technique is generally believed to be efficient with the detection rate of >85% in a single run for fragments shorter than 300 bp, some previous estimates were lower. The sensitivity of PCR-SSCP depends on several factors, including the mutation pattern in the target sequence.

Since the higher-order structure of nucleic acids is dependent on the entire sequence of the amplified fragment, the sensitivity of SSCP in detecting a given variation will vary from one fragment to another. Unlike, e.g., denaturing gradient gel electrophoresis, there is no adequate theoretical model for predicting the three-dimensional structure of single-stranded DNA under a given set of conditions. Can we still say how sensitive our SSCP analysis is for a sequence of interest?

Because the tertiary structure of single-stranded fragments depends on physical conditions such as pH, ionic strength, and temperature, these factors are likely to influence SSCP patterns and need to be controlled. Although not previously endorsed, adding glycerol to SSCP gels was found to improve detection rate by reducing the pH of the Tris-borate buffer by the reaction of glycerol and borate ion. Temperature is a particularly important variable. If not controlled, an excessive running power may generate heat, resulting in the disappearance of mobility shifts. Optimized crosslinking and polyacrylamide gel concentrations are generally recommended.

The analysis of globin, *p53,* and rhodopsin mutations suggested that the type of mutation (transition vs transversion) did not play a major role in determining whether a mutation was detected by SSCP analysis. Although the position of the base substitutions was found to be more important than the type of base substitution, it appears that the sequence flanking mutated residues plays an even more significant role. Although the sensitivity was found to vary dramatically with the size of the DNA fragments analyzed, with the optimal size fragments for the detection of sensitive base substitution at about 150 bp, subsequent studies did not support such a steep decline in sensitivity. The blind quality control study of fragments larger than 450 bp reported a detection rate of 84%, an and even higher rate was found by running fragments between 300 and 800 bp in low-pH buffer systems. Since a single base change contributes to the tertiary structure in a larger fragment less than in small one, the probability of detecting a base change in fragments larger than 300 bp is generally considered to be lower than for optimally sized fragments.

The fact that a shift of a mutated fragment is detected under certain physical conditions led the authors to suggest the use of varying running conditions. This approach is warranted together with the use of complementary methods for mutation detection of single nucleotide changes, if a high or 100% detection rate is desired. The most commonly changed variables are polyacrylamide and buffer concentrations, use of an alternative gel matrix such as the MDE gel, and changing glycerol concentration in the gel.

In practice, however, the use of too thick gels, excessive amounts of loaded DNA (sometimes owing to insufficient labeling of fragments), inappropriate pH of the gel, a high voltage leading to gel overheating, and analyzing PCR products with spurious fragments are among the most common mistakes of inexperienced users. Each of these factors drastically affects the sensitivity of detection of conformational changes in single-strand fragments. These may have been reasons behind a controversy in the estimates of sensitivity. The sensitivity is generally considered to be very high if SSCP is performed using optimal conditions.

Mutation Analysis of ATM Using PCR-SSCP

The ability of PCR-SSCP to detect mutations also reflects the size of analyzed region. The analysis of multiple PCR-amplified fragments from large genes or genomic regions may decrease the sensitivity to an unacceptably low level.

We have partially addressed this concern in the PCR-SSCP analysis of the human *ATM* gene. *ATM* is deficient in patients with ataxia telangiectasia (A-T), a multisystem recessive condition with a high risk of developing lymphoreticular malignancies. The gene contains 66 small coding exons of the average size of 253 bp spanning about 184 kb of genomic sequence. Since the size of exons is suitable for SSCP analysis, all coding exons were individually amplified using oligonucleotides primed to the flanking intronic sequence.

By analyzing cDNA prepared from A-T patients, the mutation pattern in patients' germlines was previously found to be dominated by small insertions, deletions, and point mutations, whereas most mutations were private. Assuming that A-T patients had two mutated copies of *ATM* and all mutations were in the regions covered by the oligonucleotide primers, we could estimate the detection rate of our SSCP mutation assay at 70%. This figure may be an underestimate, if the assumptions are not met. Such an estimate, however, applies to the whole gene represented by 65 amplicons. The probability of detecting a mutation in an average PCR segment (approx 1√65 of ≅ the screened region) would be 65 0.7 0.995. Such a high detection rate is likely to reflect the mutation pattern found in the germline of A-T patients, dominated by small deletions, insertions, and point mutations, changes readily identified by SSCP. The detection rate is likely to be different when analyzing genes with a distinct mutation pattern.

As the majority of SSCP changes in the germline of A-T patients result in a premature termination of the ATM translation product, the protein truncation test, is an obvious method of choice for the identification of unknown A-T alleles in the germline. However, this test may not be the most appropriate for analyzing the same gene in tumor cells. By using the SSCP analysis of tumor DNA extracted from presentation samples of patients with sporadic T-cell prolymphocytic leukemia (T-PLL), a malignancy exhibiting phenotypic similarities to a leukemia seen in A-T, *ATM* was found to be mutated in about one-half of T-PLL cases.

A variety of techniques for mutation detection have now indicated that the gene is likely to be inactivated or mutated in most, if not all, T-PLL patients. The presence of loss-offunction mutations, frequent loss of the wild-type allele in tumor cells, and clustering of missense mutation in the highly conserved 3' part of the gene suggest that *ATM* functions as a tumor suppressor gene in the develoment of T-PLL. Although mutations have not been found in all cases, the detection rate using a single pass of SSCP was found similar to that in the germline of A-T patients, suggesting that the inactivation or mutation of *ATM* is probably an essential step among genetic alterations leading to T-PLL. Although the possibility of a predisposing heterozygote change could not be excluded in T-PLL samples with mutations identical to those previously reported in the germline (normal cells were not available), the vast majority of T-PLL cases contained mutations not previously found in A-T, suggesting somatic changes. The *ATM* mutation pattern in T-PLL was found to be markedly distinct from that found in the germline of A-T patients. While the frame-shift mutations predominate in the germline, most mutations in T-PLL tumor samples were missense mutations, a characteristic type of mutation in tumor cells.

Thus, although the *protein truncation test* (PTT) appears to be a method of choice for analyzing the germline changes with reported sensitivity similar to that of SSCP, PTT alone would be unlikely to detect missense mutations that characterize the somatic mutation pattern in the same gene in tumor cells. The PTT might even miss T-PLL alterations altogether. This case illustrates the need for employing a combination of wisely selected, preferably complementing techniques, particularly in the absence of our knowledge about the mutation pattern of the analyzed gene or genomic segment.

Negative results of PCR-SSCP mutation screening need a cautious interpretation. The absence of *ATM* mutations in a large number of breast cancer samples analyzed does not exclude the presence of mutations in this malignancy. However, it is unlikely that the gene would be frequently altered in breast cancer, certainly not to an extent similar to that found in T-PLL. No somatic *ATM* mutations have been identified so far in tumor DNA isolated from breast cancer, but, given a high population prevalence of breast tumors as compared to T-PLL, it is possible that this may be the case in a small proportion of breast tumors. To address this area of question, large sets of samples will need to analyzed.

SSCP is also sensitive in detecting mutations in mixed populations of cells containing normal and mutated alleles. A study of the *p53* gene detected mutations against the background of 85–95% of the wild-type allele, a figure sufficient to identify clonal changes in tumors containing a substantial proportion of normal cells.

In conclusion, PCR-SSCP is a rapid, simple, and cost-effective scanning method for mutation detection. It is particularly useful for the initial screening of optimally sized PCR-amplified fragments for point mutations, small deletions, and insertions. It serves well as an inexpensive method of choice for screening candidate cancer susceptibility genes and in situations in which the detection rate of mutation screening is not required to be absolute. If the expected mutation pattern is not known, a combination of suitable techniques discussed in this book should provide a more sensitive and specific tool for analyzing a growing number of cancer susceptibility genes and also more accurate estimates of cancer risk conferred by genetic alterations.

Mutational Analysis of Oncogenes and Tumor Suppressor Genes

Denaturing gradient gel electrophoresis (DGGE) was introduced 20 years ago as a gel system to separate DNA fragments. The seminal principle of this methodologic conquest was that DNA molecules were not separated according to size, as in conventional electrophoresis, but rather, according to base composition and sequence-related properties. Since then, the technology has been developed into a powerful, yet still challenging, method for detection of single base changes. In combination with *polymerase chain reaction* (PCR), it has been widely used by research and diagnostic laboratories in the analysis of cancer and inherited disease.

Why use DGGE at all instead of sequencing or more simple and straightforward mutation detection methods, in particular single-strand conformation polymorphism analysis? DGGE is advantageous for several reasons. First, DGGE has a very high mutation detection rate, close to 100%, provided that the experiment has been correctly designed. Second, the behavior of DNA molecules in denaturing gradient gels can be accurately modeled by computer, which may drastically reduce the need for empirical optimization. Third, the sensitivity of DGGE is high, allowing detection of a mutant DNA species present in a low proportion in a background of wild-type DNA (down to the 5% level by conventional ethidium bromide staining). Fourth, owing to the resulting physical separation between mutant and wild-type DNA, DGGE provides a simple means of enriching the mutant DNA for further analysis. Fifth, DGGE is highly flexible, meaning that multiple PCR products with different thermal properties can be analyzed simultaneously in the same gel. This is particularly useful in diagnostic settings in which one or a few DNA samples must be scanned for mutations in an entire gene.

Despite the obvious advantages of DGGE, two matters are important to consider before deciding whether DGGE is an appropriate method for a given application: (1) the design of PCR primers to generate amplification products that are suitable for DGGE analysis may be a cumbersome process that requires computer modeling and a certain degree of personal experience; and (2) once PCR primers have been properly designed, the method is simple to perform with a relatively high throughput. Hence, generally speaking, DGGE may be considered the method of choice when primers have already been designed, or when the number of samples to be analyzed is so high that it outweighs the work involved in the phase of establishment.

Principle of DGGE

DNA melting theory

In aqueous solutions kept at a temperature below 60°C, DNA takes a doublestranded, helical conformation maintained by hydrogen bonds between base pairs on opposite strands and stacking interactions between neighboring bases on the same strand. When the temperature is raised abruptly, the two strands come apart and take a single-stranded, random coil conformation. This helix–to–random chain transition is termed *DNA melting* and may also be induced by chemical denaturants. Because the forces holding a DNA helix include both base pairing and stacking interactions, the melting temperature (T_m) of a DNA molecule is determined by the overall sequence, not just the GC content.

When a DNA molecule is subjected to gradual heating, it melts in a series of steps in which each step represents the melting of a discrete segment, termed a *melting domain*. A DNA molecule may contain several melting domains, each consisting of 25–300 contiguous base pairs, with T_m values in the range of 60–85°C. The domain that melts at the lowest temperature is referred to as the lowest-melting domain; the most stable domain is the highest-melting domain. A base substitution or other type of mutation may change the T_m of the domain in which it resides up to 1°C.

Experimental system

The DGGE system elegantly uses the melting properties of DNA and the changes that mutations impose on these properties. A standard denaturing gradient gel contains a uniform concentration of polyacrylamide and an increasing gradient of denaturants, usually a combination of urea and formamide. An increase in denaturant concentration has been shown to be equivalent to a rise in temperature, and a gradient of denaturants hence simulates a temperature gradient within the gel. Because the concentrations of denaturant alone are not sufficient to provide DNA melting, the gel is immersed in a bath of electrophoresis buffer kept at a temperature just below incipient DNA melting, usually at 56–60°C.

When a DNA molecule with two or more melting domains is electrophoresed through a denaturing gradient gel, it initially moves with a constant velocity determined by its size. At a certain point in the gel, a level of denaturant will be reached that exactly matches the melting temperature of the lowestmelting domain. This domain will be destabilized, resulting in the abrupt formation of a partially melted, three-armed intermediate that moves with a very low velocity. Small shifts in the T_m of this domain induced by the introduction of base substitutions will cause the domain to unwind at different concentrations of denaturant and, accordingly, at different positions in the gel, providing the basis for physical separation between wild-type and mutant species.

When the highest-melting domain of a DNA fragment melts, the fragment undergoes complete strand dissociation, and the resolving power of the gel is lost. To overcome this limitation, a modification was designed that involves the attachment of a GC-rich sequence, usually called a *GC-clamp*, to one of the ends of the DNA fragment. The GC-clamp introduces a new highest-melting domain and works as a "*handle*" to keep the strands together. A GC-clamp is easily added by PCR using primers, one of which has been extended by a 30- to 60-bp GC-rich sequence at its 5' end.

In rare cases in which a mutation does not affect thermostability and, therefore, cannot be visualized as a mobility shift in a denaturing gradient gel, increased resolution may be achieved by analyzing heteroduplexes, i.e., hybrids formed between wild-type and mutant DNA molecules. Under appropriate conditions, heteroduplexes are formed when wild-type and mutant DNA fragments are mixed, heated to separate the strands, and then reannealed to allow a reassortment of the single-stranded species with their complements. Four different species are expected from such reassortment: wild-type homoduplexes, mutant homoduplexes, and two different heteroduplexes composed of one wild-type strand and one mutant strand. The formation of heteroduplexes is initiated during late cycles of PCR and can be driven to completion by subsequent heating and reannealing of the PCR product. Heteroduplexes are retarded in a denaturing gradient gel at a lower concentration of denaturant than the corresponding homoduplexes, presumably as a result of the instability caused by the presence of a non-Watson-Crick base pair (mismatch).

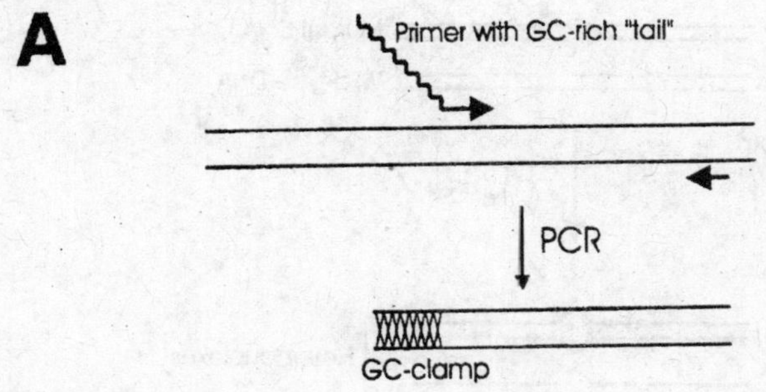

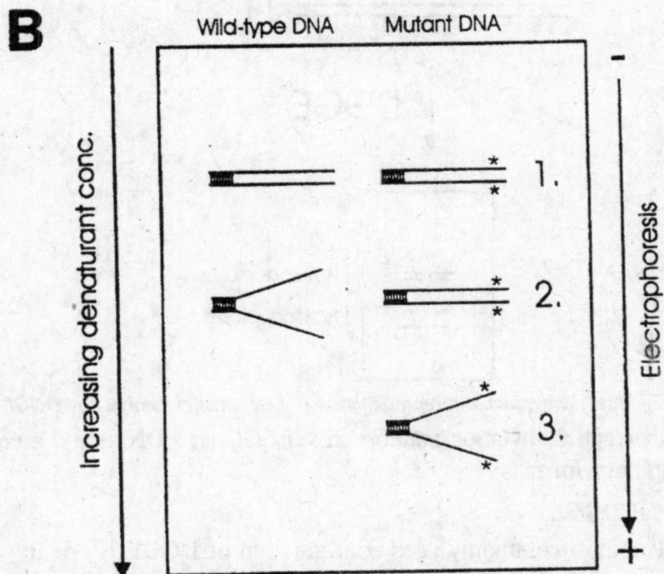

Fig. 11.2. Schematic representation of the principles of GC-clamping and resolution of mutations by DGGE. (A) PCR-mediated addition of a GC-clamp. (B) Resolution of mutations by DGGE.

Modes of Analysis

The principle of studying melting behaviors of DNA fragments in a denaturing environment for the purpose of identifying mutations has been taken into several methodologic variants. These variants include temperature gradient gel electrophoresis, in which a temperature gradient is maintained along the separation space, two-dimensional gene scanning, which is based on multiplex PCR followed by size separation in combination with DGGE; bisulfite-DGGE, for detection of mutations

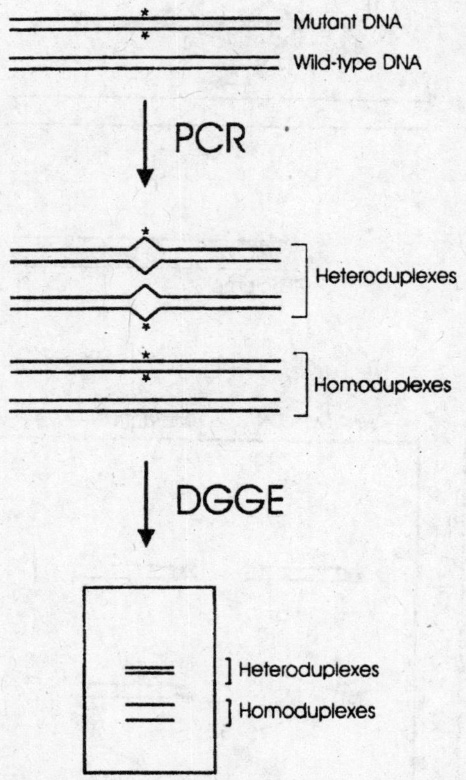

Fig. 11.3. Diagrammatic representation of heteroduplex analysis by DGGE.

and aberrant methylation patterns in very GC-rich DNA; and a variety of capillary formats.

Parallel DGGE

The most commonly used configuration of DGGE is one in which the gel contains a linear gradient of denaturants in the same direction as the applied electric field. In this configuration, a DNA molecule travels through an ascending denaturant concentration until it reaches a gradient level where its continued migration is severely retarded because of partial melting of the double helix. Loading in adjacent lanes allows analysis and comparison of multiple samples.

Perpendicular DGGE

Perpendicular gels contain a linear gradient of denaturant perpendicular to the direction of electrophoresis, and the sample is loaded in a single well spanning the entire width of the gel. In this configuration, a DNA molecule travels through a particular, unchanging denaturant concentration. The final pattern usually shows a single or multiphasic S-shaped curve, of which each steep part represents the melting of a domain. Perpendicular DGGE provides an experimental system to examine the melting properties of a DNA molecule. Although this may be valuable in the analysis of DNA fragments of unknown sequence, computer modeling is a simpler and more accurate approach to designing DGGE conditions for genes of known sequence.

Constant denaturant gel electrophoresis

Constant denaturant gels contain a uniform denaturant concentration corresponding to one of the steep parts of the profile observed by analysis of a DNA molecule in a perpendicular denaturing gradient gel. Electrophoresis at this concentration provides the optimal conditions for separation between fragments differing in nucleotide sequence in the corresponding melting domain.

Double-gradient DGGE

In double-gardient DGGE (DG-DGGE) analysis, the gel contains two colinear gradients: one of denaturant concentration and one of polyacrylamide concentration. The porosity gradient provides recompacting of homo- and heteroduplex bands, resulting in a considerable improvement in band focusing.

Broad-range DGGE

In broad-range DGGE, the gradient is typically 0–80% to accommodate different DNA fragments with a broad spectrum of melting temperatures. This approach results in considerable savings when looking for mutations in a particular gene in only one sample, but it depends on careful considerations when designing the experiment. In our laboratory, we have established DGGE conditions for whole-gene analysis for several oncogenes and tumor suppressor genes, including the *ras* genes, *p53*, *PTEN*, *Fas*, and *CDK4*.

Materials

Computer programs

MELT87 or MELT94, written in the laboratory of Lerman, can be used. These programs calculate the theoretical melting map of a known DNA sequence using the Fixman-Friere modification of Poland's algorithm for DNA melting.

PCR reagents

1. Standard PCR reagents.
2. *Taq* polymerase.

3. 5X PCR-compatible loading buffer: 0.04% cresol red, 60% sucrose.
4. Oligonucleotide primers, one GC-clamped.

Solutions

1. 50X TAE electrophoresis buffer: 2.0 *M* Tris-acetate, 0.05 *M* EDTA, pH 8.0.
2. Denaturant stock solution (0% denaturant): 6% acrylamide (acrylamide:bis = 19:1) in 1X TAE.
3. Denaturant stock solution (80% denaturant): 5.6 *M* urea, 32% (v/v) formamide, 6% acrylamide in 1X TAE.
4. Denaturant stock solution for DG-DGGE (70% denaturant): 4.9 *M* urea, 28% (v/v) formamide, 12% acrylamide in 1X TAE.
5. Photo-flo 600 solution.
6. 20% Ammonium persulfate.
7. TEMED.
8. Ethidium bromide (2 μg/mL) in 1X TAE buffer.

Gel equipment and thermoregulation

Gel systems can be commercially acquired from CBC Scientific or Bio- Rad, or they may be built from components from various sources. The system described next is routinely used in our laboratory and is based on a standard slab gel system.

1. PROTEAN II xi Cell. Modify the central cooling core by cutting out the central portion. This modification ensures uniform temperature in the gel when the electrophoresis cell is immersed in a temperature-controlled buffer bath.
2. Glass plates: 16 × 20 cm (inner plate) and 18.3 × 20 cm.
3. Spacers and combs (1 mm).
4. Glass or acrylic tank: approx 45 × 30 × 30 cm.
5. Immersion circulator that combines heating, thermoregulation, and stirring.
6. Two-chamber gradient maker and magnetic stirrer.
7. Power supply.
8. Polypropylene spheres.

Methods

Fragment design

The requirement for detailed theoretical considerations prior to PCR and DGGE analysis is at the same time the great advantage and a potential hindrance for routine use. Primer pairs have to be designed for both optimal PCR amplification and optimal melting behavior. To ensure appropriate melting temperatures of the primers, and to minimize self-complementarity and cross homologies, we recommend the use of a primer designer program. For simulation and modulation of melting profiles, the use of the MELT programs is invaluable. Although there are no strict rules that should be followed when designing experiments, and although mutations may be detected even under suboptimal conditions:

1. Aim at a fragment size of 150–350 bp (including GC-clamp).
2. Ensure that the entire sequence to be analyzed is contained within one lowermelting domain.
3. Avoid internal melting domains deviating by more than 0.2°C from the average domain temperature.
4. Ensure that the temperature of strand dissociation is higher than the melting temperature of the lower-melting domain of interest.

Melting profiles

The MELT programs generate the melting map for a known DNA sequence, i.e., a plot of the midpoint temperature at which each base pair of the sequence is in 50:50 equilibrium between the helical and melted configurations. Each melting domain of the DNA fragment appears as a horizontal line and is usually clearly demarcated from the adjacent domains on either side.

To determine the optimal position of the GC-clamp, add 40 bp of GC-rich sequence to either end of the fragment and recalculate the melting maps. The addition of a GC-clamp may have quite a dramatic impact on the melting properties of a DNA fragment, and it is not always possible to predict the optimal position of the GC-clamp solely on the basis of the melting map of the native DNA. If the unclamped end of the fragment has a lower melting temperature than the remainder of the lower-melting domain, include a short GC-clamp at this end to make the entire sequence behave as a single melting domain.

Length of GC-clamp

1. Using the MELT program, calculate for the 40-bp GC-clamped PCR product the temperature at which strand dissociation becomes significant, in practice the temperature at which log dissociation constant (*Kd*) is –5.
2. Increase the length of the GC-clamp until the temperature of strand dissociation is 0.5–1°C higher than the melting temperature of the domain of interest.

Polymerase chain reaction

As with other PCR applications, it is important that the PCR be optimized (e.g., by varying the annealing temperature and the concentrations of $MgCl_2$ and dimethyl sulfoxide). The inclusion of a GC-clamp does not appear to interfere significantly with the amplification process. Because only the GC-clamp remains double-stranded after electrophoresis, and because ethidium bromide stains single-stranded DNA only weakly, a considerable product yield is required. Unspecific bands must be avoided because they may be misinterpreted as evidence for the presence of a mutation.

Generation of heteroduplexes

Using a thermal cycler, subject the sample to a denaturation/reannealing program consisting of 95°C for 10 min, 65°C for 60 min, and 37°C for 60 min.

DGGE analysis

Preparation of gel

1. Clean glass plates carefully with ethanol and cover them with a thin layer of Photo-flo 600 solution to reduce surface tension. Assemble the gel sandwich according to the supplier's instructions.
2. From the stock solutions of acrylamide and denaturants, prepare two solutions of 14 mL each (for a 28-mL gel), corresponding to the two end points of the desired denaturant concentration range.
3. Add 50 μL of 20% ammonium persulfate and 6 μL of TEMED to each solution and mix by gently swirling.
4. Pour the two gel solutions into the gradient maker, ensuring that the solution of higher denaturant is poured into the mixing chamber. Avoid the introduction of bubbles by too vigorous mixing.
5. Open the valve interconnecting the two chambers and let some solution pass between the chambers to ensure that the connecting pipe is not blocked by air bubbles.
6. Open the outlet and introduce the gradient into the gel sandwich from the top by gravity flow or with a peristaltic pump.
7. Insert the comb gently and at an angle and let the gel polymerize for 30–45 min.
8. Remove the comb and immediately flush the wells carefully with 1X TAE buffer to remove unpolymerized acrylamide.

Running and staining the gel

1. Attach the gel sandwich to the central cooling core, fill the upper buffer chamber with 1X TAE buffer, and load the samples.

Immediately immerse the gel assembly into the temperature-controlled tank filled with 1X TAE buffer, and cover the buffer surface with polypropylene spheres to minimize evaporation. Apply the required voltage.

2. After electrophoresis, stain the gel in 1X TAE buffer containing ethidium bromide (2 μg/mL) for 10 min. Destain the gel in 1X TAE buffer if required.

Enrichment of mutant DNA for sequence analysis

1. Localize the mutant homoduplex band or one of the heteroduplex bands, and excise it from the gel with a clean scalpel.
2. Incubate the gel slice in 100 μL of H_2O overnight at 4°C.
3. Dilute the eluate 100-fold and 10,000-fold, and use 1 μL of the original eluate and 1 μL of each of the two dilutions as templates in three separate PCRs.
4. Analyze the amplification products by agarose gel electrophoresis, and use the product from the highest dilution as the template for the sequencing reaction.

Notes

1. In DGGE analysis of PCR products, polymerase-induced errors result in the production of mutant sequences that are physically separated from the correctly amplified sequences. Because the PCR-induced mutations are scattered randomly in the target sequence, the mutant amplicons will migrate to different positions in the denaturing gradient gel and result in a background smear. For detection of mutations present in a low proportion, the use of polymerases with low error rates may significantly reduce the background and improve resolution.
2. A considerable fraction of oligonucleotides synthesized by standard methods may be of incorrect length or contain nucleotide misincorporations that will be resolved in a denaturing gradient gel and result in a background smear. The number of errors increases with the length of the primer. Generally, we recommend that primers longer than 60 bp be ordered high-performance liquid chromatography- purified to be of the correct length.
3. When designing GC-clamps, avoid guanosine stretches and include a thymidine for every 20–25 bp.
4. Zero percent denaturant stock is acrylamide in 1X TAE buffer; one hundred percent denaturant is an arbitrary standard defined as 7 *M* urea (42 g/100 mL) and 40% (v/v) formamide.

5. Successful DGGE analysis depends on accurate temperature control within the gel. While the bath temperature may be set anywhere between 50°C and 60°C (depending on the melting temperature of the DNA fragment), the temperature must remain constant during the run. To avoid local temperature differences, it is important that the glass plates of the gel sandwich be in direct contact with the heated buffer on both sides, and that the buffer be constantly circulated by means of a stirring device.
6. We generally recommend that the maximum fragment length be set at 350 bp. Although DGGE has the potential to detect mutations in even longer fragments, the resolution of some mutations may be poor, the required running time may be inconveniently long, and the number of bases to be sequenced to finally identify the mutation may be inconveniently high. The fragment size must be more carefully considered when analyzing multiple different PCR products in the same gel.
7. The usefulness of DGGE for detection of mutations may be limited by the eventual occurrence of strand dissociation. The rate of strand dissociation (bimolecular melting) is determined by the equilibrium constant of dissociation at the temperature of migration arrest, which may be estimated by using the MELT program (not a facility of the commercially available MacMELT program). Detection of mutations is completely hindered if complete strand dissociation occurs at a temperature below that at which partial melting of the molecule takes place. The temperature of strand dissociation may be elevated by increasing the length of the GC-clamp. For most DNA regions with melting temperatures in the range of 60–75°C, a 40-bp GC-clamp (or even shorter) will be sufficient to prevent strand dissociation. For some sequences, however, the GC content is so high that strand dissociation cannot be prevented by means of GC-clamping. The use of a psoralen derivative to covalently link the strands may be a useful alternative for DGGE analysis of such GC-rich DNA regions.
8. Tumor specimens usually contain a mixture of cancerous cells and stromal tissue, implying that heteroduplexes will automatically be formed during PCR amplification of the target sequence. For analysis of tumor cell lines that often harbor mutations in the hemizygous constellation, it is recommended that cell line DNA be mixed with normal control DNA prior to PCR to ensure detection of all types of mutation.

9. The concentration of denaturant, x, at which a melting domain melts can be estimated by $x = (T_m - T_b)/0.3$, where T_m is the melting temperature of the domain, as determined by MELT, and T_b is the bath temperature. The choice of gradient range depends on the separation required; the narrower the gradient, the higher the resolution. Typically, a top-to-bottom difference of 30–40% denaturant centred above x gives satisfactory resolution.
10. Gels may be prepared the day before use and stored at room temperature or at 4°C.
11. The running time required for resolution of mutations may be determined by time travel experiments, preferably aided by the inclusion of control mutations. When the fragment has reached the position in the gel at which it partially melts, there will be a very small increment in migration depth, and bands will be well focused.

    For analysis of multiple different PCR products in the same gel, the running time is determined as the time it takes for all products to reach the positions in the gel at which they are retarded. For PCR products of 250–300 bp in length, typical running conditions in a 16-cm gel containing 6% polyacrylamide are 5 h at 160 V. For DG-DGGE, the running times are generally somewhat longer but much more flexible, allowing overnight runs (typically at 90–100 V) without loss of band focusing.
12. It is generally recommended that the buffer be recirculated from the tank to the cathode chamber of the gel apparatus to avoid changes in pH during the run. However, it is our experience that changes in pH do not reduce the quality of DGGE analyses in standard 5-h runs (at 160 V) or overnight runs (at 90 V).
13. If the proportion of mutated cells in a tumor specimen is very low, all mutant sequence will be used up in the formation of heteroduplexes during PCR. Therefore, the heteroduplexes must be recovered, in which the mutant DNA is present in a 50:50 ratio with wild-type DNA.

    If heteroduplex DNA is eluted from the excized gel slice, reamplified, and then subjected to another round of DGGE, all four duplexes appear, allowing recovery of the mutant DNA in a more or less pure form. For most sequencing purposes, this extra round of enrichment can be omitted because sequence analysis of heteroduplexes will be sufficient to identify the mutation.

Detection of Mutations in Human Cancer

Nonisotopic RNase cleavage assay (NIRCA) is an RNase-cleavage-based method for mutation scanning that detects mutations as double-stranded cleavage products in duplex RNA targets. A central requirement for NIRCA is the ability to produce large amounts of double-stranded target RNA by in vitro transcription of PCR products containing opposable T7 phage promoters. The target regions are amplified from genomic DNA or cDNA using forward and reverse primers with T7 promoters added to their 5' ends. The crude polymerase chain reaction (PCR) products are then converted into double-stranded RNA by in vitro transcription with T7 polymerase, in reactions containing high concentrations of all four ribonucleotide triphosphates. Transcription typically results in a further amplification of the target region of at least 20-fold.

After transcription, the reactions are heated and cooled to permit denaturation and hybridization of the complementary strands; mutations in the target region result in base pair mismatches in the duplex RNA, from hybridization of complementary wild-type and mutant transcripts. For heterozygous samples, the endogenous wild-type allele provides the reference strand needed to create the mismatch. For homozygous samples, wild-type and experimental PCR products are mixed before transcription to create the mismatches. After hybridization, the duplex RNA targets are treated with singlestrand- specific ribonucleases to cleave mismatches on both strands. The reaction products are separated by electrophoresis on native agarose gels and detected by ethidium staining. Experimental samples are scored positive for mutations if they contain smaller fragments that are not present in a no-mismatch control.

In the protocol described below, the assay is carried out by the sequential addition of reagents for transcription, hybridization, and RNase cleavage to a single tube containing the crude PCR product; no intermediate purification of the reaction products is required. Once the PCR step is complete, the turnaround time for obtaining the assay results is approx 3 h. Many recent reports describe the use of NIRCA for mutational analysis of genes involved in human cancer and other genetic disorders.

Mismatch Cleavage by RNases

Historically, RNase A from bovine pancreas was used for mutation analysis, but this enzyme is not ideal since it fails to cleave many mismatches and tends to generate a high background of nonspecific cleavage products. More recently, a bacterial ribonuclease (RNase 1 from *Escherichia coli*) and a fungal ribonuclease (RNase T1 from aspergillus) have been found to be superior to RNase A for mismatch cleavage. The mutation detection rate in NIRCA is maximized by treating the duplex RNA targets with a mixture of these two ribonucleases, which detect distinct but overlapping sets of mutations. The ability of RNase 1 and RNase T1 to cleave mismatches is dramatically increased by the use of a nonstandard reaction buffer containing intercalators and other components, which probably act on the substrate to increase the mismatch-induced helical distortion. A proprietary commercially available reaction buffer has been optimized for use with RNase 1 and RNase T1.

Sensitivity of NIRCA for Detecting Unknown Mutations

General considerations

Generation of detectable cleavage products using NIRCA requires cleavage of both strands of the duplex RNA target. The extent of cleavage of a given mismatch depends not only on its sequence but also on the context in which it occurs. Since any point mutation results in a change of two nucleotides (a base pair), each mutation generates two reciprocal mismatches, from hybridization of the wild-type sense strand to the mutant antisense strand, and from hybridization of the wild-type antisense strand to the mutant sense strand. In the basic NIRCA protocol described below, the two reciprocal mismatches are generated in a single transcription reaction, from heterozygous PCR products with opposable T7 promoters. The duplex RNA samples comprise 25% of each reciprocal mismatch and 50% of duplex RNA with no mismatch. Mutations can be detected as long as one of the reciprocal mismatches is cleaved to detectable levels. If one of the reciprocal mismatches is refractory to cleavage, the observed extent of cleavage in the mixture will be reduced. The likelihood of cleaving both reciprocal mismatches is increased by using a mixture of RNases with distinct cleavage properties (i.e., RNase 1 and RNase T1). In some cases, however, both of the reciprocal mismatches are refractory to cleavage, and these mutations will not be detected. Most microinsertion/deletion mutations are detected, but very long insertion/deletion mutations may be cleaved less efficiently, probably owing to failure to cleave the shorter strand.

Assessing the reciprocal mismatches in separate reactions

In cases in which one reciprocal mismatch is not cleaved as well as the other, the assay can be made more sensitive, but also more laborious, by assessing the reciprocal mismatches in separate reactions. In this case, each mismatch comprises 50% of the sample. To assess the mismatches in separate reactions, the two strands of the unknown sample must be separately transcribed; however, each strand of the unknown sample may be cotranscribed with the complementary wild-type strand. To cotranscribe only one strand of the unknown sample along with the complementary wild-type strand, experimental PCR products containing a T7 promoter on one or the other end are mixed with wild-type PCR products having the T7 promoter on the opposite end. The wild-type and unknown target regions are amplified in separate reactions, using appropriate primer pairs, where only one of the primers contains a T7 promoter.

Sensitivity for detecting mutations in mixed populations of normal and mutant cells

Patient samples obtained by routine methods frequently consist of tumor cells contaminated with normal cells such as lymphocytes, fibroblasts, and other stromal cells. The ability of NIRCA to detect mutations against a background of normal alleles has been assessed in a model system. In this system, a PCR product derived from a construct containing a 561-bp genomic fragment of the human *p53* tumor suppressor gene with a C > G transversion mutation was mixed with a wild-type *p53* PCR product in varying ratios, keeping the total amount of PCR product constant. These targets were assessed according to the standard NIRCA protocol, using a mixture of RNase 1 and RNase T1 for mismatch cleavage. Cleavage products resulting from the point mutation were detected when present at the level of 3% of the sample, i.e., when 97% of the sample consisted of the wild-type sequence. NIRCA has also been used to screen for *p53* mutations in bladder wash samples from patients diagnosed with bladder cancer. These samples typically consist of a mixture of tumor cells and normal cells sloughed off from the lumen of the bladder. Target regions of 561 bp (exons 5 + 6) and 765 bp (exons 7 + 8), which together account for 89% of all *p53* mutations reported in bladder cancer, were amplified and screened from each patient.

Materials

Store all reagents at –20°C unless otherwise noted. Enzymes should be stored in a nonfrost-free freezer.

PCR

1. 10X PCR buffer: 50 m*M* KCl, 10 m*M* Tris-HCl, pH 8.3, 1.5 m*M* $MgCl_2$.

2. dNTP stock solution: Mixture containing 2.5 m*M* of the sodium salts of each of the four deoxyribonucleotide triphosphates (dATP, dCTP, dGTP, TTP) in 10 m*M* Tris-HCl, pH 7.0.
3. Outer PCR primers: Mixture containing 5 μ*M* of forward and reverse primers for preamplification of the target region to be screened.
4. PCR primers with T7 promoters: mixture containing 5 μ*M*of forward and reverse primers, with the T7 bacteriophage promoter sequence added to the 5' end of each primer. The binding sites for these primers should lie within the region amplified by the outer PCR primers in item 3, if a nested PCR strategy is used.
5. Thermostable polymerase.
6. Distilled deionized water.

Transcription of the PCR product to make duplex RNA

1. 10X Transcription buffer: 400 m*M* Tris-HCl, pH 8.0, 60 m*M* $MgCl_2$, 20 m*M* spermidine HCl, 250 m*M* NaCl, 50 m*M* dithiothreitol.
2. rNTP stock solution: Mixture containing 2.5 m*M* of the sodium salts of each of the four ribonucleotide triphosphates (ATP, CTP, GTP, UTP) in 10 m*M* Tris-HCl, pH 7.0.
3. RNase-free distilled deionized water.
4. T7 RNA polymerase, 20 U/μL.
5. Hybridization solution: 50% deionized formamide, 25 m*M* NaCl, 5 m*M* disodium EDTA, pH 8.0.

RNase cleavage of mismatches

1. RNase digestion buffer.
   (a) Recommended: RNase digestion buffer. This buffer contains components required for optimal mismatch cleavage by RNase 1 and RNase T1.
   (b) Alternative: 50 m*M* NaCl, 1 m*M* disodium EDTA, pH 8.0, 10 m*M* Tris-HCl, pH 7.5. This buffer is mainly useful with RNase A.
2. 100X RNase 1 Stock Solution: 16.5 U/μL recombinent RNase 1 from *E. coli*. Recommended, RNase 1 Stock Solution.
3. 100X RNase T1 Stock Solution: 20,000 U/μL recombinent RNase T1 from aspergillus. Recommended, RNase T1 Stock Solution.
4. (Optional) 100X RNase A Stock Solution: 0.165 mg/mL of RNase A from bovine pancreas (approx 104 Kunitz units/mg protein), in 20 m*M* Tris-HCl, pH 7.5

Agarose gel analysis

1. Gel-loading solution: 3 *M* NaCl, 10 m*M* Tris-HCl, pH 7.5, 0.05% bromophenol blue, 10 μg/mL of ethidium bromide, 33% glycerol. Alternatively, High Resolution Gel Loading Solution may be used. This reagent may be stored at room temperature.
2. High-resolution agarose.
3. 10X Tris-borate EDTA (TBE): 0.9 *M* Tris-borate, 20 m*M* EDTA. Store at room temperature.
4. (Optional) Ethidium bromide stock solution: 10 mg/mL of ethidium bromide in distilled water. This solution may be stored at room temperature.

Equipment and supplies

1. Equipment for preparing and running agarose gels:
   (a) Horizontal electrophoresis box. Short, wide gel-boxes are most practical.
   (b) Power source capable of at least 80 V.
2. Ultraviolet (UV) transilluminator.
3. Gel documentation system. A digital charge-coupled device camera is recommended. Alternatively, results may be recorded on Polaroid film.

Methods

Amplification of target region

Amplify the target region, typically ranging in size from 0.5 to 1 kb, from unknown and wild-type control samples and incorporate T7 phage promoters at each end of the amplified products. The use of software for computer-aided primer design is strongly recommended for choosing the PCR primers. Reaction volumes can be scaled according to user preference; two microliters of PCR product is needed for each sample.

For a 50-μL PCR, combine the following components and amplify the target with 25–30 cycles according to standard protocols: genomic DNA or firststrand cDNA, 5 μL of 10X PCR buffer, 2.5 μL of mixture of forward and reverse primers, 2.5 μL of dNTP stock solution, water to final volume of 50 μL, and 1 to 2 U of thermostable DNA polymerase.

In vitro transcription of amplified target region

Transcribe the experimental and wild-type PCR products to make duplex RNA targets for RNase cleavage. Purification of the PCR products before transcription is not necessary, since the T7 promoter sequence in unincorporated PCR primers is single stranded, and therefore will not be recognized by T7 polymerase.

1. Prepare a transcription reaction master mix containing (by volume) 40% nuclease-free water, 15% 10X transcription buffer, 30% rNTP mix, and 15% T7 RNA polymerase. For each sample, 4 μL of transcription reaction master mix is needed. Mix thoroughly by repeated pipetting or by gently flicking the reaction vessel. Do not mix by vigorous vortexing. Spin briefly if desired.
2. Add 4 μL of transcription reaction master mix to 2 μL of each PCR product containing opposable T7 promoters. Mix gently but thoroughly.
3. Incubate for 1 h at 37°C.
4. Add 2 μL of hybridization solution to each reaction and mix briefly.
5. Heat reactions in a heat block at 95–105°C for 3–5 min. Remove the reactions and cool to room temperature (~5 min). Spin briefly if desired. This step permits complementary strands of wild-type and mutant transcripts to denature and reanneal to create the mismatches. Hybridization of the transcripts is very rapid owing to the high concentrations of the complementary transcripts and the low complexity of the reaction. If desired, the efficiency of the transcription reaction may be assessed at this point. Reactions may be stored at -20°C.

Treatment of hybridized samples with RNases

1. Prepare working solution containing RNase stock solution(s) diluted in RNase digestion buffer. The standard volume of RNase solution used for each sample is 24 μL. Standard RNase dilutions are 1:100 for each RNase. RNase 1 and RNase T1 are generally mixed in a single solution. Use RNase A alone owing to its greater tendency to cause overdigestion/nonspecific cleavage. The diluted RNase solutions may be mixed by gentle vortexing.
2. Add 24 μL of diluted RNase solution to each 8-μL transcription reaction and mix thoroughly. To conserve RNase digestion reagents, the reactions may be scaled down; for example, 4-μL aliquots of each transcription reaction may be removed to separate vessels (96-well U-bottomed microtiter plates are suggested) and treated with 12 μL of RNase solution. Microtiter plates must be covered during incubation to prevent evaporation.
3. Incubate the reactions for 30 min at 37°C.
4. Add 6 μL of gel loading solution to each sample and mix briefly.

Analyzing RNase cleavage products on agarose gel

1. Prepare a 2.5% high-resolution agarose gel in 1X TBE. Well capacity should be approx 25–30 μL. If desired, ethidium may be added to the lower buffer chamber to a final concentration of 0.5 μg/mL to improve staining of very small fragments (free ethidium runs in the opposite direction from nucleic acid, i.e., toward the cathode).
2. Load the reactions into the wells of the gel and run it at an appropriate voltage such that the dye band migrates approx 3 to 4 cm in about 30–45 min. Typically, this is achieved by running the gel at about 5 V/cm of distance between the anode and cathode, or at 80–90 V for short gel boxes. In the standard one-tube assay, the nominal final reaction volume is 38 μL, so there will be some sample remaining after loading. It is acceptable for the gel and buffer to become slightly warm, but not hot, during the run. The exact voltage, temperature, and duration of electrophoresis are not critical parameters. Restriction fragments of plasmid DNA (e.g., pUC19 cut with Sau3A) can be used as molecular size markers (the mobility of duplex DNA is very similar to that of duplex RNA on native agarose gels).
3. When the dye band has migrated about 2.5–3 cm from the well, transfer the gel to a UV transilluminator and examine it for the presence of cleavage products.
4. Replace the gel in the buffer and continue electrophoresis for about 10–15 min longer. Examine the gel again under UV light and record the results. Mutations in experimental lanes are indicated by the presence of smaller subfragments that are not seen in the no-mismatch (wild-type) control lane. When assessing results using a digital camera, the image may be electronically manipulated to aid interpretation of the data.

Notes

1. This step is often accomplished using a two-step nested PCR strategy. The firststep PCR uses genomic DNA or first-strand cDNA as template and forward and reverse primers with no extra sequences. The second PCR step uses an aliquot of the first-step PCR as template, and forward and reverse primers containing T7 promoters. The primer-binding sites for the second-step primers (or at least their 3' ends) are nested within the product amplified in the first-step PCR. The 20-base consensus T7 promoter sequence is added to 5' end of both the forward and reverse primers used

for the second-step (nested) PCR. The promoters are thus incorporated into the ends of the amplified target (this is analogous to adding restriction site sequences to the ends of PCR primers to yield amplified products flanked by desired restriction sites). The consensus T7 promoter is: 5' TAATACGACTCACTATAGGG. The last three bases of the T7 promoter (GGG) comprise the transcription initiation site, that is, these are the first three bases of the transcripts, and the 3' end of the T7 promoter may be overlapped with the 5' end of the nested primer binding site to reduce slightly the size of the nested primers. The size of the nested T7 primers is typically in the range of 35–40 bases. Keep in mind when designing primers that mismatches that occur very close to the ends of the targets may be difficult to detect, since the cleavage products will consist of one very small fragment and one large fragment very close in size to the full-length uncleaved target. For this reason, genomic targets are usually designed to contain a minimum of ~ 50 bp of intron sequence flanking the coding regions to be screened, and when large regions are screened as smaller contiguous subregions, the adjacent targets should overlap by at least 15% of their size. When screening long contiguous coding regions, a single pair of outer primers can sometimes be used to generate a product for several adjacent nested PCRs. Target regions are generally between about 0.5 and 1 kb, but longer targets have been used successfully.

It may not always be necessary to use the two-stage nested PCR procedure. In principle, a single PCR reaction can be done using primers containing the T7 promoter sequences. However, the two-step amplification strategy compensates for suboptimal yields owing to variation in the quality of the clinical/experimental samples and increases the specificity of the product when amplifying singlecopy sequences from complex mixtures (genomic DNA or total RNA). When screening for mutations in plasmids, virus, bacteria, mitochondrial genes, existing PCR products, or other high copy number, low complexity samples, a singlestep PCR step generally can be used.

2. If the experimental samples are known to be homozygous for the target region (e.g., when screening for mutations in X-linked genes from human males), 1 μL of the second-step experimental PCR product should be mixed with 1 μL of the second-step wild-type PCR product before transcription. When screening for somatic mutations in tumor samples, it is possible that mutations in

autosomal genes may be homozygous owing to loss of the normal allele (loss of heterozygosity). However, in cases of loss of heterozygosity, it is likely that the wild-type sequence needed to create the mismatch will be provided by contaminating normal cells present in the sample.

3. To assess the efficiency of the transcription reaction, run all or some of the reaction after the hybridization step on a native agarose gel. As a control, also run the amount of PCR template that will be carried over in the transcription reaction (the amount of PCR product in the transcription reaction after hybridization is 25% of the total volume). The amount of ethidium-staining material in the transcription reaction should be at least 10-fold greater than the amount of PCR product used as template. Any excess of one strand produced in the transcription reaction will be degraded in the RNase step and have no detrimental effect on the assay.
4. Optimal concentrations of the RNases for particular targets may be determined empirically. The need to optimize RNase concentration for particular targets is generally greater for RNase A than for RNase 1 and RNase T1. For A+U-rich targets or targets containing short A+U-rich regions, a reduction in RNase A concentration is usually required to prevent overdigestion. RNase 1 concentrations may need to be reduced when yields of duplex RNA are low or when screening very long target regions (>1 kb). To optimize the RNase cleavage step, a pilot experiment may be carried out on a small panel of samples containing a no-mismatch control and one or more samples with mutations. The samples should be treated with the RNase stock solutions separately and, if desired, with a mixture of RNase 1 and RNase T1. Use a range of RNase concentrations; for example, RNase stock solutions may be diluted 1:50, 1:100, and 1:300. Overdigestion is indicated by lack of all or most of the full-length duplex in the no-mismatch control, with samples running as diffuse smears. Overdigestion is more common with RNase A and RNase 1 than with RNase T1, especially if yields of duplex RNA target are low. Overdigestion with RNase A tends to generate discrete bands, whereas overdigestion with RNase 1 usually results in diffuse smears. Overdigestion with RNase T1 is rare. Some targets will show nonspecific cleavage products owing to cleavage at hypersensitive sites (e.g., A+U-rich regions). Nonspecific fragments are those seen in every sample, including the no-mismatch control, and their

presence is not indicative of a mutation. Underdigestion is suggested if there is no difference between RNase-treated and untreated samples. Typically, there is a reduction in the total amount of duplex RNA as well as a detectable background of diffuse nonspecific digestion products in RNase-treated samples, compared with untreated samples. This difference may be more pronounced for longer targets. If transcription was suboptimal, there will be very little duplex RNA, and the ethidium-staining material remaining after RNase treatment may consist of residual PCR template, which can be mistaken for uncleaved target duplex. To determine whether this is a problem, run aliquots of the RNase-treated no-mismatch control duplex, along with the amount of PCR product carried over in the reaction as a control. If the band intensities are equal, there is no duplex RNA in the treated sample, owing to poor yield of transcript or to overdigestion.

5. Short gels are more practical than long ones because less agarose is required and samples can be easily run off the end of the gel, facilitating reuse of gels. For convenience, a single standard-length casting tray (~22 cm long) can be used to prepare several gels, by spacing multiple combs along the length of the tray at intervals of about 5 cm. Teflon combs are recommended. Chilling the gel at 4°C before removing the comb may help prevent the wells from tearing. Scrubbing the comb with hot tap water and a scouring sponge immediately after removing it from the solidified gel will minimize the tendency for it to cause agarose debris in the wells the next time it is used. Any shards of agarose or precipitated TBE present in the wells should be flushed out with running buffer before loading the samples. To minimize tearing of the wells, run the gel on an UV transparent tray that can be lifted out of the gel box and placed on the transilluminator for scoring samples. The agarose gels generally can be reused for analyzing multiple sets of samples. Run the fragments from the previous experiment off the bottom of the gel at low voltage prior to reuse. The TBE running buffer should be changed fairly frequently, after about 2 h of electrophoresis per liter of buffer. If the dye band becomes diffuse during electrophoresis, the buffer should be changed.
6. The following considerations should be kept in mind when scoring samples:
   (a) Some targets will show nonspecific cleavage products owing to cleavage at hypersensitive sites, e.g., A+U-rich regions (this

is more common with RNase A). Nonspecific fragments are those seen in every sample, including the no-mismatch control, and their presence is not indicative of a mutation.

(b) Occasionally, there may be nonspecific fragments that comigrate with mismatch-specific cleavage products in experimental lanes. This is more likely to be the case when RNase A is used for digestion. Experimental samples should be scored positive if they contain subfragments that show a significantly brighter fluorescent signal under UV light, compared with similar-sized, and usually less distinct, fragments in the no-mismatch control lane.

(c) The closer the mutation is to the end of the target region, the longer the gel must be run in order to detect it. To rule out cleavage products larger than ~90% of full length, gels must be run until the dye band has migrated ~4 cm (or has run off the bottom of a short gel) and carefully examined for the presence of a doublet running at the position of the full-length fragment in the no-mismatch control lane.

(d) Large cleavage products may be obscured when the amount of full-length duplex is very high. In cases of exceptionally high yields of RNA, large cleavage products may be more easily detected by running a reduced amount of the reaction.

(e) Cleavage products of the same size that are seen repeatedly in multiple samples may be owing to common sequence polymorphisms. Mutations in experimental samples which are also heterozygous for polymorphisms can generally still be detected by the altered mobility of one fragment.

(f) Samples containing faint or poorly resolved cleavage products, barely detectable over background, should be reanalyzed in a blinded test. If they are scored "*plus-minus*" a second time, they probably contain mutations.

7. To improve detection of faint cleavage products in samples assessed using digital gel documentation systems, the image can be manipulated electronically. For example, exposure times can be integrated over longer intervals, gray-scale settings can be adjusted, and various filter options such as contour imaging can be used to make faint cleavage products more pronounced. However, to avoid false positives when electronically manipulating the image, it is important always to compare cleavage patterns of experimental samples with that of the no-mismatch control.

Mutational Analysis of the Neurofibromatosis

Neurofibromatosis type 1 (NF1) is a common autosomal dominant condition affecting approx 1 in 3500 persons. Individuals with NF1 have a small but significant risk of developing cancers, primarily derived from neural crest tissues, such as astrocytic brain tumors and malignant peripheral nerve sheath tumours. In addition, children with NF1 are at increased risk of developing malignant myeloid disorders, particularly a form of myelodysplasia termed *juvenile myelomonocytic leukemia* (JMML). Thus, NF1 may be considered an heritable cancer syndrome, a group of disorders characterized by an increased risk of developing primary cancers.

The majority of heritable cancer syndromes are caused by an inherited mutation in a single copy of a tumor suppressor gene. Tumor suppressor genes act to restrain cellular proliferation via several mechanisms including regulation of cell-cycle progression, signal transduction, and apoptosis. Classically, tumor suppressor genes behave in a recessive manner at the cellular level such that inactivation of both alleles is required for the development of a cancer. This phenomenon, referred to as Knudson's two-hit hypothesis, was first described in relation to the childhood tumor retinoblastoma. Here, a germline mutation of the retinoblastoma gene (*RB1*) confers a cancer predisposition and a subsequent "*second hit*" inactivates the other *RB1* allele, allowing the malignant clone to develop. Similarly, in NF1, individuals with a germline mutation of the neurofibromatosis type 1 gene (*NF1*) have a higher incidence of malignant neural crest tumors and JMML.

The importance of tumor suppressor genes, however, is not restricted to a small number of individuals with familial cancer syndromes. Somatic mutations of these genes are often sustained in sporadic tumors. For instance, the *TP53* tumor suppressor gene is the most frequently mutated gene in human malignancy. Other examples include the *APC* gene, inherited in familial adenomatous polyposis but frequently implicated in sporadic colon cancer, and *RB1*, which is involved in the pathogenesis of many small-cell lung carcinomas. Thus, the study of the genetics of heritable cancer syndromes has greatly enhanced our general understanding of the events resulting in tumor formation. This rationale led to our study of the *NF1* gene, in order to establish its role as a tumor suppressor gene in pediatric myelodysplasia in patients both with and without NF1. In common with other tumor suppressor genes, *NF1* has proved a difficult target for mutational analysis. *NF1* is a large gene, comprising a 12 kb mRNA that encodes 59 exons and a 327 kDa protein. Historically, conventional mutation detection methods including Southern blotting and single-strand conformation polymorphism analysis have proved relatively insensitive, detecting only 20% of *NF1* mutations in patients with an established clinical diagnosis of NF1. These problems are compounded by the fact that there does not appear to be a particular mutational "*hot spot*" in the *NF1* gene, and thus, it is necessary to analyze the entire coding sequence in the majority of patients with unknown mutations. Approximately 80% of documented *NF1* gene alterations are nonsense or frameshift mutations and would be predicted to cause premature translation termination with consequent truncation of the protein. For this reason, the in vitro transcription and translation technique (IVTT), also referred to as the protein truncation assay, has been successfully adapted for screening for mutations in *NF1*.

The protein truncation assay has been shown to be sensitive, detecting 67–70% of germline *NF1* mutations, and has a specificity approaching 100%. Because only truncating mutations are detected, there is no need for extensive investigation of rare polymorphisms in order to determine whether they are pathogenic. In addition, because total cellular RNA is used as template, detailed knowledge of the genomic organization of a gene is not necessary. Thus, the protein truncation assay has proved an efficient method for analyzing candidate genes for mutations in human disease. This approach has been successful in establishing the role of a number of tumor suppressor genes including *DPC4/SMAD4* in pancreatic malignancies and *PTEN/MMAC1* in a variety of tumors including primary glioblastomas.

The protein truncation assay was developed by two groups and originally was used for screening the dystrophin gene (*DMD*) in Duchenne muscular dystrophy and *APC* in patients with familial adenomatous polyposis. *Reverse transcriptase-polymerase chain reaction* (RT-PCR) is used to amplify overlapping fragments of the coding sequence; in the case of *NF1*, we and others have found that RT-PCR products of approx 2 kb proved optimal for analysis. The sense oligonucleotide primer is designed to encode a T7 RNA polymerase promoter sequence as well as a translation initiation sequence. Transcription and translation of the RT-PCR template can then be carried out as a coupled reaction, in a single tube, using a commercially available rabbit reticulocyte lysate mix to which a radiolabeled amino acid, such as ^{35}S-methionine, has been added. This enables in vitro synthesis of labeled polypeptides, which are then denatured and resolved by electrophoresis on a *sodium dodecyl sulfate* (SDS)-polyacrylamide gel. Truncated peptides generated from nonsense or frameshift mutations in the original coding sequence appear as additional smaller bands compared to the gene product of the normal allele. The size of the abnormal truncated protein may be estimated by comparison with a prestained protein marker; this allows the approximate position of the mutation in the coding sequence to be calculated.

RT-PCR product that gives rise to the truncated protein may then be cloned into a plasmid vector and dideoxy sequencing performed to confirm the putative mutation. However, a potential problem is that mRNAs harboring truncating mutations may be selectively degraded by various mechanisms such as exonucleolytic digestion. Consequently, this RT-PCR product may be under-represented in the cloning reaction compared with that derived from the normal allele. Binnie et al. have devised a strategy to circumvent this problem, which we have also used in our analysis of patients with *NF1* and myeloid disorders. Plasmid DNA is extracted from individual clones and subjected to a second round of IVTT. These polypeptides are analyzed by gel electrophoresis; only clones that are known to give rise to a truncated protein are then selected for sequencing. Because the position of the nucleotide alteration may be inferred from the size of the truncated peptide with reasonable accuracy (within approx 100 nt), appropriate primers can be designed, thus obviating the need to sequence the entire 2-kb RT-PCR product. We and others have found that this technique, termed second-stage IVTT, significantly reduces unnecessary sequencing of numerous plasmid clones that represent the normal allele.

In our experience, therefore, the protein truncation assay has proved an efficient method of detecting mutations in a large gene such as *NF1*. Obviously the quality of RNA extracted is crucial to the success of the assay, but we have used both fresh and frozen human blood and bone marrow mononuclear cells, as well as lymphoblastoid cell lines, with good results, despite the fact that *NF1* is not expressed at high levels in these tissues. We have also successfully adapted the assay to analyze candidate tumor suppressor genes in other hematopoietic malignancies.

Materials

Mononuclear cell separation

1. Culture medium: 90% RPMI 1640, 10% fetal bovine serum.
2. Density gradient: Histopaque-1077.

RNA preparation

1. TRIzol reagent (Gibco-BRL)
2. Chloroform.
3. Isopropanol.
4. 75% Ethanol in RNase-free water.
5. RNase-free water (add 0.01% diethylpyrocarbonate to distilled water in glass bottles, allow to stand overnight, and autoclave).

First-strand cDNA synthesis

1. SuperScript II RNase H-Reverse Transcriptase (200 U/μL).
2. 5X First-strand buffer: 250 m*M* Tris-HCl, pH 8.3, 375 m*M* KCl, 15 m*M* $MgCl_2$, supplied with enzyme.
3. 0.1 *M* dithiothreitol (DTT) (supplied with enzyme).
4. 25 m*M* dNTPs (25 m*M* each of dATP, dCTP, dGTP, and dTTP).
5. RNasin (40 U/μL).
6. Random hexamer $pd(N)_6$ (1 mg/mL).
7. Single-strand DNA-binding protein.
8. RNase-free water.

Polymerase chain reaction

1. 10X PCR buffer II.
2. 25 m*M* $MgCl_2$ (supplied with buffer).
3. 10 m*M* dNTPs (10 m*M* each of dATP, dCTP, dGTP, and dTTP).
4. AmpliTaq DNA polymerase (5 U/μL).
5. Single-strand DNA-binding protein.
6. Oligonucleotide primers (diluted to a concentration of 10 pmol/μL for each primer).
7. AmpliWax PCR Gem 100.
8. Sterile distilled water.
9. Perkin-Elmer 9600 thermocycling machine.

Agarose gel electrophoresis

1. 1X TAE buffer: 50X TAE buffer contains 242 g of Tris base, 57.1 mL of glacial acetic acid, and 100 mL of 0.5 *M* EDTA, pH 8.0; adjust to 1 L total volume with distilled water.
2. Ethidium bromide (10 mg/mL stock solution).
3. DNA-grade agarose.
4. 10X Gel-loading dye: 0.25% bromophenol blue, 0.25% xylene cyanol, 15% Ficoll-400.

5. *λHind*III DNA molecular marker (Gibco-BRL).
6. Distilled water.

IVTT reaction

1. TNT T7 coupled reticulocyte lysate system.
2. RNasin (40 U/μL).
3. EXPRE^{35}S^{35}S Translabel.
4. PCR-amplified DNA template.

Sodium dodecyl sulfate polyacrylamide gel electrophoresis

1. Reducing sample buffer: 10 mL of 1 *M* Tris-HCl, pH 6.8, 8 mL of 20% SDS, 4 mL of 2-β-mercaptoethanol, 8 mL of glycerol, 50 mL of sterile distilled water, 50 mL of 10% bromophenol blue.
2. 40% Acrylamide/bis solution (37.5:1).
3. Stacking gel buffer stock: 0.5 *M* Tris-HCl, pH 6.8. Dissolve 6 g of Tris in 40 mL of distilled water, titrate to pH 6.8 with HCl, and adjust the volume to 100 mL with water and a filter.
4. Resolving gel buffer stock: 3 *M* Tris-HCl, pH 8.8. Dissolve 36.3 g of Tris in 50 mL of distilled water, titrate to pH 8.8 with HCl, and adjust volume to 100 mL with water and a filter.
5. 2% Ammonium persulfate solution: Add 0.2 g of solid ammonium persulfate to 10 mL of distilled water.
6. TEMED.
7. 10% SDS solution: Dissolve 10 g of SDS in 100 mL of distilled water.
8. Glass plates (20 × 20 cm) with 0.75 mm spacers.
9. Running buffer (Tris:glycine:SDS, pH 8.3): For a 10X stock dissolve 30.3 g of Tris base, 144.0 g of glycine, and 10.0 g of SDS and adjust the volume to 1 L with sterile distilled water.
10. Prestained protein marker.

Fixation and development

1. Fixative solution: 30% methanol, 10% glacial acetic acid (for 1 L add 600 mL of distilled water to 100 mL of glacial acetic acid and 300 mL of methanol).
2. (Optional) Entensify, solutions A and B.
3. Gel dryer.

Cloning into Plasmid Vector/Dideoxy Sequencing

1. Low-melting-temperature DNA-grade agarose.
2. 1X TAE buffer: 50X TAE buffer contains 242 g of Tris base, 57.1

mL of glacial acetic acid, and 100 mL of 0.5 *M* EDTA, pH 8.0, adjust to 1 L total volume with distilled water.

3. Ethidium bromide (10 mg/mL).
4. 10X Gel-loading dye: 0.25% bromophenol blue, 0.25% xylene cyanol, 15% Ficoll-400.
5. λ*Hin*dIII DNA molecular marker.
6. Distilled water.
7. GENECLEAN kit or other appropriate reagents for agarose gel purification of PCR product.
8. CloneAmp kit or other suitable plasmid cloning reagents.
9. 10X Annealing buffer for CloneAmp kit: 0.2 *M* Tris-HCl, pH 8.4, 0.5 *M* KCl, 15 m*M* $MgCl_2$.
10. Subcloning efficiency DH5α competent cells.
11. SOC medium: 20 g of bacto-tryptone, 5 g of bacto-yeast extract, 0.5 g of NaCl, and distilled water to 1 L; autoclave, and add 20 mL of 1 *M* glucose and 5 mL of 2 *M* $MgCl_2$.
12. LB agar plates: 10 g of bacto-tryptone, 5 g of bacto-yeast extract, 10 g of NaCl, distilled water to 1 L, and 15 g bacto-agar; autoclave, cool to 50°C, and add antibiotics containing 100 μg/mL of ampicillin and 50 μg/mL of Xgal.

Second-stage IVTT and dideoxy sequencing

1. LB medium: 10 g of bacto-tryptone, 5 g of bacto-yeast extract, 10 g of NaCl, and distilled water to 1 L; autoclave, cool to 50°C, and add antibiotics containing 50 μg/mL of ampicillin.
2. TENS solution: 1 mL of 50X TE, 2.5 mL of 10% SDS, 1 mL of 5 *M* NaOH, sterile distilled water to 50 mL.
3. 3 *M* NaOAc, pH 5.2: 408.1 g of sodium acetate, 800 mL of distilled water, adjust pH to 5.2 using glacial acetic acid, make up volume to 1 L with distilled water, and autoclave.
4. Absolute ethanol.
5. TNT T7 coupled reticulocyte lysate system, RNasin (40 U/μL), EXPRE^{35}S^{35}S Translabel.
6. (Optional) Sequenase Version 2.0 DNA sequencing kit.

Methods

Specimens

Five to ten microliters of whole blood in EDTA or a minimum of 1 mL of aspirated bone marrow cells in a heparinized container is required. The use of preservative-free heparin is preferable. Specimens should be shipped at room temperature overnight, and cell separation ideally should be performed as soon as possible following receipt of the specimen. Frozen blood or bone marrow samples may also be used for RNA preparation; vials should contain at least 1 × 10^7 mononuclear cells and be thawed rapidly at 37°C to prevent degradation by RNases.

Mononuclear cell separation

1. Add an equal volume of culture medium to whole peripheral blood in a conical polypropylene tube. Dilute 1 vol of bone marrow with 3 vol of medium.
2. Carefully layer diluted whole blood or bone marrow onto an equal volume of Histopaque-1077 in a conical polypropylene tube, to avoid disturbing the interface.
3. Centrifuge at 2000*g* for 20 min at room temperature.
4. Using a Pasteur pipet, carefully aspirate the opaque interface ("*buffy coat*") into a clean 15-mL conical tube. Add medium to 10 mL. Centrifuge at 1000*g* for 7 min.
5. Aspirate off the supernatant and resuspend the cell pellet in 1 mL of medium. Count the cells. Cells not intended for immediate use should be frozen in an appropriate medium and stored in liquid nitrogen.

Preparation of RNA

RNA is prepared using TRIzol reagent according to the manufacturer's instructions, with minor modifications.

1. After counting, pellet the cells by centrifugation. Aspirate off the supernatant.
2. Add 1 mL of TRIzol reagent per 1 × 10^7 cells in a polypropylene tube. Using a syringe and a 25-gauge needle, aspirate the cells and TRIzol repeatedly in order to lyse the cells (seven or eight times is usually sufficient). At this point, the sample may be transferred to a 1.5-mL microcentrifuge tube if the required volume of TRIzol is 1 mL or less.
3. Incubate the lysed cells in TRIzol for 5 min at room temperature.
4. Add 0.2 mL of chloroform/mL of TRIzol and shake the tubes in order to mix the contents thoroughly. Incubate at room temperature for 2 to 3 min. Centrifuge at 4000*g* for 30 min at 4°C.
5. Aspirate off the upper aqueous phase and transfer to a clean tube. Avoid disturbing the interface, because this may result in contamination of the RNA preparation by DNA.

6. Add isopropanol to the aqueous phase (use 0.5 mL of isopropanol/mL of TRIzol used in step 2). Mix and incubate at room temperature for 10 min. Centrifuge at 4000*g* for 30 min at 4°C. The precipitated RNA should form a clear pellet at the bottom of the tube.
7. Aspirate off the supernatant and wash with 75% ethanol (use 1 mL of ethanol/mL of TRIzol used in step 2). Briefly vortex to expose the pellet to ethanol, and centrifuge at 4000*g* for 10 min.
8. Remove the supernatant and air-dry the RNA pellet for 10 min to allow any remaining ethanol to evaporate. Dissolve the pellet in an appropriate volume of RNase-free water; incubating the solution in a 55°C water bath for 10 min will facilitate this.
9. Determine the concentration of RNA in solution using a spectrophotometer at A_{260}. One A_{260} unit of single-stranded RNA corresponds to a concentration of 40 μg/mL. Pure RNA preparations should have an A_{260}:A_{280} ratio of 2.0. RNA should be stored at –70°C to prevent degradation.

First-strand cDNA synthesis

1. Add 1 μL of random hexamers (1 mg/mL of $pd(N)_6$) to an RNase-free 500-μL microcentrifuge tube, together with a volume of RNA constituting between 3 and 5 μg (to a maximum volume of 11.5 μL). Add RNase-free water to bring the total volume to 12.5 μL.
2. Incubate at 70°C for 10 min. Quench the reaction on ice for 2 min. Briefly spin and set back on ice.
3. To each tube, add 5 μL of first-strand buffer, 2 μL of 0.1 *M* DTT, 1 μL of 25 m*M* dNTPs, 0.5 μL of RNasin (40 U/μL), 1 μL of single-strand DNA-binding protein (0.5 mg/mL), and 1.5 μL of RNase-free water.
4. Add 1.5 μL of SuperScript II RNase H-Reverse Transcriptase (200 U/μL) to each tube and incubate at 37°C for 1 h. The total reaction volume should equal 25 μL.
5. Inactivate enzymes by heating to 65°C for 10 min.
6. Store synthesized cDNA at –20°C.

Polymerase chain reaction

1. Aliquot the following into a sterile 200-μL tube for each PCR reaction (total volume of 40 μL): 2 μL of first-strand cDNA template, 4 μL of 10X PCR buffer II, 3.2 μL of 25 m*M* $MgCl_2$, 1 μL of 10 m*M* dNTPs, 3 μL of forward primer (10 pmol/μL), 3

μL of reverse primer (10 pmol/μL), and 23.8 μL of sterile distilled water. A master mix using $n + 1$ (in which n is the number of samples to be analyzed) volumes of these reagents (excluding template) may be made.

2. Add one AmpliWax PCR Gem 100 to each tube, apply the caps, and incubate at 80°C for 5 min. Cool to 25°C for 10 min. Step 2 should be performed in a thermocycling machine such as the Perkin-Elmer 9600 model.
3. Make up the top mix for the hot start PCR. For each reaction use (volume of 10 μL): 1 μL of 10X PCR buffer II, 0.8 μL of 25 m*M* $MgCl_2$, 0.5 μL of single-strand DNA-binding protein (0.5 mg/mL), 0.5 μL of AmpliTaq DNA polymerase (5 U/μL), and 7.2 μL of sterile distilled water. Again, a master mix using $n + 1$ (in which n is the number of samples to be analyzed) volumes of these reagents may be made.
4. Pipet 10 μL of the top mix onto the cooled AmpliWax gem taking care not to puncture the layer. Cap the tube.
5. Perform PCR amplification in a Perkin-Elmer 9600 thermocycling machine using the following conditions: initial denaturation step at 95°C for 1 min, followed by 40 cycles of PCR at 95°C for 30 s, 62.5°C for 30 s and 72°C for 90 s with a single final elongation step of 72°C for 10 min. Cool to 15°C.
6. Visualize the amplified PCR product in all the reactions by agarose gel electrophoresis. Use a 1% agarose gel and 1X TAE running buffer. Load 5 μL of PCR product plus 1 μL of 10X gel-loading dye and include a lane containing a λ*Hin*dIII marker in order to assess the size of the product. Run at 90 V until the dark blue dye front is approximately two-thirds down the gel.
7. Stain the gel with ethidium bromide. Visualize the DNA on an ultraviolet (UV) transilluminator and photograph the gel.

IVTT reaction

1. Add 2 μL of PCR product to a sterile 500-μL microcentrifuge tube.
2. For each IVTT reaction use 4 μL of rabbit reticulocyte lysate, 0.33 μL of TNT buffer, 0.16 μL of amino acid mix minus methionine, 0.16 μL of RNasin, 1.14 μL of ^{35}S *trans*-labeled methionine (equivalent to 10 μCi/reaction), and 0.25 μL of T7 RNA polymerase. Make up a master mix using $n + 1$ volumes of these reagents, in which n is the number of samples to be analyzed.

3. Add 6 μL of the master mix to the 2-μL aliquot of PCR product in the microcentrifuge tube. Pipet to mix taking care not to introduce bubbles into the reaction.
4. Incubate in a 30°C water bath for 1 h. Reactions may be stored at 4°C for up to 24 h prior to electrophoresis.

Sodium dodecyl sulfate polyacrylamide gel electrophoresis of IVTT products

1. Make an SDS polyacrylamide (12.5%) gel for protein electrophoresis using 20 × 20 cm glass plates with 0.75-mm spacers. Set the apparatus vertically.
2. For the resolving gel, mix 9.375 mL of 40% acrylamide: bisacrylamide (37.5:1), 3.75 mL of resolving gel buffer (3 *M* Tris, pH 8.8), 0.3 mL of 10% SDS, 1.5 mL of 1.5% ammonium persulfate, and 15 mL of dH_2O. Add 0.015 mL of TEMED, swirl briefly, and pour. Layer with 0.2 mL of isobutanol. Allow the gel to polymerize (20–30 min). Rinse off the isobutanol using distilled water.
3. Mix reagents for the stacking gel (1.875 mL of 40% acrylamide:bisacrylamide [37.5:1], 5 mL of stacking gel buffer [0.5 *M*Tris, pH 6.8], 0.2 mL of 10% SDS, 1 mL of 1.5% ammonium persulfate, and 11.9 mL of dH_2O). Add 0.015 mL of TEMED, swirl, and pour. Insert the comb. Allow at least 20 min to polymerize.
4. Make up 1X running buffer from 10X stock (Tris:glycine:SDS). Remove the combs from the stacking gel and construct a vertical gel apparatus. Pour 1X buffer into the upper and lower reservoirs. Flush the wells of the stacking gel thoroughly with 1X running buffer taking care not to disrupt them.
5. Aliquot 25 μL of reducing sample buffer into sterile 500-μL microfuge tubes. Add 3 μL of the IVTT reaction product to each tube. Heat to 95°C for 5 min and then quench on ice. Spin briefly to collect the liquid at the bottom of the tubes and replace on ice. Load samples onto a 12.5% sodium dodecyl sulfate polyacrylamide gel electrophoresis (SDS-PAGE) gel immediately. A prestained protein marker should also be denatured and run on each gel in order to determine the size of any truncated protein product detected.
6. Run each gel at 30 mA of constant current until the dye front is close to the bottom of the gel. This should take approx 3.5–4 h.

Fixation and development of SDS-PAGE gels

1. Immerse the gel in a solution of 30% methanol, and 10% acetic acid for 30 min, preferably while gently agitating on a shaking table. Repeat.
2. (Optional). Enhance signal using an intensifying solution. Soak the gel in Entensify solution A, for 30 min, while shaking. Transfer the gel to Entensify solution B for 30 min, continuing to shake for the duration.
3. Affix the gel to filter paper and cover with cling film. Dry using a vacuum gel dryer at 65°C for 2 h.
4. Expose the gel to film overnight in a sealed cassette (less exposure time may be required if the signal has been enhanced). An in vitro synthesized truncated protein, if present, will appear as an additional smaller band compared to that of the full-length polypeptide.

Cloning into plasmid vector

1. Reverse transcriptase-PCR product, which gives rise to a truncated peptide by IVTT should be purified from an agarose preparative gel prior to cloning into a plasmid vector. A 1% low melting point agarose gel run in 1X TAE buffer is suitable. Run the remaining PCR product (approx 45 μL) plus 5 μL of 10X gel-loading dye and include a lane containing a λ*Hin*dIII marker. Stain the gel with ethidium bromide, visualize the DNA on a UV trans-illuminator, and excise the correctly sized band from the gel.
2. Purify the PCR product from the agarose prep gel using a suitable method. We use the GENECLEAN kit according to the manufacturer's instructions. Check the DNA yield on a 1% agarose gel.
3. Clone purified DNA into a suitable plasmid vector. We use the pAMP1 vector using the CloneAmp kit according to the manufacturer's instructions, with minor modifications. However, if this method is to be used, PCR primers will need to be designed accordingly. To 100–200 ng of DNA add 1 μL of pAMP1 vector DNA, 1 μLof uracil DNA glycosylase, 0.75 μL of 10X annealing buffer, and sterile distilled water to a total volume of 10 μL. Incubate at 37°C for up to 2 h.
4. Use 5 μL of annealing reaction mix to transform competent cells according to the manufacturer's instructions. We find that DH5α subcloning efficiency competent cells provide a satisfactory transformation efficiency.

Second-stage IVTT/dideoxy sequencing

1. Culture individual colonies overnight in 2 mL of selective medium (LB containing 50 μg/mL of ampicillin). Harvest the cells by centrifugation and prepare plasmid miniprep DNA as in step 2 or by a suitable alternative method.
2. Resuspend the cell pellet in 50 μL of supernatant. Add 300 μL of TENS and vortex. Add 150 μL of 3 *M* NaOAc, pH 5.2, vortex and spin in a microcentrifuge at 12,000 –15,000 rpm for 2 min. Transfer the supernatant to a clean tube, add 900 μL of ice-cold 100% ethanol, vortex, and spin at 12,000–15,000 rpm for 3 min. Pour off the supernatant, wash the pellet in 1 mL of 70% ethanol, air-dry, and resuspend in 30 μL of water.
3. Use 2 μL of plasmid DNA from step 2 as template for a second IVTT reaction.
4. Plasmid-derived IVTT products should be separated by gel electrophoresis and the gel examined to determine whether the resulting polypeptides comigrate with either the normal full-length or abnormal truncated protein. Only plasmid DNA giving rise to a truncated protein need be sequenced.
5. Perform dideoxy sequencing reactions using the Sequenase Version 2.0 DNA sequencing kit according to the manufacturer's instructions, or an alternative automated method. The size of the truncated polypeptide should first be estimated by comparison to a prestained protein standard. Oligonucleotide primers for sequencing may then be designed to anneal approx 100 nt upstream of the predicted mutation site and the exact nucleotide sequence of the mutation determined.

Notes

1. Regarding cDNA synthesis from a large transcript such as *NF1*, the use of random hexamers, as opposed to a gene-specific antisense primer or an oligo-dT primed reaction, appears to increase the efficiency of the reverse transcription step. In particular, we have found that this provides better representation of the 5' end of the gene. If IVTT is to be adapted for mutation screening of other genes, the method used for cDNA synthesis may need to be modified for optimal results.
2. Two exons of *NF1*, exons 23a and 48a, are known to be alternatively spliced. In some tissues or samples, greater representation of alternatively spliced isoforms is a potential source of confusion

when interpreting SDS-PAGE gels for the presence of truncated proteins.

3. Prior to embarking on second-stage IVTT and sequencing of RT-PCR products giving rise to a truncated protein, we have performed duplicate RT-PCR and primary IVTT reactions on the sample. This is done to reduce the possibility of sequence alterations generated by *Taq* polymerase error being misinterpreted as potential truncating mutations.
4. To minimize the possibility of error, we recommend confirming the presence of mutations found in cDNA sequence in patient genomic DNA. For *NF1* we used intron-based primers to amplify short sequences of genomic DNA for cloning and dideoxy sequencing. PCR products using these primers included the flanking splice acceptor and donor sequences, and in a number of our patients with NF1, this was the site of the mutation.
5. Other groups have documented the presence of abnormal RT-PCR products lacking part of the coding sequence and with breakpoints coincident with intron/exon boundaries. These products give rise to truncated peptides using IVTT, but the genomic DNA sequence from these patients is normal. They are thought to represent rare pre-mRNA species and should not be misinterpreted as mutations. We have not encountered this problem with the conditions described above for RT-PCR of *NF1* sequence. However, we have found it to be a confounding factor with other candidate tumor suppressor genes that we have analyzed. In this case, our approach has been to perform RT-PCR and IVTT on duplicate cDNA synthesis reactions from the same RNA sample. Since these aberrant pre-mRNA splicing products are rare, they are unlikely to give truncated proteins in duplicate reactions.

12

DNA Methylation of Cancer

The inheritance of information based on gene expression levels is known as epigenetics, as opposed to genetics, which refers to information transmitted on the basis of gene sequence. The main epigenetic modification in mammals, particularly in humans, is the methylation of cytosine nucleotide residue. Cytosine methylation occurs after *deoxyribonucleic acid* (DNA) synthesis, by enzymatic transfer of a methyl group from the methyl donor *S-adenosylmethionine* (SAM) to the carbon-5 position of cytosine. This enzymatic reaction is performed by one of a family of enzymes called *DNA methyl transferases* (DNMTs). This rarely discussed nucleotide is crucial for many biological processes, and its disturbance has been associated with the following diseases:

1. Autism, in which, in Rett syndrome, there are mutations in the methyl-binding protein MeCP2
2. Autoimmunity, in which patients with lupus suffer severe degrees of DNA hypermethylation
3. Neurologic diseases, in which the methylation of the fragile X mental retardation-1 (*FMR*) gene is the catalyst of the disorder of the same name
4. Atherosclerosis, in which protective cardiovascular genes are aberrantly hypermethylated
5. Immunodeficiency, in which patients with ICF (immunodeficiency, centromere instability, and facial anomalies) have mutations in a major DNA methyl-transferase

6. Cancer risk, in which germline variants of the methyl-metabolism genes affect DNA methylation patterns
7. Human imprinting, such as the aberrant methylation patterns in Beckwith-Wiedemann and Prader-Willi/Angelman syndromes
8. Animal cloning, as a result of which poor Dolly and her look-alikes have problems in establishing their appropriate DNA methylation patterns.

In mammalian cells DNA methylation occurs at the 5-position of cytosine within the CpG dinucleotide. Approximately 70% of the CpG dinucleotides in the mammalian genome are methylated, but the distribution of CpGs in vertebrate genomes is not uniform. Most of the genome is actually quite depleted of CpGs, a phenomenon termed CpG suppression. Most CpG sites in these areas are methylated during embryogenesis and remain methylated throughout the life span of the cells. By contrast, ~1% of the genome is composed of CpG-rich regions termed CpG islands. These CpG islands are usually unmethylated in all normal tissues and frequently span the 5' end (promoter, untraslated region, and exon 1) of a number of genes.

Methylation of promoter CpG islands is associated with a closed chromatin structure and transcriptional silencing of the associated genes. We can find certain CpG islands normally methylated in at least four cases: imprinted genes, X-chromosome genes in women, germline-specific genes, and tissue-specific genes. Genomic or parental imprinting is a process involving acquisition of a closed chromatin state and DNA hypermethylation in one allele of a gene (e.g., a growth suppressor gene) early in the male and female germline that leads to monoallelic expression. A similar phenomenon of reducing the gene dosage can also be invoked with regard to the methylation of CpG islands in one X-chromosome in women, which renders these genes inactive. Finally, although DNA methylation is not a widely used system for regulating "*normal*" gene expression, and we certainly have more complex and specialized molecular networks to achieve this aim, sometimes DNA methylation does accomplish this purpose (e.g., *MAGE* and *LAGE* gene families, the gene expression of which is restricted to the male or female germline and which are not later expressed in any adult tissue). A more polemic case may be postulated for the classical tissue-specific genes; some of them contain CpG islands, whereas others contain only a few CpG dinucleotides scattered throughout in their 5' regulatory region. Methylation has been postulated as one mechanism to silence these tissue-specific genes in those cell types where they should not be expressed. A well-characterized example of this type of regulation is provided by the methionine adenosyl-transferases 1A and 2A in the rodent setting. However, it is still not clear if this type of methylation is secondary to a lack of gene expression resulting from the absence of the particular cell type–specific transcription factor or is the main force behind the transcriptional tissue-specific silencing.

One question that remains to be answered is the significance of DNA methylation in areas outside the CpG islands. A possible explanation is that DNA methylation is used as a mechanism to repress parasitic DNA sequences. Our genome is littered with transposons and endogenous retroviruses acquired throughout the human history. These parasitic sequences, which account for more than 35% of the genome, can be controlled by direct transcriptional repression mediated by several host proteins; it is possible, however, that the main line of defense against expression of these sequences is inactivation through DNA methylation of their promoter regions. With time, this process has the potential to destroy many transposons.

Significance of DNA Methylation in Cancer

The phenomenon mentioned earlier changes substantially when cells become cancerous. Three major phenomena occur in cancer affecting methylation patterns: (1) there is an increase in the activity of the methylating enzymes in the malignant cells; (2) there is a global hypomethylation of the genome if we compare a tumoral versus a normal cells (this is mainly the result of a generalized demethylation in the CpGs scattered in the body of the genes); and (3) there are local and discrete regions that suffer an intense hypermethylation. Other epigenetic aberrations observed in cancer cells can be described as *loss of imprinting* (LOI) events; epigenetic lack of the repression of intragenomic parasites; and the appearance of genetic defects in chromatin-related genes. These are unique but interrelated features.

Global Genomic Hypomethylation

One of the first reports linking aberrant DNA methylation to cancer was published by Lapeyre and Becker (1979), who determined by *high-performance liquid chromatography* (HPLC) the 5-methylcytosine content from normal rat liver and hepatocellular carcinomas induced in rats by acetyl aminofluorene or diethylnitrosamine. The carcinogen-induced cancers displayed a decrease in overall genomic methylation of about 20–40% compared to normal liver. Presently, we know that the malignant cell can have 20–60% less genomic 5-methylcytosine than its normal counterpart. The loss of methyl groups is accomplished from various sources, but mainly by hypomethylation of the "*body*" (coding region and introns) of genes demonstrated, for example, in the cases of gamma-globin, gamma-cristallin, alpha-chorionic gonadotropin, *H-Ras*, and the *c-myc* genes and through demethylation of repetitive DNA sequences, which accounts for 20–30% of the human genome.

Three mechanisms can be invoked to explain the contribution of DNA hypomethylation to carcinogenesis: chromosomal instability, reactivation of transposable elements, and LOI. Undermethylation of DNA might favor mitotic recombination leading to loss of heterozygosity and promoting karyotypically detectable rearrangements. Additionally, extensive demethylation in centromeric sequences is common in human tumors and may play a role in aneuploidy. Supporting this postulate, it has been shown that murine embryonic stem cells nullizygous for the *DNA methyl-transferase* 1 (*DNMT1*) gene exhibit significantly elevated rates of genetic deletions and that patients with germline mutations in the other DNA, methyl-transferase (*DNMT3b*), have numerous chromosome aberrations. Hypomethylation of the malignant cell DNA can also reactivate intragenomic parasitic DNA: loss of methylation has been observed in L1 (*long interspersed nuclear elements*, *LINES*) and Alu (recombinogenic sequences) repeats in cancer cells. These and other previously silent transposons may now be transcribed and may even "*move*" to other genomic regions where they can disrupt normal cellular genes. Finally, the loss of methyl groups can affect imprinted genes. The best-studied case affects the *H19/IGF-2* locus in chromosome 11p15, where the disturbance of methylation may cause overexpression of an anti-apoptotic growth factor (*IGF-2*) and loss of a transformation-suppressing ribonucleic acid (RNA; *H19*) in certain childhood tumors.

Gene Hypermethylation in Human Cancer

CpG islands associated with tumor suppressor genes are unmethylated in normal tissues but often become hypermethylated during tumor formation. Growing evidence suggests that *de novo* methylation of CpG islands induces the silencing of associated tumor suppressor genes and may in fact be a critical step during tumor formation. The particular genes that are hypermethylated in tumor cells are strongly specific to the tissue of origin of the tumor. We have recently described a profile of hypermethylation among various primary human tumors; however, we do not currently know why some genes become hypermethylated in specific tumors and others, with similar properties (e.g., a typical CpG island), a history of loss of expression in other tumor types, and the absence of mutations remain free from methylation. We can hypothesize, as has been done previously with genetic mutations, that silencing of a particular gene may confer a survival advantage in some situations. The genes that undergo abnormal methylation in their 5'-CpG island in human cancer cover the whole spectrum of pathways involved in tumorogenesis from cell cycle and apoptosis to DNA repair and invasiveness ability. Tumor suppresor genes that contain highly methylated CpG islands in tumor cells affect cell cycle (*p16^{INK4a}, p15^{INK4b}, Rb, p14^{ARF}*), DNA repair (*BRCA1, hMLH1, MGMT*), cell adherence (*CDH1, CDH13*), apoptosis (*DAPK, TMS1*), carcinogen metabolism (*GSTP1*), hormonal response (*RARB2, ER*), etc.

Clinical Significance of DNA Methylation in Tumors

It is a growing hope that enumeration of the molecular alterations in cancer, particularly with respect to DNA changes, will lead to the development of new strategies for assessing cancer risk status, achieving the earliest tumor detection, monitoring prognosis, and instituting more accurate tumor staging along with the monitoring of prevention strategies. The detection of hypermethylated promoter region CpG islands may offer one of the most promising approaches to these goals. DNA methylation changes have been reported to occur early in the carcinogenesis and therefore are potentially good indicators of existing disease and even of risk assessment for the future development of disease. Four major cancer clinical areas can benefit from hypermethylation-based markers. They include neoplasm detection, tumor behavior, prediction of response to treatment, and therapies that target methylated tumor suppressor genes.

DNA Methylation as a Sensitive Biomarker for Tumor Detection

A delicate profile of CpG islands hypermethylation occurs in human tumors. The growing list of genes inactivated by promoter region hypermethylation provides an opportunity to examine the patterns of inactivation of such genes among different tumors. Usually one or more genes are hypermethylated in every tumor type. However, the profile of promoter hypermethylation for the genes differs for each cancer type providing a tumor type, and gene-specific profile. For example, gastrointestinal tumors (colon and gastric) share a set of genes undergoing hypermethylation characterized by *p16^{INK4a}, p14^{ARF}, MGMT, APC,* and *hMLH1,* whereas other aerodigestive tumor types, such as lung, head, and neck, have a different pattern of hypermethylated genes including *DAPK, MGMT, p16^{INK4a}* but not *hMLH1* or *p14^{ARF}*. Similarly, breast and ovarian cancers show methylation of certain genes, including *BRCA1, GSTP1,* and *p16*^{INK4a}. This gene hypermethylation profile of human cancer is consistent with the data of particular "*methylotypes*" proposed for single tumor types. In this way, it is possible to use the CpG island hypermethylation of tumor suppressor genes as tumor markers. One obvious advantage over genetic markers is that mutations occur at multiple sites and can be of very different types. In contrast, promoter hypermethylation occurs within the same region of a given gene in each form of cancer; thus, we do not need to test the methylation status first to assay the marker in serum or a distal site. Furthermore, the detection of hypermethylation is a "*positive*" signal that can be accomplished in a galaxy of normal cells, whereas certain genetic changes, such as loss of heterozygosity and homozygous deletions, will not be detected within a background of normal DNA.

If we wish to use these epigenetic markers in the real world, we will need to use quick, easy, nonradioactive, and sensitive ways of detecting hypermethylation in CpG islands of tumor suppressor genes, such as the methylation-specific *polymerase chain reaction* (PCR) technique (MSP). In this respect, CpG island hypermethylation has been used as a tool to detect cancer cells in all types of biological fluids and biopsies: broncoalveolar lavage, lymph nodes, sputum, urine, semen, ductal lavage, and saliva. An exciting new line of research was also initiated in 1999 when we showed that it was possible to screen for hypermethylated promoter loci in serum DNA from patients with lung cancer. Following our observation, many studies have corroborated the feasibility of detecting CpG island hypermethylation of multiple genes in the serum DNA of a broad spectrum of tumor types, some of them even using semi-quantitative and automated methodologies. Thus, DNA hypermethylation has proved its versatility over a wide range of tumor types and environments.

DNA Methylation as a Prognostic/Predictor Factor

Clinical outcome is affected by many factors, some of which are a function of the genetic composition and health status of the patient, whereas others are inherent to the malignancy itself. It is important to distinguish between predictive markers, which are associated with the relative sensitivity to specific therapeutics strategies, and prognostic markers, which are associated with treatment-independent factors such as the growth rate and metastatic behavior of the malignancy. Both of these types of stratification markers are of clinical value and can assist physicians in their choice of treatment.

As examples of DNA methylation markers of poor prognosis, we can mention that the *death-associated protein kinase* (*DAPK*) and *p16*^{INK4a} hypermethylation have been linked to tumor virulence in patients with lung or colorectal cancer. Additional candidates awaiting analysis to determine their relation to enhanced metastasizing or angiogenic activity in primary tumors include the aberrant methylation of E-cadherin (*CDH1*), H-cadherin (*CDH13*), and thrombospondin-1 (*THBS-1*), respectively.

With respect to the use of DNA methylation as predictive factors, the most compelling evidence is provided by the methylation-associated silencing of the DNA repair *MGMT* in human cancer. The MGMT protein (O^6-methylguanine DNA methyl-transferase) is directly responsible for repairing the addition of alkyl groups to the guanine (G) base of the DNA. This base is the preferred point of attack in the DNA of several alkylating chemotherapeutic drugs, such as BCNU (1,3-bis(2-chloroethyl)-1-nitrosourea), ACNU (1-(4-amino-2-methyl-5-pyrimidinyl)methyl-3-(2-chloroethyl)-3-nitrosourea), procarbazine, streptozotocin, or temozolamide. Thus, our reasoning was that tumors that had lost *MGMT* as a result of hypermethylation would be more sensitive to the action of these alkylating agents because their DNA lesions could not be repaired in the cancer cell and therefore this would lead to cell death. We have presented evidence for the principle of this hypothesis, and *MGMT* promoter hypermethylation effectively predicts a good response to chemotherapy, greater overall survival, and longer time to progression in patients with glioma treated with BCNU (carmustine).

Cases similar to that described for *MGMT* can be cited for other DNA repair and detoxifier genes that also undergo aberrant DNA methylation. For example, the response to cisplatin and derivatives may be a direct function of the methylation state of the CpG island of *hMLH1*; the response to adriamicine may be related to the methylation status of *GSTP1*, and the response to certain DNA-damaging drugs could be a function of the state of *BRCA1* hypermethylation. Contrary evidence has also been presented. An old foe of cancer treatment, the *MDR-1* gene (multidrug resistance-1), can undergo reactivation by demethylation in certain malignancies, although more studies are necessary to clarify this issue. I strongly encourage all the studies that address these issues because they may have a direct impact on clinical cancer treatment. Finally, gene inactivation by promoter hypermethylation may be the key to understanding the loss of hormone

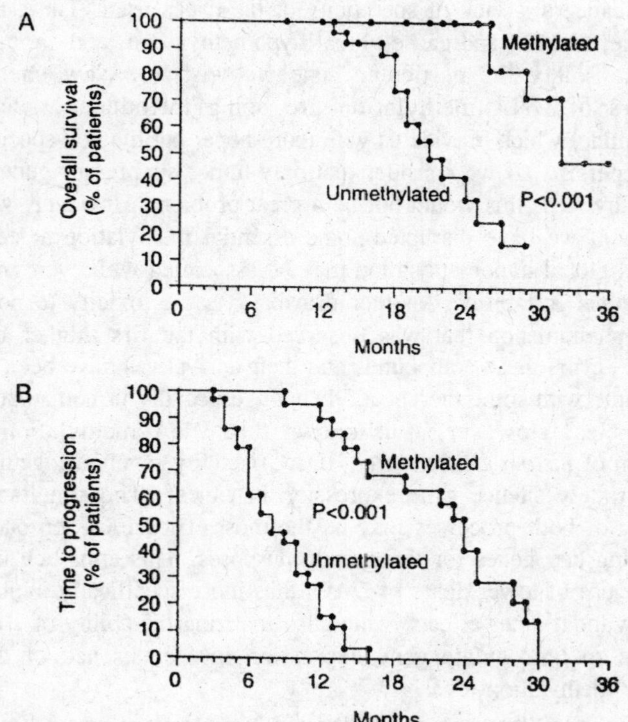

Fig. 12.1. Overall survival (A) and time to the progression of disease (B) among patients with gliomas treated with carmustine, according to the methylation status of the MGMT promoter.

responsiveness of many tumors. The inefficacy of the anti-steroids, estrogen–progesterone–androgen related compounds such as tamoxifen, raloxifene, and flutemide, in certain breast, endometrial, and prostate cancer cases may be a direct consequence of the methylation-mediated silencing of their respective cellular receptors (*ER, PR,* and *AR* genes).

DNA Methylation as a Therapeutic Target

It is increasingly apparent that many important genes can be inactivated in association with promoter hypermethylation in a single type of cancer and even in the same patient's tumor. Given that this transcriptional repression is a potentially reversible process, reactivation of the involved genes can be considered as a possible therapeutic target, and this concept is receiving increasing attention. In fact, for several years we have been able to reactivate hypermethylated genes *in vitro* using demethylating agents such as 5-azacytidine or 5-aza-2-deoxicytidine (Decitabine). One obstacle to the transfer of this technique to human primary cancers is lack of specificity of the drugs used. These drugs inhibit the DNMTs and cause global hypomethylation, and we cannot reactivate solely the particular gene we wish to. New chemical inhibitors of DNA methylation are being introduced, such as procainamide, which provide us with more hope, but the non-specificity problem persists. If we consider that only tumor suppressor genes are hypermethylated, this would not be a great problem. However, we do not know if we have disrupted some essential methylation at certain sites, and global hypomethylation may be associated with even greater chromosomal instability. Another drawback is the toxicity to normal cells, a phenomenon that was observed with the first higher doses used. However, these compounds and their derivatives have been used in the clinic with some therapeutic benefit, especially in hematopoietic malignancies. However, it is known that DNA methylation and regulation of *histone deacetylase* (HDAC) activity function together to inappropriately silence gene expression in cancer. The simultaneous inhibition of both processes may be the most efficacious approach to reactivating key genes for therapeutic purposes. This approach might allow the use of lower doses of DAC, thus more specifically inhibiting DNMT without other effects, while also realizing the ability of HDAC inhibition to up-regulate gene expression in the absence of dense promoter methylation level.

These new findings have proved very attractive to several pharmacologic and biotechnical companies, and they are now studying how to accomplish demethylation of cancer cells using novel approaches, such as antisense constructs or ribozymes, against the DNMTs. Nevertheless, we are still left with the problem of non-specificity. Other companies tackle the problem using gene therapy–like strategies in which we reactivate a targeted methylated gene specifically, but the studies are still in their infancy. Thus, a great deal of the promise remains to be fulfilled.

Methods

Although global genomic DNA methylation might have an important role in carcinogenesis, its measurement in cancer cells has little to offer as a molecular marker, either in sensitivity or in information content. Conversely, methylation levels at individual CpG dinucleotides are useful for quantifying differences at important regulatory sequences. Two alternatives are currently used to study the distribution of 5-methylcytosine residues in particular DNA sequences: nonbisulfite and bisulfite methods. The first relies on the use of methylation-sensitive restriction endonucleases combined with Southern Blot analysis or PCR detection, which sometimes means that results are limited to cleavage sites. This problem can be avoided by the bisulfite modification of the DNA, which comprises a wide range of techniques that allow the quantitative and accurate determination of the methylation status of the allele and even at the cell population level. All bisulfite-associated methods require PCR amplification of the bisulfite-modified DNA, and differences in methylcytosine patterns are displayed by methylation-dependent primer design (MSP), in conjunction with methylation-sensitive restriction endonucleases (combined bisulfite restriction analyses, or COBRA), genomic sequencing, and other approaches. Some of them even provide quantitative data about the average proportion of methylated and nonmethylated alleles in a population.

As a general rule, CpG island methylation first should be studied in great detail in cancer cell lines where the amount of material is not limited. The cell lines will also allow us to develop the demethylation and re-expression experiments using 5-azacytidine or 5-aza-2-deoxycytidine. In the case of primary tumors, techniques that allow the screening of a large number of samples, such as MSP, will be very useful, although other techniques can also be applied if a more quantitative estimate is desired.

Quantification of Global Methylation

Levels of methylcytosine occurrence in the genomic DNA can be measured by high-performance separation techniques or by enzymatic or chemical means. When separation devices are available, *high-performance capillary electrophoresis* (HPCE) may be the best choice because it is faster, cheaper, and more sensitive than HPLC. By means of labeled antimethyl-cytosine antibodies, DNA methylation can be monitored in metaphase chromosomes; in hetero/euchromatin; and, most importantly, on a cell-by-cell basis within the same sample. The latter alternative, which generally yields qualitative results, is of great interest in cancer research because it can reveal methylation differences between normal and tumor tissues in the same sample.

HPLC-Based Methods

Relative methylcytosine contents of genomic DNA can be analyzed by chemical hydrolysis to obtain the total base composition of the genome and subsequent fractionation and quantification of hydrolysis products using HPLC technologies. The degree of DNA methylation of several samples has been quantified by this method, but at least 2.5

μg DNA are generally required to quantify 5-methylcytosine with a low standard deviation for replicate samples. Sensitivity of the system can be increased with mass spectrometry detection, which has a detection limit 10^6 times the limit of absorption spectroscopy detectors.

HPCE-Based Methods

The development of HPCE techniques has given rise to an approach to research that has several advantages over other current methodologies used to quantify the extent of DNA. This method is faster than HPLC (taking less than 10 min per sample) and is also reasonably inexpensive because it does not require continuous running buffers and displays a great potential for fractionation (theoretically up to 10^6 plates). Approximately 1 methylcytosine in 200 cytosine residues can be detected by this method using 1 μg genomic DNA. To increase sensitivity, *laser-induced fluorescence* (LIF) and mass spectrometry detectors should be used.

Analyses of Genome-wide Methylation by Chemical or Enzymatic Means

As previously stated, quantifying the degree of DNA methylation by HPLC or HPCE requires access to sophisticated equipment that is not always available. The radioactive labeling of CpG sites using the methyl-acceptor assay has been developed to address this problem, but, among the technique's other drawbacks, it can only monitor CpG methylation changes, and so CpNpG methylation cannot be detected. This method uses bacterial SssI DNA methyl-transferase to transfer tritium-labeled methyl groups from SAM (S-adenosyl-L-[methyl-^{3}H]methionine) to unmethylated cytosines in CpG targets. The data obtained from a scintillation counter are used to calculate the number of methyl groups incorporated in the DNA.

In situ Hybridization Methods for Studying Total Cytosine Methylation

Global DNA methylation can also be quantified by methylcytosine-specific antibodies. An important advantage of this approach is that it may be carried out on a cell-by-cell basis rather than in a heterogeneous population. Apart from classical immunoassay detection, approaches that involve quantifying the retention of radiolabeled DNA by polyclonal antibodies on nitrocellulose filters, immunoprecipitation, gel filtration, and visualization under the electron microscope, cytosine methylation can also be detected in metaphase chromosomes and in chromatin using monoclonal antibodies combined with fluorescence staining. An alternative to fluorescence detection is to connect a colored enzyme-dependent reaction.

Nonbisulfite Methods

The most widely used methods for studying DNA methylation patterns of specific regions of DNA with no base modifications are based on the use of methylation-sensitive and *methylation-insensitive restriction endonucleases* (MS-REs). One of the restriction enzymes of the isoschizomer pair is able to cut the DNA only when its target is unmethylated, whereas the other is not sensitive to methylated cytosines. The most common isoschizomers used are the Hpa II/Msp I pair. Although these pairs of enzymes can cleave hemimethylated DNA, they do not distinguish between cytosines methylated at different positions in the pyrimidinic ring. However, there are several restriction enzymes that recognize the localization of the methyl group.

Once DNA has been digested with methylation-sensitive endonucleases, identification of the methylation status of a gene can be accomplished by Southern Blot hybridization or PCR procedures. In the former, digestion products are separated by gel electrophoresis, transferred to a nitrocellulose filter, and hybridized with a radiolabeled probe. When DNA digestion is accomplished by methylation-sensitive nucleases, the obtaining of a larger DNA fragment than expected indicates methylation at one or both restriction targets that flank the homologous region of the DNA. An mC-positive will be detected when at least 10% of the DNAs present that modification as a result of their hybridization sensitivity.

When the amount of tissue is limiting, detection of cytosine methylation can be achieved by PCR, which requires less than 10 ng DNA, whereas Southern hybridization generally needs up to 10 μg DNA. Furthermore, a methylcytosine-positive can be detected when only 0.1% of the DNA molecules present such base modification. PCR primers must correspond to flanking sequences of the restriction targets, so that the absence of methylation is revealed in the presence of a PCR band. Nonbisulfite methods for the quantification of DNA methylation patterns are simple and rapid and can be used for any known-sequence genomic DNA region. These methods are extremely specific, but their limitation to specific restriction sites reduces their value.

Bisulfite Methods

The analysis of DNA methylation changed completely with the introduction of sodium bisulfite conversion of genomic DNA. The differential rates at which cytosine and 5-methylcytosine are deaminated by sodium bisulfite to yield uracil and thymine in conjunction with PCR amplification and sequencing provides us a method to find specific methylated sequences.

Bisulfite converts all cytosines to uracil, except those that are methylated, which are resistant to modification and remain as cytosine. This reaction constitutes the basis for discriminating between methylated and unmethylated DNA. Bisulfite modification of DNA can be followed by several methods, including sequencing, methylation-specific PCR, combined bisulfite restriction assays, and others. In general, each modification leads to greater sensitivity and resolution or contributes to the development of a novel perspective on the results. All of them work with PCR, which, among other advantages, is suitable for analyzing paraffin-embedded tissues and scarce purified DNA.

Bisulfite Modification of DNA

Materials

1. Sodium bisulfite 3 M (pH 5)
2. Hydroquinone 20 mM
3. Sodium hydroxide 3 M
4. Wizard DNA purification resin (Promega)
5. Isopropanol 80%
6. Ethanol (70% and absolute)
7. Ammonium acetate 10 M

Procedure

1. Dilute 1 μg of DNA in 50 μl, mix with 5.7 μl of NaOH 3 M, and incubate at 37°C for 15 min. This first step is for DNA denaturation because only cytosines that are located in single strands are susceptible to bisulfite modification.
2. Add 33 μl of hidroquinone 20 mM and 530 μl of sodium bisulfite, both freshly prepared, and incubate at 50°C for 16–17 hr.
3. Purify modificated DNA using the Wizard DNA purification resin according to the manufacturer (Promega), and elute in 50 μl of mili Q water.
4. Complete the modification by adding 5.7 μl of NaOH 3 M, and incubate at 37°C for 20 min.
5. Add 17 μl of ammonium acetate 10 M, 1 μl glycogen 10 mg/ml, and 3 volumes of absolute ethanol, and incubate overnight at −70°C to precipitate the modified DNA.

6. Centrifuge at 12000 rpm at 4°C for 20 min, discard the supernatant, wash the pellet with ethanol 70%, and centrifuge in similar conditions.
7. Discard the supernatant, and dry the pellet in a speed vacuum.
8. Resuspend the pellet in 25 μl of mili Q water.

Bisulfite Sequencing

Sequencing bisulfite-altered DNA is the most straightforward means of detecting cytosine methylation. In general, after denaturation and bisulfite modification, double-stranded DNA is obtained by primer extension and the fragment of interest is amplified by PCR. Methylcytosine may then be detected by standard DNA sequencing of the PCR products. The most important aspect of sequencing bisulfite-modified DNA is the primers design. Three factors need to be considered in the design of PCR primers for sequencing bisulfite-modified DNA:

1. Bisulfite-converted DNA strands are no longer complementary, so primer design must be customized for each DNA chain.
2. Primers should cover several cytosines that are not part of the CpG dinucleotides in the original sequences and are therefore converted to uracils by bisulfite. Inclusion of such bases in the primer design helps to avoid amplification of any residual unconverted DNA.
3. Primers should not cover any potential sites for DNA methylation (CpG dinucleotides).

This method provides us with methylation maps of a single DNA molecule. The main disadvantage of bisulfite sequencing is that it is not useful for the screening of a large number of clinical samples.

Methylation-Specific PCR

MSP is the most widely used method of DNA methylation. It has had a significant impact on the burgeoning field of cancer epigenetics by making DNA methylation analysis accessible to a wide number of laboratories. Bisulfite sequencing is particularly useful for the quantitative or detailed analysis of 5-methylcytosine distribution, whereas MSP excels at the sensitive detection of particular methylation patterns.

The differences between methylated and unmethylated alleles that arise from sodium bisulfite treatment are the basis of MSP and are especially valuable in CpG islands as a result of the abundance of CpG sites. Primer design is a critical and complex component of the procedure. Bisulfite-converted DNA strands are no longer complementary, so primer design must be customized for each DNA chain.

Original sequence

A A C G C G G C G G T C G G C A G

Unmethylated allele

A A T G T G G T G G T T G G T A G

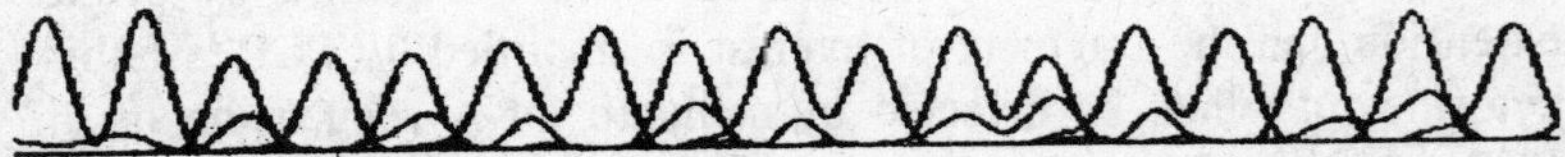

Methylated allele

A A C G C G G C G G T C G G T A G

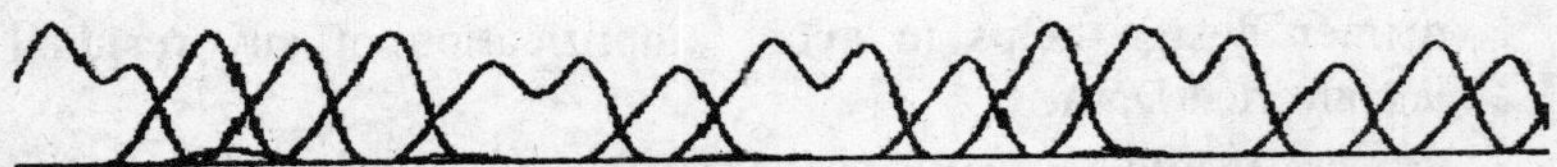

Fig. 12.2. Methylation maps of a single DNA molecule obtained by direct sequencing of Bisulfite-modified DNA.

After chemical modification, two sets of primers should be designed. One primer set (U) will anneal to unmethylated DNA that has undergone a chemical modification, and second primer set (M) will anneal with methylated DNA that has undergone chemical modification. Thus, methylation patterns of all sequences must be determined in separate reactions. To optimize the PCR amplification step, the following critical requirements must be considered when designing the primers:

1. The annealing temperature of both primers must be similar and always between 55°C and 65°C.
2. The PCR product should be between 80 and 175 bp to allow the assessment of methylation patterns in limited region and to facilitate the application of this technique to samples, such as paraffin blocks, where amplification of larger fragments is not possible.
3. Each primer should contain at least two CpG pairs.
4. The sense primer should contain a CpG pair at its 3' end.

5. To avoid false-positive results (amplification of unmethylated, unmodified DNA), primers should contain non-CpG cytosines.

The main advantages of MSP are that it is a very sensitive method, permitting the analysis of small and heterogeneous samples, it can be used on paraffin-embedded samples, it is specific for relevant CpG sites, and it avoids the use of restriction enzymes and resultant problems associate with incomplete enzymatic digestion. However, MSP tends to be a more qualitative, rather than a quantitative, accurate method.

Because of its versatility, MSP has been widely proposed as a rapid and cost-effective tool of use in the study of CpG island hypermethylation in human cancer. For example, MSP has been successfully used to evaluate the responsiveness of human cancer patients to alkalating agents or to detect tumoral DNA in the serum of patients with cancer.

Combined Bisulfite Restriction Analysis

The COBRA method consists of a standard sodium bisulfite PCR treatment followed by restriction digestion and a quantitation step. The DNA amplification products of specific loci, previously modified by bisulfite, are digested with restriction enzymes that distinguish methylated from unmethylated sequences so that the degree of DNA methylation is linearly correlated with the relative amounts of digested and undigested products. The BstU I case may illustrate this point: its cleavage site (CGCG) is resistant to bisulfite modification when it is methylated but is transformed to TGTG when it is unmethylated. Thus, DNA cleavage after bisulfite treatment only occurs if the restriction target is methylated, and, moreover, cleavage products are proportional to the degree of methylation of the analyzed sequence.

The average relative proportions of digestion products can be quantified by hybridization with 5' end-labeled oligos and Phosphorimager detection. In contrast to MSP, PCR primers should not contain CpG pairs to avoid discrimination between different methylated templates. In general, this approach can be used when absolute percentages of methylated and unmethylated alleles are required to guarantee the final diagnosis. The major drawback is that BstU I will also cut if unconverted. Therefore the use of this enzyme can lead to overestimation of methylation, so that checking conversion state with enzymes such as Hpa II is needed. This is a specific and quantitative method but requires a complete chemical modification of DNA and cannot analyze all DNA sequences because it is confined to restriction targets.

Fluorescence-Based Real-Time Quantitative PCR Analysis

Sodium bisulfite modification creates methylation-dependent sequence differences in the genomic DNA. Fluorescence-based PCR is then performed using locus-specific PCR primers flanking an oligonucleotide probe with a 5' fluorescent reporter dye (FAM) and a 3' quencher dye (TAMRA). The 5' to 3' nuclease activity of DNA polymerase cleaves the probe and releases the reporter, whose fluorescence can be detected by the laser detector of the detection system. The most striking advantage of real-time quantitative PCR analysis is its potential to allow the rapid screening of hundreds to thousands of samples and its sensitivity, making it possible to detect a single methylated allele in 10,000 unmethylated alleles. Unlike other techniques, this assay is completed at the PCR step, without the need for further gel electrophoretic separation and hybridization. The drawbacks of this method are that it requires expensive hybridization probes and calibration curves must be generated in each setting.

13

TELOMERE IN CANCER

Telomere length is now known to be directly responsible for limiting the capacity of cellular division in a number of human cell types. Comparison of telomere length in tumors and matched normal tissue from the same individual has indicated that the telomere repeat array is often shorter in tumors than in adjacent untransformed tissue. Changes in telomere length during human tumorigenesis are believed to reflect loss of terminal sequences resulting from the end replication problem during the cell divisions required for tumor formation. Although telomeres are often shorter in tumors than in matched normal tissue from the same individual, these telomeres are usually stabilized at a new length setting by the activation of the telomere maintenance enzyme, telomerase.

Telomere length is usually determined by Southern analysis of *terminal restriction fragments* (TRFs). This is technically the most simple protocol for visualizing telomere arrays. However, difficulties in interpreting the telomere length data generated from this technique arise owing to the heterogeneity in the number of telomeric repeats present at individual chromosome ends. In contrast to the discrete bands usually resulting from Southern analysis, telomeric signals appear as a smear of hybridization. The intensity of the signal is biased toward the larger telomeric fragments because these fragments contain a greater number of target sequences for hybridization. In addition, the TRFs being visualized via this method represent not only the canonical TTAGGG repeats but a variable amount of subtelomeric sequences. Recently, two additional methods for ascertaining telomere length have been developed. First, hybridization of TRFs can be done

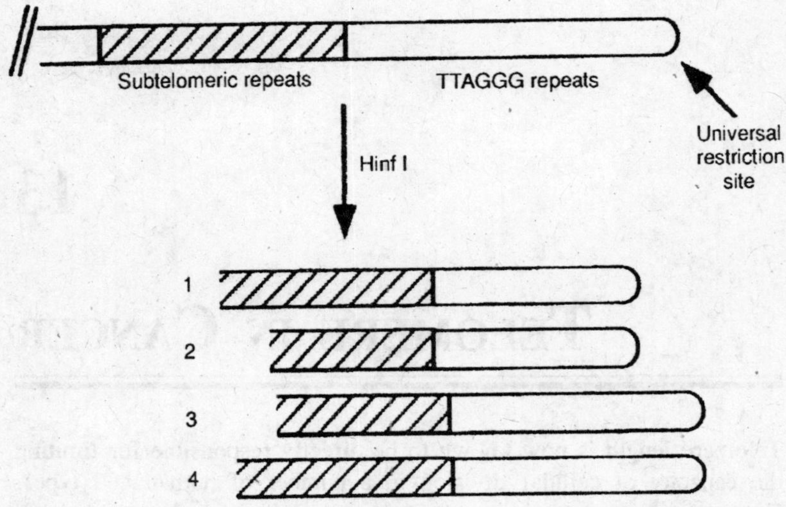

Fig. 13.1. Telomeric arrays appear as a smear rather than as discrete bands following southern analysis owing to heterogeneity in the amount of subtelomeric sequences (1 vs 2 and 3 vs 4) and in the number of TTAGGG repeats present at each chromosome end (1 vs 4 and 2 vs 3).

in solution with an oligonucleotide probe complementary to the single-stranded protrusion present at the 3' ends of chromosomes.

This method reduces heterogeneity in signal intensity owing to variable amounts of target sequence, allowing quantitation of telomere length to be somewhat simplified. However, there are several of problems associated with this technique, including the necessity of running hot gels and the care to determine that one's DNA samples do not become denatured. Second, telomere length can be determined by *in situ* hybridization using peptide nucleic acid–based probes. This technique permits accurate determination of telomere length based on signal intensity and allows investigation of telomere length on an individual chromosome basis. However, this technique requires the generation of metaphase spreads from actively growing cultures, and data collection is onerous. Thus, peptide nucleic acid-based *in situ* hybridization is not yet suitable for analysis of telomere length in large numbers of human tumor samples.

This chapter describes the analysis of human telomere length in human tumors using Southern hybridization of TRFs. This is the technique that is most widely used in the field of telomere dynamics, and where possible, we have optimized the use of commercially available reagents and kits to minimize interlaboratory variation.

MATERIALS

Preparation of Genomic DNA

1. Matched samples from tumor and normal tissue.
2. 10X PBSA: 1.37 *M* NaCl, 26.8 m*M* KCl, 106 m*M* Na_2HPO_4, 14.7 m*M* $K_2H_2PO_4$.
3. TNE lysis Buffer: 0.5 *M* Tris-HCl, pH 8.9, 10 m*M* NaCl , 15 m*M* EDTA.
4. Proteinase K (10 mg/mL).
5. Phenol (saturated with 0.1 *M* Tris/0.2% β-mercaptoethanol, pH 8.0).
6. 3 *M* Sodium acetate, pH 5.7.
7. Absolute and 70% ethanol.
8. $T_{10}E_{20}$: 10 m*M* Tris-HCl/20 m*M* EDTA, pH 7.5.
9. RnaseA (10 mg/mL).
10. 10% Sodium dodecyl sulfate (SDS).
11. Phenol/chloroform/isoamyl alcohol (25:24:1).
12. $T_{10}E_1$: 10 m*M* Tris-HCl/1 m*M* EDTA, pH 8.0.
13. Centrifuge.
14. Polypropylene tubes (15 and 50 mL).
15. Rotator.

Digestion and Quantitation of DNA Samples

1. *Hinf*I restriction endonuclease and reaction buffer.
2. Incubator.
3. Flurometer.
4. DNA quantitation kit (Bio-Rad) containing 10X TEN (100 m*M* Tris-HCl, 2 *M* NaCl, 10 m*M* EDTA, pH7.4), 1 mg/mL of calf thymus DNA, and 10 mg/mL of Hoechst 33258 (bisbenzamide). Alternatively, components for quantitation can be purchased separately.
5. Cuvets.
6. Eppendorf tubes.

Southern Blotting

1. Agarose.
2. Ethidium bromide (10 mg/mL).
3. 5X Tris-borate EDTA (TBE) buffer.
4. DNA molecular weight standards.

5. Agarose gel electrophoresis chamber and power supply.
6. 0.25 *N* HCl.
7. Denaturing solution: 0.5 *M* NaOH, 1.5 *M* NaCl.
8. Neutralizing solution: 1 *M* Tris-HCl, pH 7.5, 1.5 *M* NaCl.
9. Hybond N (Amersham).
10. Stratalinker (Stratagene).
11. Transfer apparatus (capillary or electroblot).

Probe Preparation and Hybridization

1. Hybridization mix: 0.5 *M* NaH_2PO_4, 10% BSA, 7% SDS.
2. Filter unit (500-mL, 0.45-μm) (Nalgene).
3. Hybridization setup (water bath, oven, and so on).
4. ProbeQuant G-50 microcolumns (Pharmacia).
5. T4 kinase and 5X Forward Reaction Buffer (Gibco-BRL).
6. γ^{32}P-ATP (3000 Ci/mmol).
7. $(TTAGGG)_4$ and $(CCCTAA)_4$ oligonucleotides (100 ng/μL).
8. TES: 10 m*M* Tris-HCl, pH 7.4, 1 m*M* EDTA, pH 8.0, 0.1% SDS.
9. Pyrex dish or tupperware.
10. 4X Saline sodium citrate (SSC), 0.1% SDS.
11. Autoradiographic film or Phosphorimager cassette.

Methods

Preparation of Genomic DNA

It is essential that tissue samples are pathologically evaluated to minimize cross contamination of tumor tissue with normal tissue. Tissues should be flash frozen and stored at –70°C until use.

1. Rinse approx 1 g (1 cm^3) of frozen tissue with 1X PBSA.
2. Decant the wash and finely mince the specimen (~1 g or 1 cm^3) with a razor or scalpel blade.
3. Place the minced tissue into a 50-mL polypropylene tube and add 10 mL of TNE lysis buffer supplemented with 500 μg/mL of proteinase K and 1% SDS.
4. Parafilm the cap and incubate overnight at 37°C with constant rocking.
5. Add an equal volume of phenol saturated with 0.1 *M* Tris/0.2% β-mercaptoethanol (pH 8.0), and mix gently at room temperature for 10–15 min.
6. Centrifuge at 1400*g* for 10 min.

7. Remove the aqueous phase (upper layer) with a wide-bored pipet (e.g., 25-mL disposable pipet), and transfer to a fresh 50-mL polypropylene tube. Repeat the phenol extraction as described previously until the interphase between the aqueous and organic layers is clear.
8. Transfer the final aqueous phase to a fresh tube. This solution will be very viscous, and care should be taken to slowly and gently remove the aqueous phase to limit the contamination with the phenol solution.
9. Add 0.1 vol of 3 *M* sodium acetate (pH 5.7) and 2 vol of cold absolute ethanol.
10. Precipitate the DNA by rotating gently for 5–10 min. The genomic DNA will precipitate into a white stringy clump. Loosely spool strands of DNA around a glass pipet or a yellow pipet tip and transfer to a fresh 50-mL tube.
11. Wash the spooled DNA by rotating the DNA in 25–35 mL of 70% EtOH for 5–10 min at room temperature.
12. Air-dry the DNA and place in a 15-mL polypropylene tube. Resuspend the DNA in 3 mL of $T_{10}E_{20}$ by rotating overnight at 4°C.
13. Add 100 μg/mLof RNase A (10 mg/mL stock) and incubate at 37°C for 30 min.
14. Add proteinase K and SDS to final concentrations of 200 μg/mL and 1%, respectively. Incubate for 1 h at 48°C.
15. Extract twice with equal volumes of phenol/chloroform/isoamyl alcohol (25:24:1) as described in steps 5–8.
16. Add 0.1 vol of 3 *M* sodium acetate, 2 vol of cold absolute EtOH to the aqueous phase, and spool the DNA as before.
17. Wash the DNA with 70% ethanol.
18. Air-dry the DNA and then vacuum dry the pellet.
19. Resuspend the dried DNA in 1 to 2 mL of $T_{10}E_1$ by rotating overnight at 4°C.
20. Store the DNA samples at 4°C. The concentration of the sample may be determined using a spectrophotometer at this time, but because the viscosity of the solution makes accurate pipetting difficult, these measurements are not very reliable.

Digestion and Quantitation of DNA Samples

1. Digest 5–10 μL of the DNA sample (no more than 5 μg) in a 50-μL reaction overnight at 37°C with 25U of *Hin*fI. The DNA should be pipeted using sawed-off tips to minimize shearing and facilitate

pipetting. Incubation should be carried out in an incubator rather than a water bath to minimize condensation of the reaction on the lid of the Eppendorf tube.

2. Briefly spin the tubes to collect the reaction volumes at the bottom of the tube.
3. Quantitate the amount of DNA in each reaction using the Bio-Rad fluorometer (or similar equipment) and the DNA quantitation kit.
4. Prepare sufficient 1X TEN (2 mL/sample to be quantitated).
5. Add Hoechst 33258 to a final concentration of 1 μg/mL.
6. Zero the fluorometer using 2 mL of the TEN/dye solution.
7. Calibrate the fluorometer by adding 5 μL of 100 μg/mL calf thymus DNA (equivalent to a total of 500 ng of DNA).
8. Check the calibration by adding 10 μL of 10 μg/mL calf thymus DNA to 2 mL of TEN/dye solution.
9. Determine the concentration of DNA in each digest by adding 2 μL of the reaction to 2 mL of TEN/dye solution.
10. Calculate the volumes required to load 1 μg to 2.5 μg of DNA/lane on an agarose gel.

Southern Blotting

1. Pour a 20 × 20 cm^2 agarose gel. The agarose mix is composed of 0.7% agarose in 0.5X TBE buffer supplemented with 1 μg/mL of ethidium bromide.
2. Load equal amounts of each DNA sample on the gel. We add 0.1 vol of loading dye to each sample. Also include molecular weight markers.
3. Run the gel at 30 V until the dye front has entered the gel. The gel can then be turned up to 80 V or continued running at 30 V. The gel should be run for a total of 700–1000 Vh.
4. Check the gel by observing on an ultraviolet light box. The gel should run until the 2-kb molecular weight marker is at the bottom. The majority of the genomic DNA should have run off the gel since *Hinf*I is a frequent cutter in bulk genomic DNA with resulting average sized fragments <2 kb. The intensity of ethidium bromide staining should appear equal for all lanes.
5. Take a picture of the gel with a ruler next to the molecular weight markers.
6. Incubate the gel for 15 min at room temperature with 0.25 *N* HCl on a rotator. The volume should be sufficient to cover the gel completely.

7. Treat the gel twice for 20 min each in denaturing solution on a rotator.
8. Treat the gel twice for 30 min each in neutralizing solution on a rotator.
9. Rinse the gel with ddH_2O.
10. Transfer the DNA to a Hybond N membrane by capillary transfer or using an electroblot apparatus. After transfer is complete, mark the location of the wells.
11. Crosslink the DNA to the membrane by treating in a Statalinker (Stratagene) at 1200 mJ (the "*autocrosslink*" setting). The membrane can be stored for an unlimited time or immediately be hybridized to detect the TRFs.

Probe Preparation and Hybridization

The hybridization mix is made in 500-mL aliquots and will last for months at room temperature. The solution should be incubated at 50°C overnight to ensure complete dissolution of the SDS and BSA. The following morning, the hybridization mix is filtered through a 0.45-μm filter unit. This step eliminates "*speckling*" appearing on the films. Where possible, the procedures below utilize commercially available reagents to eliminate variation from experiment to experiment.

1. Prehybridize the filter at 55°C in 10 mL hybridization mix for at least 30 min at 55°C.
2. While the filter is prehybridizing, label the oligonucleotides. We use a 1:1 mixture of the two oligonucleotides.
3. End label the oligonucleotides using T4 kinase and 20 pmol (12 μL of 3000 Ci/mmol) of γ^{32}P-ATP for 45 min to 1 h at 37°C in a final volume of 20 μL (4 μL of 5X forward reaction buffer, 1 μL of each oligonucleotide [100 ng/μL], 2 μL of T4 kinase, 12 μL of γ^{32}P-ATP).
4. Stop the reaction by adding 30 μL of TES to the reaction to achieve a final volume of 50 μL.
5. Remove the unincorporated radionuclotide from the reaction using ProbeQuant G-50 microcolumns.
6. Determine the efficiency of labeling in a crude manner using a Geiger counter. The probe should be labeled such that the counter is saturated on the most sensitive setting when the monitor is held approx 1 in. from the tube.
7. Add the probe to 7 mL of hybridization mix. Replace the prehybridization solution with the hybridization solution and incubate at 55°C overnight.

8. Wash the filter twice for 20 min each in 4X SSC/0.1% SDS at room temperature. Use a Geiger counter to monitor the filter. There should be very few counts remaining in the center of the filter and background levels of radiation at the top and bottom of the filter. If necessary, wash the filter an additional time in 4X SSC/0.1% SDS at 55°C.
9. Wrap the filter in plastic wrap and expose to autoradiographic film or a Phosphorimager cassette. The exposure time and use of intensifying screens varies with experiments and efficiency of hybridization and can range from 2 h with two screens at –70°C to 3 d with two screens at –70°C.

Notes

1. Genomic DNA can be prepared using a number of commercially available kits. We have had mixed results using kits and recommend determining the quality of DNA prepared in this manner by running 1 μL of the sample on a gel prior to digestion. Up to 50% of the genomic DNA isolated using kits may be degraded and therefore unsuitable for this type of analysis.
2. Internal telomeric fragments of approx 2 and 2.3 kb act as internal controls for loading and the integrity of DNA.
3. Because of the highly repetitive nature of telomeres, hybridization to these sequences is occasionally uneven. This is owing to insufficient quantities of probe sequence relative to target sequence, i.e., unsaturated conditions. The amount of oligonucleotide suggested in the protocol is usually sufficient to prevent this problem. However, in the event of uneven hybridization patterns, 100–200 ng of unlabeled oligonucleotides should be added to the hybridization mix.

Measurement of Telomerase Activity

Human chromosomal termini, called telomeres, consist of tandem repeat (TTAGGG) sequences and the length of this portion progressively shortens with each cell division. The terminal portions of chromosomes lose the 5' end, and, thus, since the formation of the Okazaki fragment is not accomplished, DNA does not extend toward 3'. This phenomenon was proposed by Watson in 1972 and has been designated as the end-replication problem. Telomeres in dividing cells become shortened and in somatic cells the proliferative capability ceases by decrement of telomere length at a critical level, approx 2.5 kb. Telomere shortening is observed in peripheral blood cells at a rate of 40 bp/yr and in cultured cells at 40–60 bp/cell division. This is why telomeres are referred to as mitotic clocks or mitotic bombs. Although telomere erosion occurs by division of actively proliferative cells, immortal cells, including cancer cells, become able to express telomerase activity synthesizing a *de novo* telomere DNA sequence that maintains cellular proliferative capability and, thus, avoids proliferative crisis.

Telomerase is a ribonucleoprotein that is detected in >90% of primary cancer tissues using a *telomeric repeat amplification protocol* (TRAP) assay. Recently, it has been demonstrated that peripheral blood cells and some normal hematopoietic stem cells have telomerase activity. This indicates that active proliferative cells in the component of stem cells have telomerase activity to prevent progressive shortening of telomeres resulting in cell death. However, the telomere dynamics of the most primitive stem cells, which may be quiescent, have not been clarified. Telomerase activity is not detectable in somatic cells, except hematopoietic cells and cryptic cells in the intestine and hair follicles; thus, the definition of telomerase activity in cancer cells, except for hematologic neoplasias, is easy to determine. In hematologic neoplasias, the determination of telomerase-positive cells derived from neoplastic clone can be difficult, because normal hematopoietic cells have detectable telomerase activity. This clearly indicates that caution should be exerted in the determination of telomerase-positive leukemia cells, and one should determine the telomerase activity quantitatively.

Telomere Length in Hematologic Neoplasias

Telomere structures protect chromosomal ends from illegitimate recombination. Thus, reduction of telomere length associated with cell division may induce telomeric association, e.g., the presence of dicentric chromosomes and chromosome instability. Telomere length is measurable using Southern blot analysis of *HinfI*-digested DNA. The telomeres are detected as smearlike bands, the most dense portion of which is measured and represented as a *terminal restriction fragment* (TRF). Thus, telomere length may vary among cell types and chromosomes even within a single cell, but at this time one can only define TRF as a representative telomere length. Based on this study, the reduction of TRF correlated with the number of division of cells in in vitro and in vivo conditions. When cultured cells became immortal and telomere length shortened, telomeric association became evident, however, in clinical samples telomeric association is uncommon. Since detectable cytogenetic changes in clinical samples result from clonal selection of neoplastic cells, one might not show an exact association between

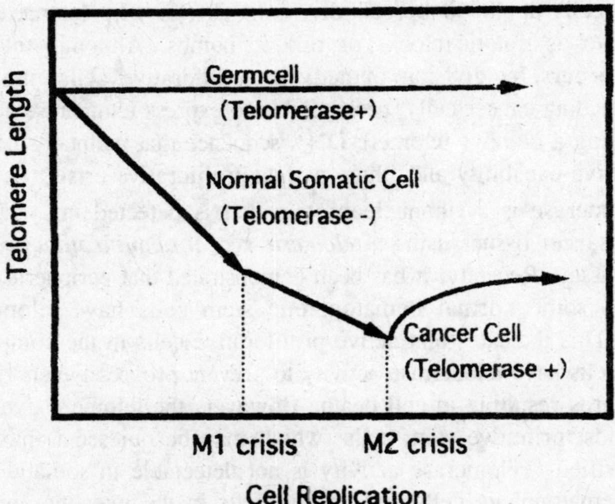

Fig. 13.2. Reduction in telomere length depends on cell division.

telomere shortening and the presence of certain chromosome abnormalities. TRFs in peripheral mononuclear cells, possibly reflecting the TRFs of the major part of normal resting lymphocytes, reduced in size with aging. As reported previously, however, the TRFs in bone marrow cells are not particularly different from those in peripheral mononuclear cells. We and other researchers have identified the formula for the reduction rate of TRF in peripheral mononuclear cells; thus, in this review the term reduced TRF means reduction in telomere length compared to this formula obtained from normal peripheral mononuclear cells. Reduction in telomere length, therefore, should be determined based on the age of each individual.

Detection of Telomerase Activity in Leukemia Cells

Detection of telomerase activity

The introduction of the TRAP assay based on a polymerase chain reaction (PCR) by Kim has made it possible to detect telomerase with a much greater sensitivity than previously. With this method, telomerase activity was demonstrated in >90% of primary tumors and almost all established cancer cell lines. TRAP assay uses a certain protein content, and dilution experiments permit the determination of inhibitor(s) for PCR. It is easy to count blood mononuclear cells, including leukemia cells; therefore, we counted the number of cells and used them for the TRAP assay. This allows us to calculate the telomerase activity easily. Moreover, as reported previously, hematopoietic stem cells and peripheral mononuclear cells in younger individuals have detectable telomerase activity; thus, we modified the TRAP assay to detect telomerase activity semiquantitatively, called fluorescence- based TRAP assay. On the other hand, Tatematsu et al. developed a "*stretch PCR assay*" also to detect telomerase activity semiquantitatively.

Fluorescence-based TRAP assay

To semiquantitate telomerase activity, we use fluorescence end-labeled CX and TS primers, an internal control, and an automated laser fluorescence DNA sequencer. This technique allows us to determine telomerase activity in real time and to calculate relative telomerase activity without using a photocapture system. We first calculate 2000 blood mononuclear cells and extract protein from the sample using a previously reported method. Telomerase activity was assessed according to the method of Kim et al. and Piatyszek et al. with modifications using the TRAP-eze detection kit (Oncor), and an automated laser fluorescence DNA sequencer. The TRAP assay procedure was performed according to the supplier's instruction and the report by Holt et al.. The frozen cell pellets were dissolved in 10–30 μL of 1X CHAPS lysis buffer, incubated on ice for 30 min, and then centrifuged at 10,000*g* for 30 min at 4°C. The supernatants were collected, and the protein content was determined using standard procedures (BCA protein assay).

Briefly, 2 μL of the cell extract (equivalent to 3 μg of protein) was added to a 48-μL reaction solution consisting of 10X TRAP buffer, 50X deoxynucleotide triphosphates (dNTPs) mix, 10 pmol of fluorescein isothiocyanate–labeled TS primer 5'-AAT CCG TCG AGC AGA GTT-3' (5'- end labeling using FluorePrime), TRAP primer mix already including a 36-bp internal standard, 2 U of *Taq* polymerase, and distilled H_2O. The mixture was incubated at 30°C for 10 min and then was heated at 90°C for 90 s. The PCR conditions were 30 cycles of 94°C for 30 s, 55°C for 30 s, and 72oC for 1.5 min.

The PCR products (1.5 μL) were subjected to 12% denaturing electrophoresis in an automated laser fluorescence DNA sequencer II and analyzed by the Fragment Manager program. To compare the relative amount of telomerase activity between samples, a ratio of the 36-bp internal standard to the telomerase peak was calculated. To confirm that the sample contained telomerase activity, multiple periodic 6-bp peaks of telomerase signal had to be detected, and preincubation of the extract with heat (95°C, 1.5 min) or RNase eliminated the periodic peak.

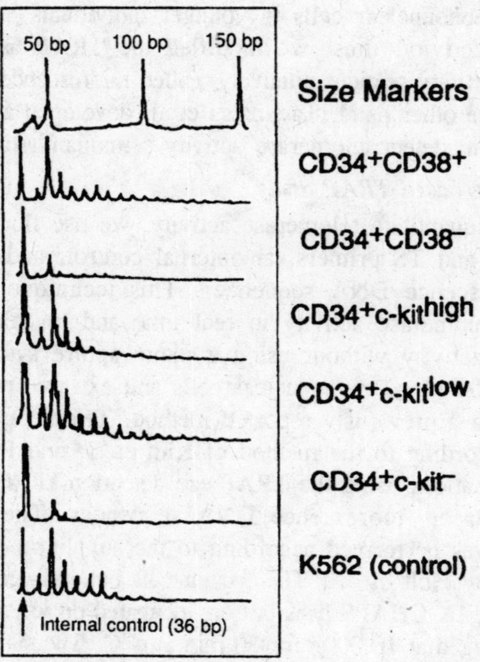

Fig. 13.3. Fluorocurve of the fluorescence-based TRAP assay. Each 6-bp peak corresponds to telomerase activity.

Telomerase Activity in Normal Hematopoietic Cells

Telomerase activity in hematopoietic stem cells

Human hematopoietic stem cells are considered to be enriched in CD34$^+$ cells' population, although in the mouse most primitive stem cells exist in the CD34$^-$ fraction, and it is still controversial whether or not human hematopoietic stem cells exist in the CD34$^-$ fraction. In the CD34$^+$ cell fraction, cells with CD38 antigen have more committed characteristics with elevated telomerase activity compared with the CD34$^+$/CD38$^+$ population. Engelhardt et al. confirmed this evidence that telomerase activity in CD34$^+$/CD38$^+$ cells exceeds levels in CD34$^+$/CD38$^-$ and CD34$^-$ cells. They also demonstrated that telomerase activity is highest in bone marrow CD34$^+$ cells followed by peripheral blood and umbilical cord blood. It is noteworthy, that they did not observe any particular difference in telomere length between bone marrow CD34$^+$ cells and peripheral blood (7.6 kb vs 7.4 kb), but that cord blood cells had long telomeres (10.4 kb). Moreover, they found a correlation between telomerase activity, cell cycle status, and the expression of cyclin D1 and cyclin A. Other investigators also confirmed these observations. Chiu et al. demonstrated that early progenitors ($CD34^+/CD71^+$) expressed telomerase activity at a higher level, which was subsequently downregulated in response to cytokines, and that primitive hematopoietic stem cells ($CD34^+/CD71^{low}/CD45RA^{low}$) had low levels of telomerase activity. Moreover, c-kit negative cells in the $CD34^+$ fraction are considered to contain the most primitive stem cells within the $CD34^+$ fraction.

Regarding telomerase activity, $CD34^+$/c-kit$^-$ cells carry very low telomerase activity, whereas those with $CD34^+$/c-kit$^-$ apparently have telomerase activity. This clearly indicates that most primitive hematopoietic stem cells might be low or negative for telomerase activity, and after they enter the cell cycle they become telomerase positive. Thus, most primitive stem cells may not have telomerase activity since they are quiescent, and it is currently demonstrated that cells in the G0 phase do not express telomerase activity. When a part of them enters a proliferative population, telomere erosion starts and telomerase activity may be upregulated.

The telomere-telomerase relationship allows us to speculate that there is a certain controlling mechanism or mechanisms that upregulate telomerase activity. Therefore, all these results supported the concept that purified hematopoietic stem cells show dramatic functional differences in turnover time and the ability to produce cells with stem cell properties.

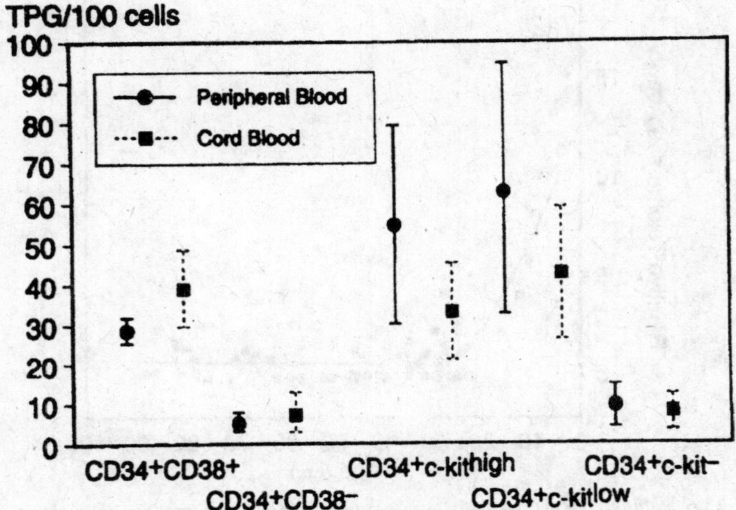

Fig. 13.4. Telomerase activity in hematopoietic stem cells sorted.

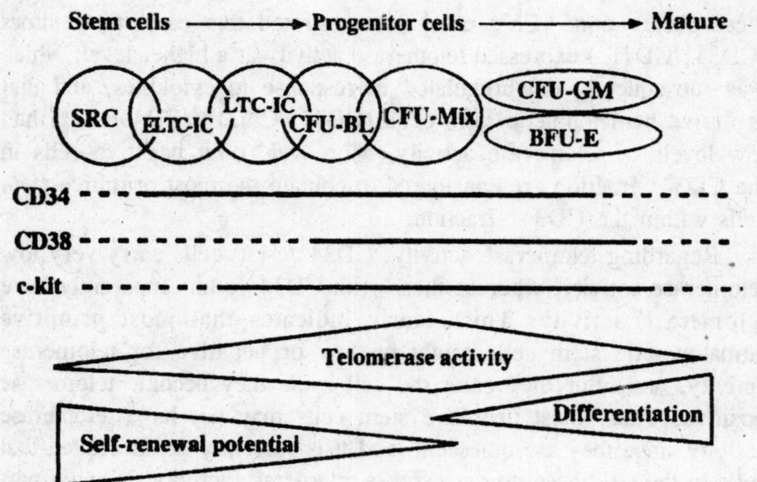

Fig. 13.5. Schematic presentation of differential level and expression of telomerase activity in hematopoietic stem cells.

Telomerase activity in normal peripheral blood cells

Peripheral blood mononuclear cells obtained from normal individuals show detectable telomerase activity. As Tatematsu et al. demonstrated, peripheral leukocytes from younger individuals show detectable telomerase activity, whereas those in older individuals do not. The

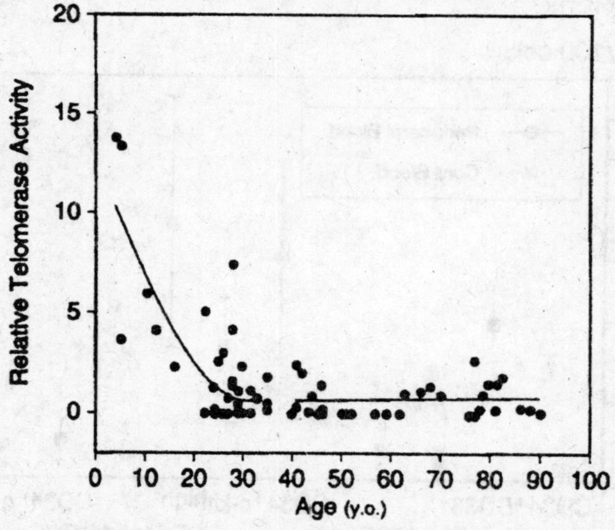

Fig. 13.6. Relative telomerase activity in peripheral blood mononuclear cells obtained from normal individuals of various ages.

exact mechanism of downregulation of telomerase activity with aging is obscure. Our study demonstrated that about half of the samples of peripheral mononuclear cells obtained from subjects older than 40 yr did not have detectable telomerase activity and the remaining samples had very low telomerase activity. By contrast, all samples obtained from subjects younger than 20 yr have detectable telomerase activity and show relatively high telomerase activity when compared with those age 20 yr. Thus, telomerase activity in normal individuals younger than 40 yr progressively declined with increased age, whereas those age 40 yr or older had a very low level or no detectable telomerase activity that was stably maintained. In peripheral granulocytes, however, no telomerase activity was detectable.

Upregulation of telomerase activity after cytokine or mitogen exposure

Most primitive bone marrow progenitors expressing telomerase activity showed downregulation of activity after cytokine exposure; Yui et al. demonstrated that telomerase activity was up-regulated after culturing purified hematopoietic stem cells ($CD34^{+}/CD71^{low}/CD45RA^{low}$) with stem cell factors, interleukin-3 and Flt3-ligand, but not with a combination of stem cell factor and Flt3-ligand, indicating that IL-3 is a key cytokine in the differentiation of hematopoietic stem cells. Engelhardt et al. also found that telomerase activity was upregulated within 48–72 h after culturing with IL-3, IL-6, erythropoietin, and granulocyte colony-stimulating factor, decreasing to baseline after 3 to 4 wk.

It is well known that mitogen-stimulated lymphocytes show upregulation of telomerase activity: circulating T-lymphocytes and B-lymphocytes in peripheral blood have telomerase activity. In T-lymphocytes, telomerase upregulation was noted by stimulation of not only anti-CD3 monoclonal antibody but also Ca ionophore and phorbol myristate acetate, which were considered to be the stimulants that bypass T-cell receptor signaling. It was also demonstrated that telomerase activity is induced in the B-lymphocyte activation of the antigen-specific immune response.

Telomerase Activity in Acute Leukemia

Telomerase activity in freshly obtained acute leukemia cells

Most acute leukemia cases have reduced telomere length, and this may represent active cell division. It has been demonstrated that leukemia cells have a short telomere length at the time of diagnosis and that their length returns to within the normal range during the complete remission state. This trend is particularly common in *acute myelogenous leukemia* (AML) and acute lymphoid leukemia. Although Takeuchi et al. reported that t(8;21) acute leukemia had a significant short telomere length at the time of diagnosis, other investigators did not confirm this change. In acute leukemia, a significant overlapping of telomerase activity between acute leukemia cells and normal peripheral mononuclear cells has been reported. In some patients with acute leukemia, telomere length decreases, but the shortening of telomeres might not reach the critical level for upregulation of telomerase activity, whereas some leukemia patients may have normal TRFs that may result from upregulation of telomerase activity. This is supported by the finding that the length of TRFs and level of telomerase activity in each patient did not show any particular correlation.

Thus, we should determine both TRF length and telomerase activity in leukemia patients. In previously reported studies, about 70% of acute leukemia patients had elevated telomerase activity at the time of diagnosis, and the remaining patients had detectable telomerase activity but within the agematched normal range. By using a stretch PCR assay, Tatematsu et al. demonstrated that most AML patients in their study had telomerase activity. At the time of relapse, higher telomerase activity was noted compared with that at the time of diagnosis. This may partially support the concept that relapsed leukemia cells have more malignant characteristics. Nevertheless, although most acute leukemia patients have shortened TRFs, some acute leukemia patients hve telomeres that might not reach the critical point for reactivating telomerase activity. It has been demonstrated that telomerase activity in myeloid leukemia cells is downregulated during the process of cellular differentiation. AML is categorized into several subtypes based on morphologic and cytologic characteristics (M0–M7), and some of them have cellular differentiation mimicking either normal or catastrophic differentiation. This suggests the possibility that telomerase activity in certain leukemia cells showing differentiation potential may be downregulated. Another key point is that telomerase activity in leukemia cells may be controlled by the cell cycle; quiescent cells (e.g., cells in the G0 phase and most primitive stem cells) have downregulation of the expression of telomerase activity. It is well known that a part of the population of *de novo* leukemia cells enters the G0 phase. These observations may indicate that telomerase activity

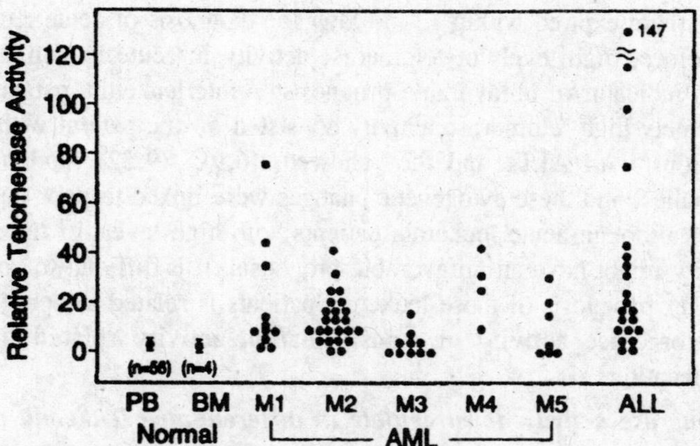

Fig. 13.7. Relative telomerase activity in acute leukemia patients. Patients with AML-M3 had low but detectable telomerase activity.

in leukemia cells may depend on the population of leukemia cells in certain cell-cycle phases and with cellular differentiation, in addition to controlling the mechanism of the telomere-telomerase relationship.

Zhang et al. demonstrated that acute leukemia patients with high telomerase activity are significantly frequent among in patients showing –7/7q– and 11q23 anomalies, and high telomerase activity indicates an extremely poor prognosis. As already discussed in a study by Ohyashiki et al., about 30% of acute leukemia patients had telomerase activity within the normal range. About 10% of the acute leukemia pateints had high levels of telomerase activity (equivalent level of telomerase activity in solid tumors), and they had a significantly poorer outcome:

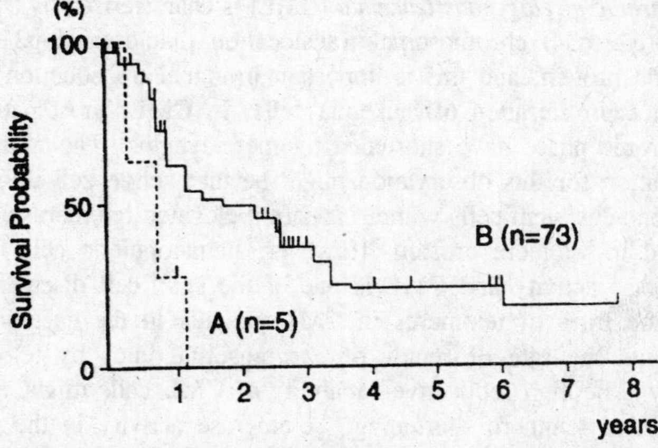

Fig. 13.8. Survival probability of acute leukemia patients depends on telomerase activity.

all of them expired within 12 mo after the diagnosis of acute leukemia. Therefore, high levels of telomerase activity in acute leukemia might be an indicator of unfavorable prognosis. Acute leukemia patients with extremely high telomerase activity consisted of one patient with AML and four with ALL, and they showed t(6;9), t(9;22), and t(17;19) anomalies, and these cytogenetic changes were linked to poor outcome. Thus, although acute leukemia patients with high levels of telomerase activity might have an unfavorable prognosis, it is difficult to conclude whether prognosis of those leukemia patients is related to upregulation of telomerase activity or transformation activity related to gene translocation.

Telomerase activity downregulate in differentiated leukemia cells

In patients with acute promyelocytic leukemia (FAB-M3), telomerase activity is not elevated compared with other types of leukemia. In a differentiation experiment using an AML cell line, HL-60, cells differentiated using all-*trans*-retinoic acid had reduced telomerase activity. However, some differentiated cells without proliferative capability maintain elevated telomerase activity, indicating that the signaling pathway that affects cellular differentiation may also reduce telomerase activity independently. Although some solid tumors with differentiation have relatively low telomerase activity compared with those with undifferentiated tumors, the level of telomerase activity is not simply related to differentiation stage of cancer cells.

Telomere Dynamics in Chronic Leukemia

Telomerase activity in chronic myeloid leukemia

Chronic myelogenous leukemia (CML) is characterized by a specific t(9;22)(q22;q34) chromosomal translocation that creates $p210^{BCR/ABL}$ chimeric protein, and this is important in signal transduction, which promotes proliferation of leukemia cells. In CML, most patients in the chronic phase have shortened telomere lengths. The most likely explanation for this observation might be that active cell division of hematopoietic stem cells without apparent elevated telomerase activity resulted in telomere erosion. However, hematopoietic cells possess telomerase activity and CML is one of the stem cell diseases, thus, reduction rates of telomeres in CML patients in the chronic phase overcome the rate of repair of chromosomal ends by telomerase activity. The high replicative capability of CML cells might result in progressive telomere shortening. Telomerase activity in the chronic phase of CML is enhanced. There is no significant difference in telomerase levels between peripheral mononuclear cells from normal subjects (resting lymphocytes) and mononuclear cells (myeloid cells) of CML cells. However, granulocytes from normal individuals do not express telomerase activity; upregulation of telomerase activity in CML myeloid cells might represent neoplastic characteristics. Telomerase activity in granulocytes in CML patients might be downregulated during the process of granulocytic differentiation, as reported by Zhang et al. using myeloid leukemia cells. Thus, the telomerase activity in the granulocytes of CML patients might not exactly reflect telomerase activity in the stem cells of CML patients. Blast crisis in some CML patients is accompanied by additional cytogenetic anomalies, and blastic transformation is considered to result from genetic alterations and clonal selection.

Telomere dynamics in CML in the chronic phase

In the chronic phase of CML, low, but detectable, telomerase activity is demonstrated. Telomere length in the chronic phase varies and some patients show normal telomere length (i.e., TRF length within the normal range). We have demonstrated that CML patients with normal TRF lengths at the time of diagnosis responded well to interferon-alpha treatment, and they had a favorable prognosis. This indicates that telomere length in CML patients may reflect disease severity and further suggests that measurement of telomere length might provide an indicator for interferon-alpha treatment. When CML patients were divided into two groups according to TRF length, CML patients with normal TRF length had significantly low levels of telomerase activity compared with those with shortened TRF length at the time of diagnosis.

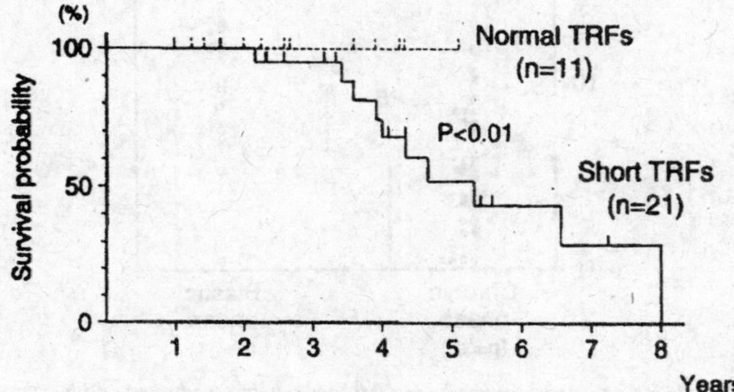

Fig. 13.9. Survival probability of CML patients depends on telomere length. CML patients with telomere length within the age-matched normal range had a significantly better outcome compared with those with shortened telomere length.

It is possible, therefore, that CML patients with short telomere length with elevated telomerase activity might reflect the excess amount of myeloid progenitor cells and be related to disease severity.

Telomerase activity in CML in the blastic phase

In blast crisis, telomerase activity is significantly elevated compared with that in the chronic phase. It is still controversial whether elevated telomerase activity in the blast phase reflects blast clones in the chronic phase or whether it is owing to reduction in telomeres. We have reported a relationship between reduction in telomere length and reactivation of telomerase activity during the process of establishing leukemia cell lines. In the chronic phase, reduction in telomere length was not remarkable, but telomeres became shortened to the critical point, and high telomerase activity was evident when they developed blast crisis. If the short telomeres and high telomerase activity reflect blast cells that exist in the chronic phase (preexisting as a minor clone), how can one explain why they show very short TRFs in the blast phase? The blast cells in both the chronic and blast phases carry the Ph translocation and they may have transforming potential. Thus,

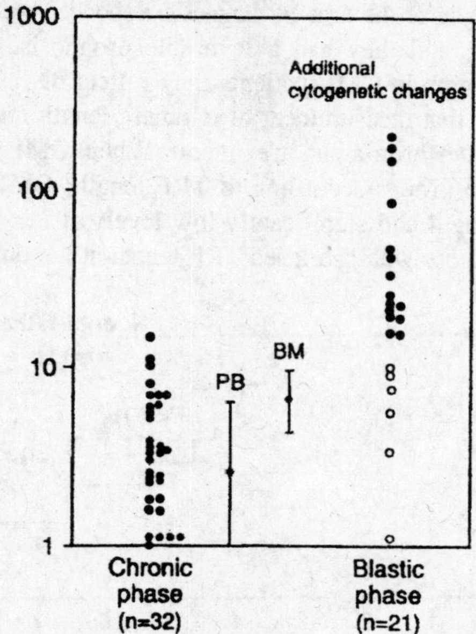

Fig. 13.10. Relative telomerase activity in CML patients in the chronic and blastic phases. A significant elevation of telomerase activity was noted in the blast phase, and most patients with high telomerase activity showed additional cytogenetic changes.

the most plausible explanation for the telomere dynamics in CML might be that Ph chromosome-positive cells, including CML stem cells, have a high proliferative potential in the chronic phase that may overcome telomerase activity, resulting in progressive erosion of telomeres.

CML stem cells that can produce blast crisis (actually present in the chronic phase) may be quiescent. Thus, they may keep telomere length without the presence of upregulated telomerase. However, we do not have any evidence that blast cells in the chronic phase are quiescent until blast crisis is clinically detectable. One can speculate that additional genetic changes cause the quiescent blast cells to "*wake up*," and then the blast cells obtain high proliferative capability resulting in the telomere length becoming shorter and shorter. Furthermore, this process may upregulate telomerase activity. According to this hypothesis, telomere dynamics in the chronic phases and blast phase might not be similar events. This aspect might be clarified by detecting telomerase activity at each cell level in the chronic and blast phases.

Telomerase activity in chronic lymphocytic leukemia

In *chronic lymphocytic leukemia* (CLL), Counter et al. telomerase activity was reported to be undetectable in the stable phase, whereas in the blast phase telomerase is upregulated. The important evidence for this is that telomerase activity in the CLL-stable phase is undetectable; thus, it is lower than in normal peripheral blood cells. This indicates that telomerase activity is not related to the mass of neoplastic cells but is linked to the population of quiescent cells.

In CLL patients, active production of CLL cells is present, but once the cells (CLL cells in the peripheral blood) become quiescent, they lose their telomerase activity, indicating that telomerase activity in neoplastic cells could also be downregulated. When CLL cells actively proliferate (terminal phase), they restore or show upregulation of telomerase activity. Therefore, it is easy to consider that upregulation and downregulation of telomerase activity can be coexistent not only in the same patient but also in the same tumor.

Telomere Dynamics in Myelodysplastic Syndromes

Myelodysplastic syndrome (MDS) encompasses a heterogeneous category of diseases showing cytopenia in the peripheral blood and characteristic dysplastic morphologic features. Approximately 30% of MDSs develop into leukemia, but some of them suffer from "*bone marrow failure*." We reported an association between the disease progression pattern and reduction of telomeres in the developmental process of disease in MDS patients.

The likely explanation of the genetic change during the process of disease progression is the genetic instability that was demonstrated by microsatellite alteration. Although the question of any correlation among cytogenetic changes, microsatellite alteration, and telomere reduction in MDS patients is obscure, this may be partially owing to the heterogeneous category of this disease entity. Chromosomal changes related to telomere reduction are also rarely seen in MDS with disease progression. Therefore, we focused on the disease progression pattern in MDS and cytogenetic changes or telomere length. Some MDS patients showed telomere reduction and karyotypic progression with disease progression, whereas some had telomere shortening before disease progression with multiple chromosomal changes. Telomere shortening was evident in all subtypes of MDS; thus, the replication history in each MDS patient that depends on telomere erosion is not related to the percentage of blast cells. There have been no reports regarding telomerase activity in MDS patients. Further studies in this field might disclose a possible association between telomere dynamics and the outcome of MDS patients.

Telomere length in myelodysplastic syndromes

As mentioned below, telomerase activity in MDS patients is detectable but not as elevated as in those with *de novo* acute leukemia, and telomere length is correlated with disease severity. About 70% of MDS patients had shortened TRF length. This might be owing to the insufficient upregulation mechanism of telomerase. MDS patients with shortened TRF length had a significantly high incidence of cytogenetic abnormalities, multiple cytopenias, and marrow blast percentage. Patients with shortened TRF length were frequently seen in the *International Prognostic Scoring System* (IPSS) highrisk group ($p < 0.01$). MDS patients with shortened TRF length had a very poor prognosis ($p < 0.01$), suggesting that telomere dynamics may be linked to clinical outcome in MDS patients. Thus, an abnormal mechanism of telomere maintenance mechanism in subgroups of MDS patients may be an early indication of genomic instability. This study demonstrates that telomere stability is frequently impaired in a high-risk group of MDS patients and suggests that in combination with the IPSS classification system, measurement of TRFs may be useful for risk stratification and, in the future, management of the care of MDS patients.

Conclusion

Telomeres are very important structures that protect chromosomal ends from recombination, but the structure itself induces irreversible reduction without the presence of telomerase activity. Researchers are now collecting evidence of telomere dynamics in clinical samples, but we are still far from being able to discuss telomere dynamics and chromosomal changes in such materials. Although there is a growing body of evidence that telomerase might be a very important key enzyme to obtain immortality, and possibly oncogenesis, other pathways for immortal characteristics are currently being reported. Moreover, we do not have any evidence at hand to indicate whether quiescent cells, especially most primitive stem cells, have telomerase activity or not.

MATERIALS

Preparation of Cell Lysate

1. Wash buffer: 10 m*M* HEPES, pH 7.5, 1.5 m*M* $MgCl_2$, 10 m*M* KCl, 1 m*M* dithiothreitol.
2. Lysis buffer: 10 m*M* Tris-HCl, pH 7.5, 1 m*M* $MgCl_2$, 1 m*M* EGTA, 0.1 *M* phenlymethylsulfonyl fluoride, 5 m*M*β-mercapto-ethanol, 0.5% CHAPS, 10% glycerol.

Amplification

1. Fluorescence-labeled CX reverse primer: 5' CCC TTA CCC TTA CCC TTA CCC TTA 3'.
2. Ampliwax.
3. 1 *M* Tris-HCl, pH 8.3.
4. 50 m*M* $MgCl_2$.
5. KCl.
6. Tween-20.
7. 0.1 *M* EGTA.
8. Deoxynucleoside triphosphates: 2.5 m*M* each.
9. Fluorescent-labeled TS forward primer: 5' AAT CCG TCG AGC AGA GTT 3'.
10. T4 gene 32 protein (Boehringer Mannheim).
11. Bovine serum albumin (BSA).
12. *Taq* DNA polyerase.
13. RNase.
14. Thermal cycler.

Analysis

1. Long Ranger polyacrylamide gel mix.
2. 1X Tris-borate EDTA (TBE): 45 m*M* Tris-borate, 1 m*M* EDTA.
3. Loading buffer: 90% formamide, 10% blue dextran.
4. Fluorescent size markers (100, 150, and 200 bp).
5. ALF automated DNA sequencer II.
6. ALF Fragment Manager Program.

METHODS

Preparation of Cell Lysate

1. Resuspend 1×10^7 cells from either fresh samples or dimethylsulfoxide-free samples stored at –80°C in 1 mL of ice-cold wash buffer, and centrifuge at 16,000*g* at 4°C for 1 min.
2. Resuspend the cell pellets in 100 μL of ice-cold lysis buffer.

Amplification

1. Lyophilize 0.1 μg of fluorescence labeled CX reverse primer in a microtube, and seal with Ampliwax.
2. Add 50 μL of TRAP reactions above the wax barrier containing 20 m*M*Tris-HCl, pH 8.3, 1.5 m*M* $MgCl_2$, 63 m*M* KCl, 0.005% Tween-20, 1 m*M* EGTA, 50 μ*M* deoxynucleoside triphosphates, 0.1 μg of fluorescence labeled TS forward primer, 1 μg of T4 gene 32 protein, 0.1 mg/mL of BSA, 2 U of *Taq* DNA polymerase, and 5 μg of the CHAPS cell extract. For RNase treatment, incubate 5 μg of extract 1 μg of RNase for 20 min at 37°C before PCR amplification. For standardization of telomerase activity, we used internal telomerase assay standard generating the 150-bp product or internal standard (TRAP-eze kit) generating the 36-bp product.
3. Place the prepared microtube at 22°C for 10 min for telomerase-mediated extension of the TS primer. Heat-inactivate the reaction mixture at 90°C for 90 s.
4. Perform the PCR in a thermal cycler under the following conditions: 27 cycles of 94°C for 30 s, 50°C for 30 s, and 72°C for 90 s.

Analysis

1. Prepare an 8% denaturing gel containing 6 *M* urea according to the supplier's instructions. Use glass plates for the ALF DNA sequencer II.
2. Add 1X TBE running buffer to the gel apparatus of the sequencer.

3. Mix 1 μL of the PCR product with 1 μL of loading buffer.
4. Denature for 1 min at 95°C, and then chill quickly on ice. Load the samples on the 8% denaturing gel. Use 100-, 150-, and 200-bp fluorescent size markers.
5. Run the DNA sequencer.
6. The fluorescent gel data obtained by the ALF DNA sequencer II are collected and analyzed automatically by the Fragment Manager Program. Each fluorescent peak is quantitated in terms of size (base pair), peak height, and peak area.

14

Detection and Prevention of Cancer

Evolving Scope of Molecular Diagnostics

There is widespread agreement that insights into the molecular biology of human cancers will make their most rapid impact in the area of cancer diagnosis. Implementation of cancer prevention is not only impeded by our limited knowledge of the complex causes of cancer, but also by a host of socioeconomic factors. The development of molecular-based cancer therapies is also hampered by scientific as well as general factors. In contrast, translation of research results into routine diagnosis is underway and is favored by scientific and general factors.

1. Other than in cancer therapy, the techniques used in research laboratories can be applied in diagnostic laboratories with relatively little additional effort. In general, techniques need to be further standardized and additional controls must be introduced. Often, procedures are developed to make them amenable to automatization.
2. The translation of molecular biology results into diagnostic procedures can built on the existing infrastructures provided by pathology and clinical chemistry laboratories in the clinic. These laboratories are already accustomed to performing biochemical and immunochemical assays and are now adding molecular biology techniques to their repertoire.
3. Similarly, the production of standardized and validated reagents for molecular diagnostic techniques has been taken up by companies

that have previously marketed diagnostic kits for immuno-histochemical or biochemical assays or by new biotech companies.

4. Molecular biology techniques fit well into an ongoing trend towards individualized therapy.

Molecular biology techniques can be applied for a wide range purposes in cacer diagnosis.

Table 14.1. Applications of molecular diagnostic techniques for cancer detection and classification

Purpose
Detection of cancer predisposition
Detection of preneoplastic changes
Cancer detection
Tumor staging
Tumor grading
Differential diagnosis
Subclassification
Prognosis of spontaneous clinical course
Prognosis of response to therapy

Tumor Staging, Grading, and Differential Diagnosis

The first applications that come to mind concern differential diagnosis of tumors before therapy. Here, assays for proteins and nucleic acids in body fluids and tissue samples supplement diagnostic procedures relying on imaging techniques and '*classical*' histopathology. Routine histopathology increasingly makes use of molecular markers at the protein, RNA and DNA level. After all, it is not a big leap from traditional staining methods for tissue samples to immunohistochemistry to detect specific protein markers, RNA-in-situ-hybridization to detect specific mRNAs, or fluorescence-in-situhybridization to detect chromosomal aberrations. Nevertheless, a new specialty is emerging, labeled '*molecular pathology*'.

It is important to be aware that, as developments in molecular biology are changing histopathology, developments in physics and information technology are revolutionizing imaging techniques. Modern computing power, e.g., allows the reconstruction of virtual dynamic 3D images from tomography data to detect and precisely localize very small tumors by non-invasive techniques. The combination of modern imaging techniques with molecular markers, such as labeled antibodies, is a rapidly developing field of applied medical science. This combination may eventually be used to localize even micrometastases consisting of a few tumor cells, to monitor the distribution of therapeutic molecules, and to improve the targeting of radiotherapy.

While modern imaging techniques can excellently circumscribe the extent of a tumor and thereby help to determine its stage, they yield little information on its histology and its biological properties, which determine its further clinical behavior. This information is also required for the choice of therapy. Traditionally, the tumor subtype was determined by its morphology, usually determined by staining of tissue sections. More recently, immunohistochemistry, e.g. for cell type-specific cytokeratins in carcinomas or CD surface proteins in leukemias, has entered routine practice and improved differential diagnosis. In general, the precise identification of the tumor type already provides a great deal of information on the likely future course of the disease (i.e. the prognosis of the patient) and a basis for the choice of the most appropriate treatment. In routine histopathology, additional information on the aggressiveness of a tumor is obtained by grading, which relies on subjective estimates of the degree of tissue disorganization as well as cellular and nuclear atypia.

Like the determination of the tumor type, this estimation of its '*character*' has in many cases been improved by the use of antibodies. These can help, e.g., to measure the proliferative fraction of the tumor or to ascertain the intactness of the basement membrane separating a questionable carcinoma in situ from the underlying connective tissue. In spite of these improvements, classification, staging and grading of many tumor types by current methods are far from perfect in predicting prognosis and the response to specific therapies. Molecular diagnostic techniques will thus be helpful for the determination of tumor stage, e.g. by allowing detection of tumor cells in the blood or in the bone marrow.

Cancer Subclassification

A major impact of molecular diagnostic techniques is expected in the subclassification of tumors with respect to prognosis and response to therapy. In several cases, particularly in hematological cancers, molecular analyses have revealed that a disease which appeared uniform by morphological criteria can be further differentiated. In other instances, e.g. renal cancers or breast cancer, molecular classification has corroborated previous suspicions that different subclasses of the disease exist and may need different treatments. Yet another situation is found in some cancers that are morphologically and molecularly similar, but in which progression depends on specific molecular alterations. For instance, mutation of *TP53*, as detected by accumulation of the mutant protein in the tumor cell, may predict a worse prognosis in several cancers, including Wilms tumors and bladder cancer.

Prediction of Response to Specific Therapies

The advent of cancer therapies directed against specific molecular targets has advanced these developments one step further. Previously, cancer therapy was directed against one type of cancer in general, e.g. against breast cancer, exploiting what was seen as general properties of cancer cells, such as increased DNA synthesis or increased sensitivity to ionizing radiation. As therapy increasingly targets specific molecular changes which are present in a subclass of cancers of one histological type, diagnosis has to follow suit. So, increasingly, molecular diagnostics is required to determine which cancers express the targets for specific molecular therapies. In this way, the introduction of molecular diagnostics into the clinic strengthens the already established trend towards individualized cancer therapy.

Early Detection

Although imaging and histopathology have become more sophisticated, they are limited by the size of a cancer. Molecular diagnostics holds the promise of detecting cancers at even earlier stages. This can be applied in several circumstances, particularly in cancer prevention and screening. Another application is in the monitoring of therapy efficacy and of recurrences.

Detection of Predispositions

Specifically, molecular diagnostics can be used to identify populations at risk for the development of a cancer. This is often not possible by traditional methods. Importantly, the definition of risk conferred by inherited mutations is unique to molecular diagnostics.

Molecular Diagnosis of Hematological Cancers

Arguably, molecular diagnostics is presently best established in hematology, of all subspecialties within oncology. Molecular techniques are used to ascertain the initial diagnosis and to determine the exact subtype among morphologically similar leukemias and lymphomas as a basis for prognosis and therapy selection. They are applied to assay autologous bone marrow and stem cell transplants for residual tumor cells and to match allogenic donor transplants to the recipient patient. During and after therapy, they are employed to monitor its success and to detect residual tumor cells and recurrences at an early stage.

Since many hematological cancers are characterized by specific cytogenetic aberrations, typically translocations, cytogenetic techniques are well suited for differential diagnosis. In addition, detection of surface markers by antibody staining is used, since cells at various stages and sublineages of the hematopoetic lineage express specific cell membrane proteins.

Burkitt lymphoma (BL) invariably carries one of three translocations which bring the *MYC* gene under the control of immunoglobulin gene enhancers. These translocations can be detected by karyotyping of tumor cell metaphases, which is best performed on cultured tumor cells. For the direct investigation of tissue sections, interphase two-colour FISH is more convenient. Tissue sections are hybridized with two DNA probes, one each from the *MYC* locus at 8q and an immunoglobulin locus (initially for *IGH* at 14q, which is most often involved), labeled by different colours. In normal cells, the loci are on distinct chromosomes and located at some distance from each other in an interphase nucleus. Even in BL cells, one pair of signals corresponding to the normal chromosomes 8 and 14 remains apart and serves as an internal control. In contrast, the signals from the translocation chromosome appear close to each other. While this apposition may occur by chance in an occasional cell, its regular appearance in a lymphoma tissue proves the presence of this particular translocation chromosome and confirms the diagnosis of Burkitt lymphoma.

This kind of technique can be used in general to detect translocations, including those in *chronic myeloid leukemia* (CML). However, while the translocations in BL cause the overexpression of MYC mRNA and protein, whose structures are not necessarily altered, the characteristic translocation in CML generates a novel fusion gene, *BCR-ABL*, with a transcript and a protein that are unique to tumor cells. This provides further opportunities for detection. The rearrangement creating the *BCR-ABL* gene can be detected by Southern blot or PCR analysis. In principle, translocations in BL could also be detected by these methods, but the detection is more straightforward and reliable in CML, since the breakpoints occur within restricted regions in both genes. They therefore create a limited number of different mRNA forms, none of which is present in a cell without a translocation. All can be detected by RT-PCR using a few pairs of PCR primers, one primer each from the *BCR* and *ABL* gene. This detection can be performed qualitatively to verify the diagnosis or quantitatively to estimate the number of tumor cells. Moreover, RT-PCR can be made extremely sensitive by nesting and real-time techniques allowing the detection of one tumor cell in a billion. Therefore, this method is much more sensitive than cytogenetic or morphological detection of tumor cells.

Thus, owing to the development in molecular diagnostics, CML therapy can be monitored at several levels by a set of techniques with different sensitivities. '*Clinical remission*' remains an important criterion. The improvement of symptoms in a treated patient and the disappearance of morphologically detectable tumor cells ('*hematological remission*'), however, are not sufficient to predict whether a recurrence will occur. Indeed, in some cases with clinical improvements and lack of obvious tumor cells, cytogenetic techniques can still detect translocation chromosomes indicative of '*minimal residual disease*'. Without additional therapy, such patients as a rule relapse. The prognosis is much better, if '*cytogenetic remission*' is achieved and no cells with translocation chromosomes can be detected. However, some of these patients still experience recurrences. Indeed, RT-PCR analyses can detect residual tumor cells in the bone marrow and even in blood. In fact, these methods can be made so sensitive as to detect tumor cells in every treated patient and even in some healthy individuals. Therefore, quantitative methods are employed and cut-off values are defined to determine which patients are very unlikely to experience recurrences.

Molecular monitoring in CML is not only important to determine the efficacy of treatment. It is also helpful in the choice of therapy, particularly to decide which patients need stem cell transplantation, and when. This treatment can have serious side-effects, such as graft-versus-host disease. Therefore, the definitive exclusion of residual disease by molecular diagnostic techniques can identify those patients for whom transplantation can be deferred. Of course, the selection of donors and cells for transplantation is also aided by molecular techniques.

In a similar fashion, molecular diagnostics can help in the choice of *acute promyelocytic leukemia* (APL) therapy. Cytogenetic or molecular diagnostics can identify patients that carry the t(15;17) (q22;q21) translocation generating the *PML-RARA* fusion gene. These can then be treated with all-trans retinoic acid, which has little effect in other acute myeloid leukemias and even in some cases of APL that are not caused by this particular translocation.

Unfortunately, the predominance of *MYC* translocations in BL, of *BCR-ABL* fusion genes in CML, and of *PML-RARA* fusions in APL are the exception rather than the rule in hematological cancers. More often, acute leukemias and lymphomas with similar phenotypes can be caused by several different genetic alterations, i.e. different translocations or other characteristic chromosomal alterations. Moreover, not all leukemias and lymphomas are characterized by specific single chromosomal changes or gene mutations. In carcinomas, this is the rule. Phenotypically similar diseases caused by different translocations can exhibit large differences in their spontaneous clinical course and in their response to specific treatments. So, determining the correlation between specific translocations and clinical behavior is a continuing effort in hematological oncology that leads to a steady progress in adapting the treatment to the individual patient's cancer.

The problem is of course exacerbated in those hematological cancers that do not show specific chromosomal aberrations. Such cases represent a significant fraction of acute lymphocytic leukemia. Here, advances are expected from '*gene expression profiling*'. Initial studies using these techniques showed that is feasible to distinguish ALL from AML (*acute myeolid leukemias*) by analysis of mRNA expression patterns. This is rarely a problem in the clinic, because protein markers for the myeloid and lymphatic lineage can be used, if the morphology of the tumor cells is not already distinctive. Indeed, the mRNAs that showed the most pronounced differences in the expression profiles were those encoding such protein markers. More importantly, the technique can distinguish different subtypes among AMLs lacking conspicuous chromosomal changes.

Another pressing clinical problem is the distinction between different subtypes of follicular lymphomas and large cell lymphoma. They exhibit similar morphological and biochemical markers, but some subtypes are rather indolent, while specific ones are aggressive, and therefore require a different therapy. This distinction can also be made by expression profiling. In other cases, expression profiling has suggested new protein markers for detection of minimal residual disease of specific subtypes.

Molecular Detection of Carcinomas

Molecular diagnostics of carcinomas is less straightforward than that of leukemias and lymphomas. The first additional complication lies in obtaining material for analysis. For leukemia diagnostics, blood samples are in many cases sufficient to detect the presence of a leukemia and even establish an initial differential diagnosis. In some cases or later in the diagnostic procedure, bone marrow aspirates or other biopsies are additionally required. Even solid types of lymphomas often present as relatively accessible swellings.

In contrast, samples from carcinoma can often be obtained only through more invasive procedures, which may carry a risk of inadvertently spreading tumor cells, e.g. in the peritoneum. So, often, only limited amounts of useful material from a carcinoma are available until surgery has been performed. This may be one reason why molecular biology of human carcinomas is not as advanced as that of hematological cancers. Another reason is that molecular alterations in carcinomas are often more complex and more heterogeneous than in hematological cancers.

Table 14.2. Important criteria in the use of molecular diagnostic assays in the clinic

Criterion
Minimal sample required
Applicable with samples obtained by non-invasive or minimally invasive methods
Speed of result
Stability of molecule assayed
Cost effectiveness
Reliability
Specificity
Sensitivity
Reproducibility
Compatibility with existing expertise, procedures, and equipment

A diagnostic assay applicable in a clinical setting has to fulfil several requirements. (1) It should require as little material as possible, e.g. from biopsies. This is a strong point of many molecular assays, in particular of PCR techniques. (2) Ideally, an assay should be able to use samples obtained by non-invasive methods. Saliva, sputum, urine, and stool samples can be obtained by completely non-invasive routes. Blood samples also present few problems. In some organs, e.g. the urinary bladder, washes can be performed which yield '*lavage*' fluids containing cells and molecules from tumors. (3) PCR techniques have also, in general, made molecular assays more rapid, which is a further requirement in many clinical situations. (4) A more problematic requirement is the stability of the molecule to be assayed. Some proteins and RNA in general are not very stable in tissue samples, unless these are quickly frozen or fixed. Therefore, assays based on DNA or on more stable proteins are generally preferable. RNA instability is even more of a problem, if quantitation is required. This is one factor withstanding the use of expression profiling techniques in clinical routine. (6) Another factor in this case, as in general, is cost-effectiveness. Cost, however, is relative. Using an expensive assay to determine the correct therapy in a small number of patients is a different issue from using an assay for screening a large population. (7) Assay sensitivity and specificity are of course crucial, although again, the required levels depend on the intended use. (8) Last not least, an assay has to be reliable, which means that it measures the parameter it is supposed to measure, not only in a laboratory situation, but also with clinical samples.

Specificity and cost are the major hurdles when a molecular assay is designated for screening larger groups or populations. Such assays also have to be essentially non-invasive, i.e. no more invasive than taking a small blood sample. In the application of molecular diagnostic techniques for carcinomas in the clinic, sensitivity and cost effectiveness most often represent the crucial issues. It is at these points, where the complexity and heterogeneity of molecular alterations in carcinomas become relevant.

The problem of sensitivity arises mainly, because there are only few instances, in which a single molecular alteration is found in every cancer of one type. This is particularly true for carcinomas. For instance, while almost every colon carcinoma shows constitutive activation of the WNT pathway, these are brought about by different genetic changes. In most cases, both copies of the *APC* gene are inactivated, while in a smaller fraction activating mutations in *CTNNB1* (β-Catenin) are responsible. In still another, albeit small fraction of colon carcinomas, neither of these genes is affected. This would probably not compromise sensitivity overly. More problematic is that the alterations in *CTNNB1* and *APC* are not homogeneous, either. Mutations that activate β-Catenin are restricted to a small region of the protein, but are not uniform. *APC* inactivation is worse, since it occurs by different mechanisms which include small and large deletions as well as point mutations at many different sites in the gene. Since most lead to a truncated protein, alternatively a protein assay could be envisioned that employs an antibody against the carboxy-terminus of the APC protein. This assay could be applied to colon cells obtained by biopsies or from faeces. This method would miss the (rare) cases with missense mutations, in addition to all those not caused by APC mutations. More problematic is that this is a '*negative marker*' assay. Assays that detect the disappearance of a marker tend to yield lower sensitivities and specificities. Hopes are placed in a microarray technique that detects all possible mutations in *APC* and *CTNNB1* (and perhaps *AXIN1*).

In contrast to loss of a protein, point mutations in DNA represent '*positive*' markers that can be detected in spite of a background of DNA from non-tumor cells in samples obtained by non-invasive methods (e.g. stool samples). Therefore, some approaches for the molecular detection of colon cancer have pursued detection of *KRAS* mutations. While these occur only in 40-60% of all colon cancers, they are strictly limited to the three codons 12, 13, and 61. These mutations can be highly sensitively detected by appropriate PCR techniques. Of course, as *KRAS* mutations mostly develop during the progression of colon cancers, this assay would detect carcinomas rather than adenomas. In theory, then, a sensitivity of 40-60% could be achieved, with a specificity approaching 100%. In practice, neither figure has been reached. The reasons for this disappointing outcome are under investigation. One might speculate that sensitivity is limited by the amount of tumor DNA entering the gut lumen and surviving the passage. There are furthermore indications that specificity is lowered by an unexpectedly high fraction of false positives, i.e. mutations detected in persons without carcinomas. Perhaps, mutations in *KRAS* sometimes occur in normal cells or arise in DNA as it travels through the gut.

A straightforward place to look for molecules originating from a cancer is blood. A number of serum protein markers are employed for the detection and monitoring of specific cancers.

Some carcinomas, including those of the colon, can be detected by increased levels of *carcino-embryonic antigen* (CEA) in the blood. This protein marker can be determined very reliably and at moderate cost by a routine immunoassay. Unfortunately, the assay is not very sensitive, since only a fraction of cancers express this oncofetal antigen, and not very specific, a.o., because several cancer types express CEA. However, once a cancer has been found to express CEA, the marker can be used to monitor the success of the therapy.

A similar immunoassay for *prostate-specific antigen* (PSA) is used to monitor prostate cancer therapy. Detection of PSA has several advantages that have led to its almost ubiquitous use. (1) Prostate epithelial cells are the only significant source of PSA in males.

Therefore, any increase in serum must be due to a process in this tissue. (2) Only few prostate carcinomas cease to synthesize the protein, often only at a very late stage when this is no longer clinically important. (3) The PSA level is roughly related to the tumor volume. Following removal of the prostate harboring the cancer, PSA declines. Ideally, the protein should become undetectable (<0.1 ng/ml) and stay so, if the cancer has been cured. A nadir in the ng/ml range typically indicates that the local tumor has not been completely removed. In that case, one would consider adjuvant radiotherapy or anti-androgenic therapy. Recurrences caused by micrometastases are usually announced several years in advance by a slow increase of serum PSA from zero levels. In late stage systemic disease, values >1000 ng/ml may be reached.

PSA levels can also be employed in clinical and experimental studies. The presence and size of primary and metastatic tumor masses is an important parameter to determine the efficacy of a new drug or the significance of a molecular marker. However, metastases in prostate cancer can often only be detected with difficulty, least their size be measured. So, in prostate cancer the success of a new therapy is often monitored via the PSA level, which is used as a '*surrogate parameter*' of cancer extension. In general, a 50% decrease is taken as evidence of remission. While PSA assays are thus helpful, they do have downsides, on the scientific as well as on the psychological side. On the scientific side, PSA synthesis is induced by androgens. Therefore, treatments that influence androgen signaling may decrease PSA levels much more than they affect tumor growth. On the psychological side, as PSA plays such a dominant role in the treatment of prostate cancer, not only patients, but also doctors and scientists are tempted to ascribe more value to a PSA level than it is worth.

While PSA is an excellent marker for monitoring of prostate cancer, its specificity for the initial detection of the carcinoma is limited. Here, additional molecular diagnostic assays might be helpful, which detect cancer cells in prostate biopsies or blood, or cancer-specific markers in blood, urine, or ejaculate.

As in colon cancer, genetic alterations in prostate cancer are heterogeneous, if anything, much more so. In some patients, tumor cells can be detected in the blood, e.g. by an RT-PCR assay for prostate-specific mRNAs such as PSA mRNA. Detection of PSA mRNA is a more specific indication of cancer than detection of PSA protein, because the protein is secreted, whereas its mRNA can only be dectected if prostate epithelial cells are present in the circulation. These are in most cases cancer cells. For a while, this method was even thought to be useful for the distinction of metastatic from organ-confined cancers, i.e. for '*molecular staging*'. However, this may not prove to be true.

Other assays are based on DNA alterations in tumor cells. In many tumor patients, increased levels of DNA are found in blood plasma, which is cell-free. Its source is not entirely clear, but much of it appears to be derived from tumor cells, perhaps released from cells dying in the circulation. Typical mutations present in cancer tissues can also be detected in this circulating DNA, e.g. *KRAS* mutations from a colon or pancreatic carcinoma.

In prostate cancer, specifically, no characteristic mutations occur regularly enough to be exploited for this kind of assay. However, alterations of DNA methylation are highly prevalent, in particular hypermethylation of the *GSTP1* gene, which may occur in >80% of all prostate carcinomas. Since DNA hypermethylation affects CpG-islands which are unmethylated in normal tissues, its detection is very specific and sensitive because of a negligible background from normal tissues. Moreover, while hypermethylation of some genes is also found in aging tissues or early preneoplastic lesions, the hypermethylation of *GSTP1* appears to be cancer-specific, or at least restricted to late preneoplastic lesions in addition. So, detection of *GSTP1* hypermethylation in blood or prostate fluid may provide a valuable technique to supplement PSA assays.

DNA hypermethylation is also found in many other cancers and similar assays are being developed for their detection. Unlike in the case of prostate cancer and *GSTP1*, in most cancers, hypermethylation assays must be performed for several genes, since each is hypermethylated in only a fraction of cancers. Moreover, hypermethylation of *GSTP1* is relatively specific to prostate cancer. It is otherwise only found in a smaller fraction of renal carcinomas and hepatomas. These cancers are relatively straightforwardly excluded in prostate cancer patients. In contrast, another gene, *RASSF1A*, is hypermethylated in prostate cancer, but also in many others and even some precursors. This property could make *RASSF1A* hypermethylation useful as a general sensitive tumor marker, but limit its specificity.

Tumor DNA in plasma can also be assayed for mutations or for allelic imbalances. As in general, the sensitivity of these assays is limited by the heterogeneity of genetic alterations within the tumor type. Some current research therefore aims at developing assays which detect every mutation in one gene, e.g. in *TP53*. These assays would, however, still miss alternative pathways of TP53 inactivation, such as MDM2 over-expression. The sensitivity of assays for allelic imbalances is in addition limited by the extent to which tumor DNA is diluted in the plasma by DNA originating from normal cells.

A hotly debated question in the use of plasma DNA for tumor detection is how its overall presence and amount relate to tumor stage. A similar question pertains to the issue of tumor cells found to circulate in the blood. If DNA from a tumor is present in blood, it appears to have gained access to the circulation, which is almost certain, if tumor cells are encountered in blood outside the tumor tissue. So, while early stages of tumor development can perhaps not be discovered by assays using blood samples, the detection of tumor-specific DNA alterations or even of tumor cells may yield information on how far the cancer has advanced. This approach may therefore yield a chance to achieve a '*molecular staging*'. Alternatively, the type of mutations and allelic imbalances might be used for '*molecular staging*', if they can be assigned to specific stages of tumor development.

Molecular Classification of Carcinomas

Detection of a cancer is only the first step towards therapy. Whether and which therapy is administered, depends on a further, more precise classification of the cancer. Traditionally, cancers were assigned to different histological subtypes by their morphology and further classified by stage and grade by imaging techniques and histopathological examination. Experience and carefully collected observational data were used to assess the prognosis of the cancer and select the most appropriate therapy.

The criteria underlying tumor staging, in particular, are not arbitrary, but have usually been chosen to correspond to those steps in tumor progression, at which the prognosis and accordingly, the most appropriate treatment changes. Such steps may be evident, such as beginning invasion of outer layers in a tissue or growth beyond an organ, or they may have to be determined by careful follow-up of large numbers of patients. For instance, renal carcinomas rarely metastasize unless they exceed a certain volume, but are as a rule incurable, once metastases have developed. Accordingly, the criteria for staging of renal carcinomas have been changed back and forth based on observational data relating the course of disease to the diameter of the tumor. In this case, prognosis additionally depends on the specific histological subtype, with some histological subtypes metastasizing more readily than others. Therefore, knowledge on the histological type of the tumor is important for the determination of prognosis. More recently, identification of characteristic chromosomal alterations for each subtype of renal carcinomas has been introduced to aid in the classification of ambiguous cases.

There are many carcinomas, in which the '*classical*' trias of histology, staging, and grading does not consistently yield sufficient information for optimal selection of therapy. It is not at all exceptional for carcinomas with identical stage, grade, and histology to take divergent clinical courses. The most severe problem in general is that micrometastases escape detection by current imaging methods. Therefore, staging is not really precise and the extension of the primary tumor as well as its histology and grade only yield an estimate on the presence of micrometastases. These are responsible for recurrences and patient death, even if the primary tumor can be completely removed or destroyed. Thus, the decisions on how to deal with the primary tumor and whether to apply an adjuvant therapy (and which, if there is a choice), are based on probabilities rather than definitive information. A large set of empirical data has been collected for each cancer type which can be used in these decisions. In some cancers, algorithms and nomograms taking all known relevant parameters into account have been introduced as a help for patients and doctors. Nevertheless, the overall situation is far from satisfactory.

In a sense, progress in therapy has aggravated this dilemma. Since a larger choice of treatments has become available, criteria are needed to determine which patients will respond to which therapy. In addition, therapies differ with respect to their side-effects and their costs, which can often not be neglected.

For these reasons, improvements in the classification of carcinomas are a major goal of current molecular research. Breast cancer may represent a major carcinoma, where this type of research is advanced and is translated into the clinic at a rapid pace. Molecular assays are increasingly used in this cancer as supplements to staging, grading and histology.

As in other carcinomas, prognosis in breast cancer depends on tumor size, tumor grade, and the histological subtype. Neither unusually, breast cancers in young patients tend to be more aggressive. More specific to breast cancer, prognosis and therapy differ before and after menopause. The single most significant prognostic factor in this cancer is the extent of lymph node involvement. Less than 30% of cancers without detectable tumor cells in the lymph nodes recur, whereas >75% of cancers with several positive lymph nodes have progressed to systemic disease and will recur, if only the primary tumor is destroyed. So, almost all patients with lymph node involvement receive adjuvant therapy. Moreover, since recurrent breast cancer is rarely curable, chemotherapy or anti-estrogenic therapy is also administered to most of the patients with no positive lymph nodes as well, unless additional favorable factors are found, such as small tumor size or low grade, or a rarer less aggressive histological subtype is present. This means that overall ≈60% of breast cancer patients unnecessarily receive an unpleasant and toxic therapy, but it is difficult to determine, whether this is so for each individual patient.

Some molecular markers are already in routine use to help with this decision. Low concentrations of the plasminogen activator uPA and its inhibitor PAI-1 indicate a favorable prognosis, at least in cancers that are well or moderately differentiated. Patients with cancers designated ER+/PR+ that express both the estrogen and progesterone receptors also fare better, as a rule. More recently, determination of the ERBB2 status by immunohistochemistry and FISH analysis has been introduced. In general, breast cancers with ERBB2 overexpression caused by gene amplification are more likely to have metastasized. However, determinations of the ER/PR and ERBB2 status are employed primarily for the choice of therapy rather than for the determination of prognosis. Cancers that are ER+/PR+ tend to respond well to anti-estrogenic therapy, whereas cancers that do not express the steroid hormone receptors or that overexpress ERBB2 do not. Instead, some cancers with ERBB2 over-expression can be treated more successfully by a combination of chemotherapy, including anthracyclins, and an antibody directed against ERBB2, trastuzumab.

Overall, >100 individual molecular markers for the prognosis of breast cancer have been suggested over the last years. Promising candidates that may make it into clinical routine are the proliferation markers Ki67 and PCNA, which are also useful in several other cancers. They can be detected in a semi-quantitative manner by immunohistochemistry. Similarly, the cell cycle regulator Cyclin E is overexpressed in more aggressive breast cancers, and $p27^{KIP1}$ is accordingly down-regulated.

It is generally presumed that no single clinical or molecular parameter may be sufficient for an optimal prognosis of breast cancer.

Rather, several are already in use and further ones are being added. Considering appropriately all the known factors and their complex relationships becomes increasingly difficult. Therefore, algorithms and nomograms have been introduced that help to take into account the relative importance of each information obtained, including histology, staging, grading, patient age, and various molecular markers, and their relationship to each other. These can help in the choice of therapy, which ultimately rests with the doctor and the patient. As more and more interacting factors become known and can be assayed, computer programs are being developed that calculate the risks associated with each treatment strategy. Learning algorithms and neuronal networks are particularly suited to this task, as they can improve with their 'own' experience and integrate information from new clinical studies.

In a sense, therefore, expression profiling using microarrays is a logical continuation of a development that is already underway in breast cancer diagnosis. Analysis of the expression levels of a large number of genes indeed allows to classify breast cancers into ER+ and ER- types. It distinguishes previously unrecognized luminal cell-like and basal cell-like subtypes, with ERBB2+ cancers representing a distinct subclass within the basal-cell-like subtype. Cancers arising in patients with inherited mutations in the BRCA genes also exhibit characteristic profiles. Most importantly, metastatic cancers appear to show distinct expression patterns from those still growing locally.

The next step therefore will be to verify these profiles in larger groups of patients in prospective studies. A large population study of this kind is underway in the Netherlands. If these studies are successful, the technical and cost problems that currently prohibit routine use of expression profiling in the clinic are likely to not present serious obstacles in the long run. In parallel with these studies, much smaller sets of genes that are decisive for the distinctions provided by microarray data will be assayed for their potential as prognostic markers. For prostate cancer, e.g., a set of just four genes has been proposed for this purpose. Expression of all four can be followed by immunohistochemistry, facilitating the introduction of these markers into routine laboratories.

Prospects of Molecular Diagnostics in the Age of Individualized Therapy

The examples of breast cancer and leukemia described in the previous sections illustrate a general development in cancer diagnosis and therapy. Cancer therapy has moved towards individualization. This development began actually quite independently of the availability of adequate molecular markers and any in-depth understanding of the molecular basis of cancer pathophysiology. Already, surgery, chemotherapy and radiotherapy are administered contingent on histopathological parameters and on the patient's general state of health and psychosocial circumstances. A vast amount of empirical data can serve as a basis for the decision in each individual case ('*evidence-based medicine*'). This individualization helps to achieve optimal therapeutic results, to minimize suffering not only from the cancer, but also from the treatment, and to avoid unnecessary expenses. In this situation, molecular markers come in handy to continue an ongoing development in all subdisciplines of oncology.

However, the potential of molecular markers in the diagnosis of cancer goes beyond providing better distinctions between subclasses of one cancer and serving as prognostic markers. It is captured in the novel notions of '*pharmacogenetics*' and '*pharmacogenomics*'.

In a sense, pharmacogenetics is also a continuation of an existing trend, since it has been known for quite a while that individual patients can react very different to some drugs.

NAT2

'*Slow*' and '*fast*' acetylators, e.g. not only metabolize carcinogenic arylamines at a different rate, but also a variety of drugs in medical use. Therefore, this phenotype influences susceptibility to cancer as well as the response to therapy. The '*slow*' and '*fast*' acetylator phenotypes are due to polymorphisms in genes encoding N-acetyl-transferases, mostly in *NAT*2.

UGTA1

Individuals with Gilbert syndrome, like slow acetylators, are otherwise asymptomatic, but excrete certain drugs more slowly than others. These can therefore accumulate to dangerous levels. The molecular basis of Gilbert syndrome is a polymorphism in the promoter of the *UGTA1* gene encoding UDP-glucuronyl-transferase A1. The promoter contains a variable number of TA repeats. The allele *UGT1A1*1* with six repeats yields maximum expression, whereas a frequent polymorphic allele containing seven repeats, *UGT1A1*28*, is associated with diminished expression. The UGTA1 enzyme transfers glucuronic acid to hydroxyl groups of endogenous or exogenous compounds, which increased their solubility in aquous solution and facilitates their excretion. In cancer therapy, this polymorphism is most relevant for the metabolism of irinotecan, a topoisomerase inhibitor used a.o. in the treatment of colorectal and lung cancers. Severe toxicity of the compound is observed predominantly in persons homozygous for the *UGT1A1*28* allele.

TS

The promoter of the *TS* gene encoding thymidylate synthetase is likewise polymorphic. It contains either two or three repeats of a 28 bp tandem repeat. The respective alleles are designated *TSER**2 and *TSER*3*. The *TSER*3* alleles lead to increased expression of the enzyme that is crucial for the synthesis of dTTP required for DNA replication. Increased expression of TS diminishes the effect of inhibitors, such as 5-fluoro-uracil, which are employed in the treatment of many different cancers.

TMPT

Thiopurine methyltransferase (TPMT) metabolizes and detoxifies purines containing a thiol group, especially the drug azathioprine, which is used in the chemotherapy of leukemias. About 1% of all individuals lack enzyme activity due to a genetic polymorphism. In these persons, administration of thiopurine drugs at the standard dose can be lethal. Heterozygotes for the *TPMT* polymorphism tolerate intermediate doses.

ATM

Sensitivity to radiotherapy, likewise, is influenced by genetic polymorphisms, as exemplified by individuals heterozygous for mutations in the *ATM* gene. This gene encodes a protein kinase controlling the cellular response to DNA damage by ionizing radiation, but also to other forms of DNA damage. Pharmacogenetics, thus, is the systematic study of all genetic variation that determine the individual response to drugs. Of course, pharmacogenetics is not restricted to drugs used in cancer therapy, and as indicated by the case of *ATM*, genetic polymorphisms are also relevant to therapies other than drugs.

In current clinical practice, pharmacogenetics is rarely used explicitly. Rather, it is implicit in the way drugs are administered. Patients are asked about known hypersensitivities and are observed for adverse reactions known to occur with specific compounds. New drugs are monitored for side effects while being developed and are continued to be monitored for side effects after their introduction to the general market. This latter monitoring is important, since some polymorphisms are present in only a few individuals or are only prevalent in specific subpopulations. Drug trials can never be comprehensive in this respect. While these general procedures are well established, specific genetic analysis for polymorphisms influencing drug sensitivity are currently only used in selected circumstances. For instance, some institutions have an *TPMT* assay set up routinely.

The reasons for this are practicability and cost to a much greater extent than a lack in understanding of individual variabilities in the reaction to drugs. For many drugs in current use, the mechanisms underlying different toxicities are in fact well elucidated. However, the genetic polymorphisms underlying individual variabilities are often complex and assaying them is currently more expensive than relying on careful observation in a trial-and-error fashion.

The '*slow*' and '*rapid*' acetylator phenotypes, e.g., are brought about by quantitative interactions between >10 different *NAT2* alleles. To predict the phenotype from the genotype, a range of polymorphisms must be tested. So, observing the patients or monitoring the excretion of a test drug dose, is more practical. Similarly, individuals with low UDPGTA1 expression can usually be identified by a slight elevation of serum bilirubin in the absence of other signs of liver disease, as determined by routine clinical chemistry. A molecular genetic assay is preferred for assaying *TPMT*, because the genotype/phenotype relationship is straightforward and the polymorphisms are relevant for a clearly defined class of drugs administered for selected diseases.

This situation may change radically in the future. One factor driving the change is the continuing automatization of techniques for molecular genetic analysis which reduces expenses. Many in the field envision a chip-based assay, which at one stroke detects all polymorphisms relevant for drug metabolism in an individual. This analysis could be performed once and for all for each person and drugs could be prescribed accordingly. However, not everybody is enthusiastic about this scenario, for diverse reasons. One concern is safeguarding of individual genetic data. It is one thing to determine the genetic properties of an individual responsible for the sensitivity to one particular drug administered against a deadly disease, but it is another to record many polymorphisms influencing the response to a variety of medical and other drugs. There are also purely scientific concerns. As the example of the acetylator phenotype shows, the relationship between genotype and phenotype is often not straightforward. The individual reaction to most drugs is determined by several factors, of which only some are determined by the DNA sequence assayed in molecular tests. Even if genetic factors predominate, several genes may be involved and their interactions can be complex.

The issue is different, if not adverse reactions, but positive response to a drug or treatment are at stake. A substantial number of otherwise efficacious drugs have failed in early clinical trials (i.e. in phase I or phase II) or have not even proceeded to being tested in humans (i.e. to phase I) because they display intolerable sideeffects. Others seem efficacious in a subset of patients too small to warrant their further development for the general market. If one could predict which patients tolerate or respond, respectively, to such drugs, they could still be used in selected patients. This would extend the range of individualisation of therapy.

The notions of '*pharmacogenetics*' and '*pharmacogenomics*' are still pretty fresh and are often used rather loosely, so some confusion has arisen. In fact, prediction of positive responses to therapy is one area in which pharmacogenetics and pharmacogenomics meet and overlap. The precise distinction should be that pharmacogenetics deals with the patient's reactions to specific therapies, whereas pharmacogenomics considers the therapeutic targets specific for a disease. A broad definition of pharmacogenomics would therefore encompass almost the entire molecular biology of human cancers. In everyday use, the term '*pharmacogenomics*' more specifically denotes the investigation of drug targets in specific cancers.

A good illustration of the purpose of pharmacogenomics is the case of ERBB2. In a specific subclass of breast cancers, ERBB2 is overexpressed, typically as a result of gene amplification. Determination of ERBB2 expression and of amplification of its gene gives a very good indication of whether cancers will respond to an antibody directed against the protein. This may sound like an issue for pharmacogenetics, but it is a genetic property of the particular tumor and not the individual patient that provides the basis of the treatment.

As more and more therapeutic agents become available that are targeted to specific molecules in specific tumors, pharmacogenomic testing will become more important.

Moreover, other than in pharmacogenetics, prediction of the response of a cancer to a drug typically relies on an molecular assay. Obviously, the response of a breast cancer patient to an anti-ERBB2 antibody cannot be predicted from her previous experience with everyday drugs. Similarly, the simple strategy of applying the drug and monitoring the response is inefficient and costly, since the treatment is expensive and is efficacious in only a fraction of the patients. So, the molecular assay has to precede the application of the drug. The necessity of pharmacogenomic tests is underlined by failed efforts to extend the use of ERBB2-targeted therapy to other cancers. Amplification and over-expression of ERBB2 are rare in prostate and bladder cancers and clinical trials with the antibody directed against the protein were by and large unsuccessful.

In contrast, imatinib, an inhibitor of the BCR-ABL protein kinase, was found to induce remissions not only in chronic myeloid leukemia, which is driven by this fusion protein, but also in other cancers. In gastrointestinal stromal tumors, its effect could be related to the inhibition of the KIT receptor tyrosine kinase, already known as an alternative target of the drug from in vitro assays. However, among these, only those cancers in which KIT was activated by a mutation responded. This experience makes a strong argument in favor of pharmacogenomical approaches to therapy. However, further cancer types, without KIT activation, have responded to imatinib. In these, the effect of the drug is ascribed to inhibition of the receptor tyrosine kinase PDGFR (*platelet-derived growth factor receptor*).

Pharmacogenetics and pharmacogenomics are two specific areas which may be representative for the overall direction that molecular diagnostics in oncology is taking. It is expected that molecular diagnostic techniques will supplement the established methods of tumor diagnosis, rather than replace them. The main impact of innovation will be to better tailor therapy to each individual patient and to each individual cancer.

Prevention of Cancer

Less than 60% of all cancers can be cured by current therapies, even though these are often burdensome with serious side effects. Therefore, the best strategy would seem to prevent cancers in the first place. Moreover, strategies focusing on cancer prevention could circumvent the increasing economic problems in the health systems of Western industrialized countries, where treatment costs are felt to have become exuberant and ressources are strained. In some developing countries, with health care budgets of down to $1 per person and year, cancer preventive strategies are plainly the only realistic option.

While these arguments are in principle conceded by everybody, in practice cancer prevention measures are slowly implemented. The scientific literature, too, rarely yields the impression that cancer prevention is high on the list of research priorities. The reasons for this discrepancy are manifold. Political and socioeconomic factors may be dominant. More pertinent to the theme of this book, the science behind prevention is also anything but trivial. Cancer prevention requires a multidisciplinary approach with contributions from many fields, from molecular biology, infectiology, and pharmacology through psychology to health system economy. The scientific basis for successful prevention is not convincing for many cancers. Nevertheless, many programs have already been successfully implemented and further developments are underway. The prime task of molecular biology research in this context is to identify the causes of cancers as precisely as possible and to define the most appropriate stage and optimal means for intervention. Both are different for different cancers. Moreover, in many cases the implementation of cancer prevention hinges on progress in diagnostics and therapy. Several different types of cancer prevention are distinguished, mostly according to the stage of cancer development at which they are applied.

Table 14.3. Types of cancer prevention

Type of cancer prevention
Primary prevention (avoidance of exposure to carcinogens)
Chemoprevention
Dietary changes
Detection of preneoplastic changes and early cancer stages
Prevention of cancer after preneoplastic changes
Prevention of recurrences and second cancers
Prevention in individuals with inherited high-risk predisposition to cancer

Primary Prevention

Ideally, a cancer can be prevented by eliminating or avoiding the responsible carcinogens. These can be chemical compounds such as aromatic amines in bladder cancer, physical agents such as UV radiation in skin cancer, or biological agents such as the virus HBV in liver cancer and the bacterium *H. pylori* in stomach cancer. Obviously, cancers arising overwhelmingly from endogenous processes, which may include many cases of colorectal cancer and prostate carcinoma, will require a different approach for prevention.

Even in those cancers, in which a responsible carcinogen has unequivocally been identified, the implementation of prevention is not generally straightforward. Arguably, the most tragic case is that of tobacco smoking and lung cancer. A causal relationship has been established at every conceivable level from epidemiological data down to the molecular detail of detecting major carcinogens from cigarette smoke covalently bound to precisely those bases in the *TP53* gene of bronchial epithelial cells, at which mutations are most often observed in lung cancers. Moreover, while addiction to tobacco smoking is difficult to heal in many afflicted persons, tobacco use is not necessary for human life and could principally be avoided. The inability to prevent a large fraction of lung cancers (and others caused by tobacco smoke carcinogens) is hardly due to a lack of scientific insight.

Not all these arguments apply to UV radiation, which is the established major cause of different types of skin cancer. The relationship between the carcinogen and the disease can be considered proven. An important piece of molecular evidence is that mutations in *TP53* and other tumor suppressor genes like *PTCH1* in skin cancers bear the signature of induction by UV radiation. However, while unreasonable exposure to UV radiation during leisure activities might be avoided, complete avoidance of the carcinogen is not realistic for people with outdoor occupations. Even more importantly, up to a certain dose sunlight with its UV component is beneficial and even necessary for human health.

The critical level, at which danger surpasses benefit, differs between individuals and populations. It depends strongly on genetic polymorphisms that determine the intensity of skin pigmentation. In addition, a smaller number of individuals are oversensitive to UV radiation or sunlight, e.g. as a consequence of defects in DNA repair in xeroderma pigmentosum patients. Thus, skin cancer prevention requires an individualized approach. It is pursued by a combination of campaigns aiming at the general public and individual counseling by general practitioners and dermatologists.

A different dilemma is posed by chemical carcinogens in the workplace, illustrated by the case of aromatic amines causing bladder cancer in humans. Like in the above cases, the relationship is well established and consequences have been drawn. Today, a situation like that encountered by Ludwig Rehn when he went to investigate why so many of his patients developed bladder cancers, is - hopefully – not found anywhere anymore. Yet, it was not a century ago, when one third of the employees in another German chemical plant manufacturing benzidine developed bladder cancers. However, after a retreat battle vividly described by Robert Proctor in "*Cancer Wars*", these experiences have led to the establishment of strict regulations in the production and use of chemicals that are established or likely carcinogens in man. Unfortunately, many carcinogenic chemicals are necessary and cannot reasonably be eliminated completely. Therefore, it is in the end a political decision which amounts should be produced and which levels should be accepted. Chemical plants and laboratories can be fitted to minimize the risk for those working there, whereas the environment and the population at large cannot. Therefore, the acceptable levels of chemical carcinogens are not only determined from the angle of occupational risk, but also by their presumed impact on the environment and the general population.

In many cases, however, the responsible carcinogens are not known sufficiently precisely for intervention. For instance, epidemiological studies consistently demonstrate an increased risk of bladder cancer in the plastics and rubber industry, but it is not entirely clear which compounds are responsible and which measures could be taken to avoid exposure to them.

Another complication stems from the fact that most cancers have different and potentially interacting causes. Consider the (realistic) case of a bladder cancer patient, who has been employed in a tire factory, has been a long-time smoker, is an amateur painter, and regularly takes (too much) phenacetine against his recurrent headaches. This person has likely been exposed to four different sources of chemical carcinogens that each could cause bladder cancer, and it is not unlikely that they synergize. With the exception of smoking, none of these exposures is completely preventable in a real world.

As in the case of UV exposure, there are substantial differences in the way individuals react to chemical carcinogens. In the case of exposure to aromatic amines, several polymorphisms in enzymes responsible for their activation, metabolism, and excretion have been found to modulate a person's risk of cancer and other adverse reactions. Their combined effects are not small. Thus, among the employees that developed bladder cancer after occupational exposure to benzidine-related compounds, the vast majority where '*slow acetylators*', while few '*rapid acetylators*' were affected. These phenotypes are due to polymorphisms in the *NAT2* gene.

In the general population, all different combinations of such polymorphisms are represented. It is tempting to select more resistant persons from this heterogeneous group for the inevitable production of arylamines needed for dyes and drugs by testing for their *NAT2* and further genotypes. There are, of course, serious ethical problems associated with this approach, since it might lead to a sort of '*genetic selection*'. Proponents point out that this approach is already used in protecting more sensitive persons, e.g. pregnant women are prohibited from working with radioactive materials. Certainly, one would not like to expose an over-sensitive person to a dangerous chemical compound either? On the other hand, a person's genotype can be considered a part of his or her privacy. If it is revealed to employers, who else could be barred from that information? In addition, choosing a vocation is certainly an important constitutent of individual freedom. A general concern is that genetic testing for susceptibility to carcinogens in the workplace might lead to a lowering of the established standards for prevention of occupational carcinogenesis and might eventually endanger the population. Clearly, this issue requires a public consensus as a basis for political decisions. It also requires solid data and excellent counseling for informed choices to be made.

The problem of balancing economic necessities with disease prevention reemerges in the wider context of exposure of the entire population towards chemical carcinogens. Unlike in the workplace, special protective measures are not feasible here. Moreover, the population is even more heterogeneous than the employees in a chemical plant, encompassing not only healthy adults, but also children or people with disabilities or largely increased susceptibilities. Moreover, while the release of synthetic chemical compounds into the environment can often be controlled, many natural sources of carcinogens cannot. It is hardly surprising, therefore, that issues such as the allowable levels of carcinogenic benzene in fuel or of carcinogenic arsenic in drinking water have not only stirred up scientific but also political debates.

These two cases illustrate different kinds of problems that complicate the scientific evaluation of such issues. Benzene causes leukemia after being oxidized to phenolic and quinoid metabolites in the bone marrow. Its carcinogenicity appears to be limited by the activity of a specific quinone reductase, NAD(P)H:quinone oxido-reductase 1 (NQO1). The *NQO1* gene is polymorphic in man, and $<2\%$ of Central Europeans, but $\geq 20\%$ in some Asian populations are homozygous for an allele encoding an unstable and essentially inactive enzyme. These homozygotes are likely more susceptible to the carcinogenic effect of benzene. So, which level of sensitivity should be chosen?

Arsenic, too, is established as a human carcinogen by epidemiological data and case studies. It causes primarily cancers of the skin and the bladder. Its mode of action, however, is not at all clear, so all estimates of its impact have a large error margin. It does not induce point mutations, but appears to cause epigenetic changes and perhaps acts by indirect mechanisms as a clastogen, e.g. it favors chromosomal instability. Moreover, the uncertainty is exacerbated by evidence pointing to substantial differences in arsenic metabolism between individuals, whose molecular basis is neither elucidated.

While many controversies surround the issue of prevention of chemical carcinogenesis, prevention of carcinogenesis by infectious agents is almost unanimously accepted. Theoretically, elimination of the infectious agents by chemotherapy or vaccination could have major effects. Its potential is illustrated by the geographical differences in the incidence of liver cancer (more precisely: hepatocellular carcinoma) caused by HBV or HCV and the decline of stomach cancer in industrialized countries, which is ascribed largely to the decreasing prevalence of *H. pylori*.

Indeed, vaccination programs against HBV appear to be highly effective. For instance, in countries where the virus is endemic, such as Taiwan, even children develop hepatocellular carcinoma. Since the introduction of vaccination for young children, the incidence of such cases has plummeted. Hopefully, this trend will continue in the future. Since HBV appears to act synergistically with aflatoxins from contaminated food in countries with a humid climate, protection against viral infection might be complemented by programs improving the quality of food storage. Like the actual implementation of vaccination programs, however, this may be less of a scientific than of an economic problem.

The RNA virus HCV is likewise implicated as a cause of liver cancer and could be the next target for a vaccination campaign. In Western countries, where this virus is responsible for a slow, but persistent increase in the incidence of hepatocellular carcinoma, efforts are made to advertise a recently developed vaccine against HCV in risk groups.

Several other viruses, mostly DNA viruses, are implicated in human cancer. The relevance of the papovaviruses SV40, BK, and JC for human cancer is controversial, although (or perhaps, because) chronic infection with BKV, in particular, is highly prevalent. The herpes virus EBV is very likely involved in some human cancers, but its mode of action is unclear and the majority of the population lives without adverse effects. Apparently, its cocarcinogenic effect is mostly exerted in immuno-comprised persons. This is almost certainly so for another member of the herpes virus family, HHV8/HKSV, which is the causative agent in Kaposi sarcoma. For both viruses, preventing or improving the immunodeficiency seems the most practical strategy.

Therefore, the current prime candidates for cancer prevention by antiviral vaccination are the oncogenic strains of *human papilloma virus* HPV. Vaccination against HPV is expected to lead to a huge decrease in cervical cancer incidence, but it might also diminish the incidence of other cancers, notably of squamous cell carcinomas of the head and neck.

The most clear-cut case of a bacterium causing cancer in humans is that of *H. pylori* in stomach cancer. Quite certainly, the continuous decrease in stomach cancer incidence in most Western industrialized countries is in part due to eradication of the bacterium by antibiotic treatment and increased hygiene. Other factors have very probably contributed. They include lower exposure to nitrosamines from smoked and pickled foods and the increased availability and consumption of protective fruit and vegetables. Since it is considered difficult to eradicate *H. pylori* completely, progress in prevention of this cancer, which worldwide remains one of the most lethal diseases, may also come from improvements in general hygiene and nutrition. There are some concerns that in the absence of accompanying measures, the eradication of *H. pylori* by antibiotic treatment or vaccination might result to some extent in a shift of cancers from the lower parts of the stomach to the cardia and the esophagus.

How strongly pathogenic *H. pylori* acts in an individual person depends on genetic variation among the bacterial strains and on genetic polymorphisms in the host. Together, these determine whether the bacterium behaves as a symbiote protecting against reflux disease (and perhaps other infections and obesity) or as a carcinogenic agent. In an ideal world with unlimited ressources, one would like to understand these interactions as fully as possible, determine the genotypes of bacterium and host alike and then choose how to proceed for each individual. This is, however, not even practical in a rich industrialized country, least in a $1 per year and person health system. A more realistic strategy is targeting of high-risk strains of *H. pylori* in populations known to carry a high risk overall. Another approach relies on the assumption that carcinogenesis in the stomach can be reversed even at the stage of gastritis and intestinal metaplasia by antibiotic treatment against *H. pylori*. This is in fact the approach that is now pursued, more or less deliberately, in countries with a well-functioning health system. Strictly argued, this type of strategy does not fall into the category of '*primary prevention*'. Instead it is a case of '*secondary prevention*', because the primary carcinogen is eliminated only after carcinogenesis has begun, but at an early stage.

Cancer Prevention and Diet

In most human cancers, carcinogens are not so clearly defined that they can be eliminated or avoided. Even the carcinogens discussed in the previous section are not the only causes of the respective cancers. Thus, more careful exposure to sunlight will prevent many, but not all skin cancers. Vaccination against HBV (and eventually HCV) is expected to prevent liver cancers resulting from chronic viral infection, but not those resulting from alcohol-induced cirrhosis. Only a fraction of bladder cancers is prevented by strict regulations of arylamine use in the workplace. Nevertheless, primary prevention in these cancers is feasible and is successfully pursued.

Among the four major lethal cancers in Western industrialized countries, in only one, lung cancer, a large fraction of the cases is associated with exposure to a clearly defined exogenous agent, i.e. tobacco smoke. As mentioned above, primary prevention in lung cancer has proven frustratingly difficult in spite of the evident relationship between carcinogen and cancer. In the other three major cancers, colorectal carcinoma, breast cancer and prostate carcinoma, there is certainly no single major exogenous carcinogen. Therefore, early dectection of localized tumors and preneoplastic lesions is the main option for reducing their mortality.

However, in epidemiological studies, all three cancers show associations with a more or less clearly defined '*Western life-style*'. While several aspects of this lifestyle have come under scrutiny, the most convincing arguments point to diet as a major factor. This is not to say that the Western diet is thought to contain a high level of contaminating carcinogens. Rather, diet appears to modulate the risk for these three cancers by affecting endogenous carcinogenic processes. The potential for prevention by changes in the diet is illustrated by the order of magnitude difference in the incidence of prostate cancer between East Asia and North-West Europe, and even more impressively, by the same difference emerging in successive generations of Asian immigrants into the USA. The incidences of the three cancers in Southern Europe and in the Near East are typically intermediate, so a '*Mediterranean life-style effect*' has been postulated. Of note, diet may be only one of several factors responsible for these differences.

The difficulty with prevention at the level of life-style is illustrated by the case of tobacco smoking. If prevention of a cancer caused by a clearly defined recreational drug is frustrating, prevention of cancers by insufficiently defined factors in the everyday diet could prove impossible.

This difficulty may be one reason, why much research on prevention of these major cancers has focussed on single components in the diet. Ideally, one might be able to identify one responsible dietary component that could be added as a supplement to staple foods (e.g. folate to flour) or offered as a drug (e.g. soy extracts). This '*micronutrient*' component could either be low in the Western diet or be specifically present in East-Asian foods. In fact, candidates for both types of factors have been proposed.

Compared to '*Westerners*', East Asians eat on average fewer calories. This difference in absolute calories is relatively small, whereas the difference in calories provided by animal fat is huge. Typical '*Western*' diets are reach in red meat, which has a high fat content, and in dairy products. In contrast, typical '*Eastern*' diets provide a higher fraction of calories from grains and legumes. There are also differences in the amount and type of vegetables and fruit consumed as well as in the proportion of fish in the diet. These differences are, however, almost as large within the '*East*' and '*West*' each as between these regions, and do probably not account for the difference in cancer incidence in general. There are more factors of this sort. For instance, selenium deficiency predisposes to several cancer types in some regions of China as well as some in Europe. Selenium deficiency compromises protection against reactive oxygen species, since enzymes such as glutathione peroxidase require this trace element for their catalytic activity.

Among the components discussed to be lacking in the typical Western diet are some that are thought to protect against reactive oxygen species. Carotenoids and related compounds are contained in many vegetables and fruits, and their levels in blood correlate with the consumption of yellow/red vegetables. According to such measurements carotenoid supply may indeed have been low in more traditional Western diets. In particular, the main carotenoid of tomatoes, lycopene, has been proposed as a major protective factor in the Mediterranean diet. Several large prospective longitudinal cohort studies, which are among the most reliable tools of epidemiology, have indeed confirmed the presumed relationship between consumption of vegetables and risk for the major cancers. Variously, significant decreases in cancer risk were found between consumption of vegetables overall, of yellow/red or green vegetables. In contrast, intervention studies using pure β-carotene were unsuccessful and in some cases even increased the rates of cancer. Taken together, these results could mean that a combination of compounds rather than a single compound in vegetables and fruit protects against cancer.

Several further compounds contained in fruits and vegetables may synergize with carotenoids to protect against cancer. Vitamin C (*ascorbate*) and vitamin E (*tocopherol*) are also antioxidants. Unsaturated fatty acids contained in vegetable oils and seeds are essential for cell membrane function and the synthesis of paracrine factors regulating tissue homeostasis and function as well as immune responses.

Table 14.4. Dietary components proposed to influence cancer risk

Increasing risk	*Decreasing risk*
High fat (saturated animal fat)	Carotenoids (e.g., β-carotene, lycopene)
High total calory intake	Vitamin C (ascorbic acid)
Alcohol consumption	Vitamin E (tocopherol)
Pickled and salted foods	Vitamin B_{12}
Smoked and burnt meats	Folic acid
Phytoestrogens	Unsaturated fatty acids
Mold toxins (e.g., aflatoxins)	Phytoestrogens
	Flavonoids, isoflavonoids (e.g. genistein, resveratol, epigallo-catechin-3-gallate)
	Sulphoraphane

Flavonoids and isoflavonoids are also antioxidants, but may exert additional effects. Some are weak estrogens and may modulate hormone metabolism. This may influence the development of breast cancer and prostate cancer, although the evidence is vague. Some of these compounds are kinase inhibitors and, at least at pharmacological doses, are capable of inhibiting the proliferation of tumor cells or induce apoptosis. Genisteine from soy beans, resveratol from grapes and wine, and epigallocatechin-3-gallate (EGCG) from green tea belong to this group. Flavonoids and isoflavonoids are present at higher levels in East Asian and Mediterranean diets than in typical Western diets. Accordingly, quantitative, albeit not striking differences in their blood levels are observed between different geographic regions.

It is nevertheless unlikely that concentrations of such compounds sufficient to inhibit a receptor tyrosine kinase are reached by consuming typical Eastern or Mediterranean diets. It is also questionable whether consuming these compounds as purified dietary supplements will prevent cancer. More likely, in a well balanced diet they may synergize to impede the early development or progression of cancers. Notably, these compounds are excellent '*leads*' for the development of specific cancer drugs.

Dark green vegetables contain specific compounds, in addition to carotenoids, which could affect cancer development. For instance, sulforaphane contained in several kinds of cabbages, especially in broccoli and brussel sprouts, is a potent inducer of glutathione transferases and other phase II enzymes of xenobiotic metabolism. Induction of such enzymes would be thought to accelerate the inactivation of electrophilic carcinogens from exogenous and endogenous sources and prevent mutagenesis.

Dark green vegetables are also an important source of bioavailable folic acid, which is limited in some traditional Western diets and in modern low-quality ('*junk*') foods. Deficiencies in folic acid are known to synergize with deficiencies in vitamin B_{12}, with deficiencies in methyl group donors such as choline and methionine, or with extensive consumption of alcohol to cause cardiovascular disease and developmental defects such as spina bifida. These deficiencies may also advance the development of several human cancers.

Folate deficiency acts by two related pathways. Folate is an essential coenzyme for one-carbon metabolism, prominently for the biosynthesis of thymidine and of purine nucleotides. In an initial reaction, the hydroxymethyl-group of serine is transferred to *tetrahydrofolic acid* (THF) yielding N^5,N^{10}-methylene-THF. This is used in the *thymidylate synthase* (TS) reaction to derive dTMP from dUTP. The TS reaction is rate-limiting for dTTP biosynthesis and under some conditions for the synthesis of DNA. This is exploited in chemotherapy by 5-fluorouracil and related compounds. In the absence of cytostatic drugs, the thymidylate synthase reaction can be suboptimal, when folate or methyl group donors are insufficiently available. As a result, more dUTP becomes incorporated into newly synthesized DNA. Uracil in DNA is removed by uracil glycohydrolase and replaced by thymine via short-patch repair. So, as a consequence of folate deficiency, the number of DNA strand-breaks and the potential of errors during DNA replication increase. An alternative reaction catalyzed by *methylene tetrahydrofolate reductase* (MTHFR), directs N^5,N^{10}-methylene-THF towards the '*methyl cycle*'. Its product is N^5-methyl-THF. This can be used by methionine synthase to regenerate the otherwise essential amino acid methionine from homocysteine in a reaction that also requires coenzyme B_{12}. Following conversion to *S-adenosylmethionine* (SAM) by SAM synthetase, the methyl group can be used in a variety of methyltransferase reactions, including the methylation of lipids, RNA, proteins and DNA. In each case, S-adenosylhomocysteine (SAH) is formed, which is hydrolyzed to adenosine and homocysteine by SAH hydrolase, thereby completing the '*methyl cycle*'. SAH is a product inhibitor of methyltransferase reactions, including the DNA methyltransferases. Therefore, the efficiency of DNA methylation depends on the SAM:SAH ratio. Deficiencies in folate, vitamine B_{12}, methionine or other methyl group donors can therefore compromise the correct establishment of DNA methylation patterns, and perhaps also the methylation of RNA and of proteins.

The extent to which such deficiencies become relevant also depends on genetic factors. Several enzymes involved in one-carbon metabolism and in the '*methyl cycle*' are polymorphic in man, most prominently MTHFR. Among several polymorphisms in the *MTHFR* gene, the most prevalent is an exchange of alanine for valine at codon 677. Since the valine variant is less stable, MTHFR activity varies between individuals. Depending on the genotype, limited amounts of methylene tetrahydrofolate are therefore shuttled preferentially towards nucleotide biosynthesis or towards the methyl cycle, thereby compromising either DNA synthesis or DNA methylation. Indeed, the *MTHFR* genotype and folate deficiency have been shown to synergize in causing defects in DNA replication and DNA methylation. Moreover, several epidemiological studies have shown cancer risk to increase, e.g. in the colon, most strongly in individuals with specific *MTHFR* genotypes who consume a diet deficient in folate and vitamin B12 and consume large amounts of alcohol.

Popular accounts of these studies and others demonstrating similar interactions for cardiovascular disease have labeled this effect '*methyl magic*'. There is, in fact, little magic involved. A diet with a good supply of folate and vitamin B_{12} is all that is needed. Current nutritional recommendations such as '*Take 5*' (meaning: per day servings of fruit and vegetables) are based on the insights into methyl group metabolism, antioxidant action, and effects of other plant ingredients described above.

In some countries, folate is even added to staple foods. Recommendations such as these could lead to a gradual decrease of the incidence of major cancers, even more when they are supported by overall changes in life-style. For instance, immigrants from Southern Europe and the Near East have introduced a greater variety of Mediterrean fruits and vegetable dishes into the Central European diet. Tomatoes, e.g., are now common in the 'Western'diet. Because of the complex interactions involved, the precise causes of changes in cancer incidence that result from such cultural developments will be very difficult to trace.

While individual ingredients of the diet certainly influence cancer risk, and may synergize with each other, the most consistent difference between '*Eastern*' and '*Western*' diets is the amount of saturated fat consumed, particularly of animal fat. For breast and prostate cancer each, and to a lower degree for colon cancer, the cancer incidence in a country is proportional to the amount of saturated fat consumed. The molecular basis of this relationship is not understood. Conspicuously, the risk for these three cancers, among all malignancies, also increases in adipose (obese) persons. Obesity is caused by an interplay of genetic predisposition, cultural factors, overnutrition and lack of exercise that in itself is extremely complex. Even *H. pylori* may feature in this relationship by influencing the levels of hormones secreted by the stomach that regulate satiety. So, the relationship between adipositas and cancer is not expected to be straightforward.

An important component in this complex relationship may be insulin-like growth factors. While IGF2 acts mostly locally as a paracrine factor, IGF1 circulates as a hormone in the blood, supporting the growth of several tissues. It also regulates glucose metabolism, but much less so than insulin, which in turn is a weaker growth factor. Increased expression of IGFs is thought to contribute to a wide range of human cancers, including breast and prostate cancers. Normally, IGF1 levels in blood peak during the adolescent growth phase and decline later on. They remain significant, however, and are regulated by nutrition and by exercise, similar to those of insulin. So, in adipose persons, insulin levels are often enhanced, leading to a pre-diabetic state and often to diabetes, but IGF1 levels too are supraphysiological. Indeed, the level of IGF1 in mid-life has been found to predict the risk of prostate cancer which appears several decades later. The action of IGFs is controlled by binding proteins (IGFBPs). These are likewise subject to regulation by nutrition and by insulin. The levels of IGFBPs in serum also appear to correlate with the risk for breast and prostate cancers. While these relationships are intriguing, they are certainly only part of a complex relationship that needs to be elucidated to define the best approach to addressing obesity as a cause of cancer.

Prevention of Cancers in Groups at High Risk

Recommending dietary changes such as 'Take 5!' is a cancer prevention strategy that addresses the overall population. This strategy is unproblematic. No adverse effects are to be feared and the same changes in diet supposed to decrease the risk of major cancers very likely diminish the risk of cardiovascular disease and diabetes, to a perhaps even greater extent. It is similarly unproblematic to pursue cancer prevention by vaccinating an entire population against HBV or HCV, which likewise has the additional benefit of preventing acute and chronic liver disease. There are risks involved in vaccination, since a few individual show adverse reactions, but they are much lower than the risks associated with actual infections. Moreover, as HBV does not seem to possess an animal reservoir, there is hope that this virus may not only be contained, but eventually be exterminated by vaccination. No foreseeable downside would be associated with its demise.

A bit more problematic is the handling of *H. pylori*, since many strains of the bacterium may actually constitute symbiotes rather than pathogens, even though others present a considerable risk to susceptible humans. Therefore, a vaccination strategy would have to take these considerations into account. As described above, one way out of this dilemma is to restrict anti-bacterial treatment to the susceptible part of the population and/or to those carrying high-risk strains. Ideally, one would identify these persons by molecular diagnosis, but more realistically, patients with gastritis will be identified and treated before ulcers and cancer have a chance to develop.

This is an example of identifying a population at increased risk for a specific cancer. In the case of stomach cancer associated with *H. pylori* infection, there is the added advantage that treatment is available and can usually be admitted without severe side effects and at moderate cost. Moreover, it is not too difficult to identify a precancerous state, viz. gastritis or ulcers, because it is symptomatic. Each of these factors is generally important for the successful prevention of cancers in risk populations, i.e. straightforward delineation of the population at risk, availability of an achievable specific treatment with few or no side effects, and easy identification of preneoplastic or early tumor stages by symptoms or simple and affordable assays. Unfortunately, instances such as stomach cancer associated with *H. pylori* infection represent the exception rather than the rule.

Table 14.5. Prerequisites for successful cancer prevention in risk groups

Criterion
Clear identification of population at risk
Sensitive, specific, reliable, and inexpensive assay
Detection of significant preneoplastic or early cancer stage
Efficient and affordable treatment with acceptable side effects

Important tasks during cancer prevention in populations at risk are monitoring and – as in the case of stomach cancer – education and information of health professionals and the affected population. This can be very successful, if the population exposed to a specific cancer risk is clearly defined, e.g. in the workplace. In occupations with hazards from radiation or chemicals, regulations aiming at minimizing exposure are put in place and controlled, regular instruction meetings are instituted, and regular examinations are performed to detect early signs of cancers such as aberrant cells in the blood or urine. Monitoring in such instances can be improved by molecular-based techniques for the early detection of cancers or preferably of preneoplastic changes.

Like exposure to defined carcinogens, inheritance of mutations in high-risk genes predisposing to cancer is a risk factor in a specific part of the population. Insights from molecular genetics now allow a better definition of this population by identification of those individuals within affected families who carry high-risk mutations. Since monitoring is likewise warranted in these persons, techniques for early detection of cancers are being developed. One might feel intuitively that preventing inherited cancer today should be a straightforward task. It is unfortunately not, for a variety of reasons.

One complication is encountered in cancer syndromes inherited in a recessive mode. These are typically rare diseases caused by mutations in genes involved in DNA repair and become manifest during childhood or during adolescence. This means that familial clustering occurs only to a limited extent. In most cases, only siblings of the first child affected (the '*index patient*') are also at risk, unless the family belongs to a religious or ethnic group with frequent intermarriage. These diseases often comprise a wider range of symptoms, some of which may precede the manifestation of cancers. This can provide an advantage in so far as monitoring for cancers can be begun after the disease has been identified by other symptoms and has been confirmed by molecular genetic diagnostics.

The major problem then is how to avoid and treat the cancers that develop. In spite of being aware of the risk, and even of understanding the involved mechanisms as precisely as in the hypersensitivity of xeroderma pigmentosum patients towards UV, this can be exceedingly difficult. Another problem may arise during therapy, because patients with these afflictions may be hypersensitive to commonly used treatments such as radiation therapy (in ataxia teleangiectasia) or to crosslinker cytostatic drugs such as cis-platinum (in *Fanconi anemia*). So, each case requires a careful, individualized approach. As a practical consequence patients with this sort of diseases are often referred to specialized centers. There, experience can be gathered and therapy can be improved with each case. Some diseases in this group are candidates for gene or stem cell therapy, e.g. *Fanconi anemia*, where predominantly the hematopoetic system is at risk for cancer.

The second, larger group of inherited cancers comprises autosomal-dominantly inherited diseases with an increased incidence of benign and malignant tumors, typically in young adults or in middle age. Cancer predisposition in these cases is not necessarily associated with conspicuous symptoms characteristic of a syndrome. Instead, the diseases often run within families, affecting not only siblings of an '*index*' patient, but also second and third degree relatives. Almost all are caused by an inherited mutation in a tumor suppressor gene. *Familial adenomatous polyposis coli* (FAP) predisposing to multiple colorectal adenomas and eventually carcinoma and hereditary breast cancer are prominent examples.

The first hurdle encountered when trying to prevent cancer in affected persons can be awareness. FAP is very distinctive and the emergence of multiple polypous adenomas typically precedes the development of a cancer. Therefore, patients are usually identified, even if the familial background is unknown. A familial background in a disease like FAP may seem hard to overlook, but as families become smaller and mobility increases, family history is not always trivial to ascertain.

This problem is more severe in patients with hereditary breast cancer, since malignancies are generally the first manifestation of the disease, except in patients with more generalized cancer syndromes, e.g. *Cowden disease*. Awareness of hereditary breast cancer may have increased since the discovery of the *BRCA* genes was widely reported in medical journals and in the lay press. Perhaps, the following controversies about how to apply the new knowledge may have increased awareness further. These controversies relate to the most crucial problems in cancer prevention within selected groups mentioned above, viz. delineation of the population at risk, availability of achievable specific treatments with few or no side effects, and the identification of preneoplastic or early tumor stages.

FAP is not only phenotypically distinctive, but is also essentially a homogeneous disease at the genetic level. Almost all cases are caused by mutations in the *APC* gene and many of these occur in hot spots within the gene. So, molecular genetic confirmation of the disease is feasible at moderate cost. Within a family, the mutation identified in one person can be specifically sought in relatives, or closely linked genetic markers, e.g. microsatellites, can be used. Moreover, a reasonably good correlation exists between the location of the mutation and the severity of the disease. So, molecular diagnostics can be helpful to choose an appropriate preventive approach.

Nevertheless, problems remain. The first one is ethical. Diagnosing the disease in one person reveals an information on all relatives, particularly if diagnostics is performed by linkage analysis. In the case of FAP with its very high penetrance, this is mostly a problem concerning children, since asymptomatic adults are rare. Nevertheless, people have a right to to know or not to know. So, adequate counseling is absolutely necessary. Because of the nature of the disease in FAP, this issue is not as problematic as in some other diseases, including breast cancer.

In everyday practice, the most serious problem is how to proceed after an *APC* mutation has been verified. One option is preventive surgery by partial colectomy, i.e. removal of the segment of the gut most susceptible to adenomas and carcinoma, usually in young adults before multiple polyps have developed. This diminishes the cancer risk, but does not exclude cancers in other parts of the colon and rectum. Thus, monitoring for carcinomas is regularly performed.

More recently, chemoprevention has been introduced. Non-steroidal antiinflammatory drugs, i.e., inhibitors of COX2 such as celecoxib, diminish colon cancer risk not only in patients with inflammatory bowel diseases, but also appear to be efficacious in FAP patients.

Thus, overall early diagnosis of FAP allows to diminish the risk of lethal cancers and extends the life of affected individuals. This is achieved with considerable effort and costs, in life quality of the patient and in economic terms. Similar, but also additional issues are to be considered in the prevention of hereditary breast cancer. One additional problem is the identification of the population at risk. Unlike FAP, hereditary breast cancer has no distinctive morphological features and worse, no distinctive precursor stage preceding actual cancer. So, before the advent of molecular techniques, it was not possible to discern whether a familial clustering of breast cancers was accidential or caused by a pre-disposition inherited in the family.

This distinction can now often be made, but the disease is genetically heterogeneous. While the majority of hereditary cancers appears to be caused by inherited mutations in *BRCA1* or *BRCA2*, some cases are due to mutations in other known genes. However, a sizeable fraction of familial cases cannot be ascribed to a specific gene. Most likely, no single '*BRCA3*', but several genes are involved.

So, verifying a hereditary predisposition toward breast cancer in a family with several '*index*' cases can still constitute a considerable problem. Moreover, the *BRCA* genes are pretty large and germ-line mutations are spread throughout the genes. The task of identifying mutations is in some cases facilitated by the occurrence of other cancers in a family. For instance, frequent ovarian carcinomas suggest *BRCA2* as the prime candidate. Also, in some populations founder effects have caused a predominance of specific mutations whose presence or absence can be tested before a larger screening procedure is undertaken. In clinical routine, if a mutation is found in a *BRCA* gene in a member of a family, a hereditary predisposition can be assumed, if none can be found, it cannot be excluded. This is rather unsatisfactory for everybody involved.

If a *BRCA* mutation is detected, the next problem arises from another difference towards FAP. While the penetrance of FAP is generally very high and the exceptional cases with attenuated disease can be defined with some certainty (i.e. by mutations at the 5'-end of the gene), considerable differences have been observed in the penetrance of hereditary breast cancer caused by various mutations in BRCA genes. Unfortunately, very few of these differences are consistent enought to allow a prediction of the risk for an individual patient. This means that – by and large – patients with a life-time risk of 20% for development of breast or ovarian cancer have to be treated like those with a life-time risk of 80%. Again, this is not satisfactory for anybody involved, the more so, since the options for cancer prevention are also rather limited.

As in FAP, surgery is the primary option and has been shown to diminish the risk substantially. Oophorectomy not only strongly diminishes the risk of ovarian cancer, but also that of breast cancer, likely because estrogen levels are decreased. Mastectomy in various forms can be performed. An important issue is when to perform these operations. Obviously, one would like to delay them as long as possible without incurring the risk of a cancer having metastasized. Likewise, the extent of mastectomy must be balanced between risk of cancer and risks of the procedure, which are physical as well as psychological. Standard recommendations are available, but the actual decision should be made by the patient after counseling.

Monitoring can detect some breast cancers at comparatively early stages, but is not straightforward, especially in younger women. For instance, mammography has been critized as being unreliable in women below the age of 50. There is no good molecular marker for breast cancer yet, which could be used with serum or with nipple aspirates. However, research on this issue is very active.

Brighter prospects emerge from newer developments. Chemoprevention appears to be efficacious in breast cancer as well and specifically in hereditary breast cancer caused by *BRCA* mutations. NSAIDs are also tried for the prevention of breast cancer. In addition, although BRCA-associated cancers normally do not respond well to anti-estrogenic therapies, SERMs such as tamoxifen or the newer raloxifene may also be active in their prevention. However, they may delay the manifestation of the disease rather than prevent it. These drugs can have side effects, because they interfere with the normal functions of estrogens in protection of the cardiovascular system and regulation of the balance of resorption and osteogenesis in the bone. Moreover, older SERMs increase the risk of endometrial cancer.

In summary, therefore, prevention of cancers caused by inherited mutations is rarely simple and typically only to some extent efficacious, in spite of considerable efforts and costs. Not least, the quality of life is often compromised. Clearly, the task for molecular research remains to better understand the underlying pathophysiological mechanisms in order to identify more specific targets for prevention, and to improve diagnostic techniques, in particular for the early detection of cancers arising in persons at risk.

Prevention of Prostate Cancer by Screening the Aging Male Population

There can be little doubt that the considerable efforts to prevent or at least delay cancers is appropriate in small populations at high risk, such as families with inherited cancer syndromes. Likewise, drastic measures such as surgical removal of organs or long-term treatment with anti-hormonal drugs are accepted in persons known to run a high risk of developing a lethal cancer. Such measures would certainly not be acceptable for the whole population, even though one third of the population in a typical Western industrialized country will develop some kind of cancer in their life-time and one fifth will die of it. However, many different cancers in different organs contribute to this morbidity and mortality and no universal prevention scheme is at hand.

Nevertheless, for some cancers, screening of the entire population or a susceptible subpopulation could make sense, if certain requirements are met. They are similar to those defined in high-risk populations, viz. the part of the population at risk needs to be clearly defined, an affordable and reliable assay for detection of preneoplastic or early tumor stages must be at hand, and an efficacious treatment with acceptable side-effects and – in a large population – affordable costs must be available. There is a continuing debate for which cancers these requirements might be met. Obviously, the four major cancers, lung cancer, colon cancer, breast cancer, and prostate cancer are prime candidates for population screening. While according developments are underway for each of them, they are most advanced in the case of prostate cancer.

Screening for prostate carcinoma is basically a realistic option. (1) It is very prevalent with a life-time risk of up to 10% in the male population and a considerable mortality (≈3% of the male population). (2) Prostate cancer is extremely rare before the age of 50, increasing exponentially thereafter. In males over 75, the disease often takes a slower course and/or surgical treatment is not advisable. This restricts the population to be tested to males aged between 50 and ≈75. (3) A routine biochemical assay for prostate specific antigen (PSA) in serum can detect most tumors while they are still restricted to the organ. This assay has acceptable sensitivity, although its specificity is only moderate. In most cases, a definite diagnosis of prostate cancer can be achieved by further molecular assays, by imaging and by histological investigation of biopsies. (4) Organ-confined prostate cancer can be successfully treated by surgery or radiotherapy. In advanced cases, progression can be delayed by anti-hormonal treatment.

For these reasons, PSA screening of the male population starting from the age of 50 has been introduced in several countries. In smaller regions within Austria or Canada systematic attempts have been made to screen the entire male population and treat all those with detectable cancers. Indeed, the mortality rates of prostate cancer and meanwhile even its incidence have declined. Not all Western countries have followed suit, however, again for several reasons.

1. Prostate cancer is biologically heterogeneous. While a sizeable fraction of prostate cancers take an aggressive course, many remain relatively indolent, and will not cause clinical symptoms, least death in the age group at risk. In contrast, treatment by surgery or radiation can cause considerable morbidity such as incontinence and impotence and carries even a (low) risk of mortality. Moreover, while the introduction of PSA assays has dramatically reduced the fraction of cases that have metastasized at the time of detection, some still are and cannot be cured.

   At present, while a combination of biochemical and morphological parameters can predict the prognosis of a specific patient quite well, the distinction between indolent, aggressive, and already metastatic cases can rarely be made with certainty. This means that on one hand a fraction of patients are unnecessarily treated, while on the other hand in some cases treatment is useless. As one might expect, the debate on the relative sizes of the three fractions rages. A study in Scandinavia, where '*watchful waiting*' rather than therapeutic intervention is the favored strategy, has suggested that radical prostatectomy prolongs life in only one out of seventeen patients treated. This is likely an underestimate. Nevertheless, it raises doubts about the usefulness of a population-wide screening and intervention approach. Moreover, opponents of screening point out that the incidence and mortality of prostate cancer are also declining in countries where no screening/intervention has been introduced. One way out of the dilemma would be the development of molecular markers that allow to stratify prostate cancers into groups with very high, moderate and low risk.

2. PSA screening is more expensive than it looks at first sight. The PSA assay itself is relatively inexpensive, but is not highly specific. While it yields relatively few false negatives, i.e. misses few

cases of prostate cancer being present, it has a relatively high rate of false positives. Specifically, men with benign prostatic diseases such as prostatitis or extensive benign hyperplasia often test positive. In these cases, further diagnostics has to be performed and - although some of these men may indeed have to undergo treatment for their benign diseases - there are considerable costs associated with the diagnostic procedure. Because taking of biopsies is an invasive procedure, a slight risk of serious infections is incurred. All this would not matter much in a small population at risk, but if an entire population of older males is screened, costs are magnified and very slight risks become significant. Consider an assay with 95% specificity (which is an excellent value) used in a population of one million males over 50. It means 50,000 men having to undergo the following more extensive diagnostical procedures unnecessarily. Combined with the uncertainty on the clinical significance of a cancer detected in an individual, this leaves room for doubt.

3. Moreover, if 10% of all males eventually develop clinically significant prostate cancer and are all detected at an early stage, can they all be treated by current methods? In the fictious example population, 100,000 men would be diagnosed with prostate cancer. Currently, many cases are only detected, after the cancer has progressed. Before the advent of PSA assays, most cancers were highstage, often metastasized and incurable. With optional PSA assays, cases are more often diagnosed at an organ-confined stage at which they can be cured. Not so rarely, they are diagnosed in men older than 75 years or suffering from other - typically cardiovascular - diseases prohibiting surgery. In many of these men, rather slow-growing prostate carcinomas are not limiting life expectation, although the patients may eventually require palliative treatments. If screening was efficiently performed in younger men, e.g. at the age of 60, one could not predict by current methods whether many cancers detected would cause severe clinical symptoms years later or limit life expectancy. Since few males at 60 are nowadays not fit enough for surgery or radiotherapy, most of them would therefore need to be treated right away. This may be feasible in selected regions like Tyrol or Quebec, but in larger populations the ressources would simply not be available. Again, a better definition of the population at risk, more precisely, a classification of the cancers detected by PSA screening and subsequent diagnostic procedures, is required to solve this dilemma.

Evidently, an alternative approach would be chemoprevention rather than definitive therapy in men with suspicious serum levels of PSA. Anti-hormonal treatment is an option, but is problematic because of its side effects. Moreover, there are concerns that applying anti-androgenic treatment early on might spur the early development of androgen-resistant cancer cells, leaving no options if the disease recurs after surgery. Moreover, androgen independence in prostate cancer is typically associated with a more invasive and metastatic phenotype and therefore anti-androgen chemoprevention might prevent the development of less malignant cancers, while promoting the more aggressive ones. A compromise in this situation is being tried by using inhibitors of 5α-reductase. This enzyme catalyzes the formation of the more active dihydro-testosterone from testosterone in the prostate. Therefore, its inhibition has fewer side effects than anti-androgenic treatments by androgen receptor antagonists or LHRH agonists. Moreover, the less active androgen testosterone remains present to exert beneficial effects in other tissues. As often in prostate cancer research, acquiring definitive data on the value of this approach will take many years. Intriguingly, preliminary results suggest indeed a decrease in prostate cancer incidence at the expense of a shift towards less differentiated cases.

Other Types of Prevention

Detection of prostate cancer by PSA assays can, of course, not be considered strictly as cancer prevention. PSA levels in serum increase, after the prostate epithelium has become disorganized and epithelial cells release some of their secretory products into the mesenchyme. This presupposes invasion and therefore a carcinoma by definition. Ideally, however, the cancer is detected at an early stage, while it can still be cured and systemic disease is prevented.

This is the aim of many attempts at detecting cancers early on by molecular markers. Ideally, one would detect a preneoplastic state allowing prevention of the actual malignancy. If that is not possible, detection is aspired at a stage where a cure remains possible with minimal harm to the patient.

One step further, viz. following successful therapy of a cancer, e.g. removal by surgery, another type of prevention aims at diminishing the risk of further cancers of the same type. This is prevention of secondary cancers. In contrast, adjuvant therapy by drugs or irradiation aims at eliminating residual cells of the primary cancer that might lead to recurrences.

The distinction between prevention of secondary cancers and preventing recurrences of the first cancer is clear in the prostate, which is completely removed during surgery for prostate cancer. So any cancer appearing later must have been present at the time of surgery, having spread beyond the organ.

In organs that cannot be completely removed this distinction is more difficult to make. The issue is further complicated by '*field cancerization*' occurring in many tissues. For instance, carcinomas of the oral mucosa tend to recur. Nevertheless, surgery in this sensitive enviroment must be kept as limited as possible. Therefore, in the standard procedure the cancer is removed with a margin of several cm of morphologically normal tissue around it. Some cancers recur in distant places and indeed can be shown to harbor distinct genetic alterations.

Other cancers recur close to the surgical margin in tissue that was morphologically normal at the time of initial surgery. As a rule, they contain the same genetic alterations as the initial cancer. In such cases, prevention of second cancers and adjuvant therapy tend to overlap. Importantly, in each case, patients need to be closely monitored to detect recurrent as well as second independent tumors.

The main difference between adjuvant therapy and prevention of secondary cancers lies in the type of treatment used. Adjuvant therapy aims at killing tumor cells that have not been eliminated by the primary treatment, i.e. surgery or irradiation. Prevention aims at keeping normal or partially transformed cells from becoming malignant. So, it is certainly prevention to convince a bladder cancer patient treated by local surgery to stop smoking, whereas installing the moderately toxic cytostatic drug mitomycin C into the bladder is really adjuvant therapy.

In other cases, this distinction is even more blurred. For instance, anti-estrogenic therapy after partial mastectomy for breast cancer aims at both residual tumor cells and prevention of independent cancers.

Nevertheless, the distinction between prevention and adjuvant therapy is not only theoretically important. If there is a serious concern that tumor cells are still present after an attempt at definitive therapy, the side-effects of cytostatic drugs will have to be accepted. If the aim is prevention of a second cancer, they will not. For instance, if there is a concern that a bladder cancer has not been completely removed or may have metastasized, systemic therapy based on the more toxic cis-platinum will be used rather than local application of mitomycin C. Likewise, if breast cancers have spread beyond a certain stage, e.g. cancer cells are detected in multiple lymph nodes, cytostatic therapy rather than anti-estrogenic treatment will be considered.

There are several further organs, in which independent second cancers occur frequently, e.g. the skin, particularly in patients with increased susceptibilities, the epithelia of the mouth and throat, particularly in smokers, and the colon, most strongly in patients with inherited susceptibilities. Beyond regular monitoring and general preventive recommendations, such as to avoid smoking and eat a healthy diet, chemoprevention is being developed as an option for these patients. Vitamin mixtures or specific antioxidants such as β-carotene have been tried for several different tumors. For prevention of secondary colon cancers, non-steroidal antiinflammatory drugs are now the treatment of choice and they are also tried for cancers of other organs. Another group of compounds investigated for the purpose of chemoprevention are retinoids and related compounds.

INDEX